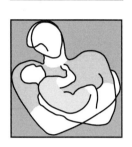

Complementary

Therapies

for Pregnancy

and Childbirth

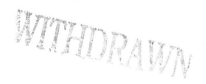

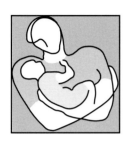

Complementary

Therapies

for Pregnancy

and Childbirth

edited by

Denise Tiran

SRN, SCM, ADM, MTD, PGCEA

Pathway Director for the Diploma in Professional Practice,
Faculty of Health, University of Greenwich

and

Sue Mack

BA, CQSW, Dip Counselling

Counsellor & Trainer in Women's Health

 Baillière Tindall

LONDON PHILADELPHIA TORONTO SYDNEY TOKYO

<u>Baillière Tindall</u>   24-28 Oval Road
W. B. Saunders   London NW1 7DX

The Curtis Center
Independence Square West
Philadelphia, PA 19106-3399, USA

Harcourt Brace & Company
55 Horner Avenue
Toronto, Ontario, M8Z 4X6, Canada

Harcourt Brace & Company, Australia
30-52 Smidmore Street
Marrickville
NSW 2204, Australia

Harcourt Brace & Company, Japan
Ichibancho Central Building
22-1 Ichibancho
Chiyoda-ku, Tokyo 102, Japan

The tables in Chapter 9 (as listed below), are taken from material © Barbara Geraghty BA (Hons) Lic.LCCH RSHom, 1993, with permission:

   1 – Carpal Tunnel Syndrome
   2 – Haemorrhoids
   3, 4, 5, 6 – Labour
   7, 8 – Recovering from Operative Procedures in Obstetrics
   9, 10 – Breast-feeding and Breast Problems
   11 – Ophthalmia Neonatorum
   12 – Colic

A catalogue record for this book is available from the British Library

ISBN 0-7020-1795-7

Typeset by Columns Design & Production Services Ltd, Reading
Printed and bound in Great Britain by Butler & Tanner Ltd., Frome, Somerset.

Contents

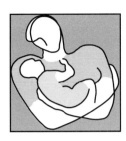

Contributors *vii*

Acknowledgements *ix*

Foreword *xi*

1   **Introduction** Denise Tiran *1*

2   **An Overview of Complementary Therapies for Pregnancy and Childbirth** Denise Tiran *13*

3   **Massage and Aromatherapy** Denise Tiran *35*

4   **Reflexology in Midwifery Practice** Denise Tiran *71*

5   **Complementary Therapies for the Relief of Stress** Sue Mack *91*

6   **The Uses of Hydrotherapy in Today's Midwifery Practice** Dianne Garland *113*

7   **Shiatsu** Elise Johnson *127*

8   **Women as Midwives and Herbalists** Helen Stapleton *153*

9   **Homeopathy for Pregnancy and Childbirth** Bridgit Cummings *181*

10   **Acupuncture** Sarah Budd *217*

11   **Osteopathy During Pregnancy** Penny Conway *243*

12   **Attitudes to Complementary Therapy** Sue Mack *265*

Conclusion *283*

Glossary *285*

Useful Addresses *289*

Index *294*

The colour plates are located between pages 180–181.

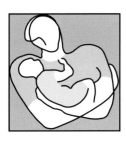

Contributors

Sarah Budd RGN RM
Dip Ac.B. Phil (Complementary Health Studies) MRTCM
Midwifery Sister/Acupuncturist
Maternity Unit
Freedom Fields Hospital
Plymouth, Devon PL4 7JJ

Penelope Conway
Osteopath
14 Eversley Park Road
Winchmore Hill
London N21 1JU

Bridgit Cummings
Homeopath
The Derryleigh
Skibbereen
West Cork
Eire

Dianne Garland SRN RM ADM PGCEA
Senior Midwife – Practice and Research
Mid Kent Health CT
Maidstone Hospital
Hermitage Lane
Maidstone
Kent ME16 9QQ

Elise M Johnson BSc BAc MRTCM MRSS
Shiatsu Practitioner
27 Poplar Drive
Hutton Poplars
Brentwood
Essex CM13 1YU

Sue Mack BA CQSW Dip. Counselling
Counsellor and Trainer in NHS and Private Practice
83 Glenesk Road
London SE9 1QS

Helen Stapleton RM MSc MNIMH
Independent Midwife/Medical Herbalist
2 Ulysses Road
London NW6 1EE

Denise Tiran SRN SCM ADM MTD PGCEA
Pathway Director for the Diploma in Professional Practice,
Faculty of Health
University of Greenwich
Elizabeth Raybould Centre
Bow Arrow Lane
Dartford DA2 6PG

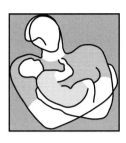

Acknowledgements

Chew Yeen Lawes for her contribution on T'ai Chi.

Chris Mack of Starlight Productions for the photographs of osteopathy and Shiatsu.

Nursing Times for the use of photographs of Denise.

Carola Beresford-Cooke for the boxed quotation at the foot of p. 132.

Beverley Peck (midwife) and Clifford Andrews (Shiatsu practitioner) for the case study on p. 144.

Rowan McConegal for the photographs of herbs.

Barbara Geraghty for the homeopathy charts in Chapter 9.

All the midwives, mothers and doctors who gave their help and especially those who agreed to be photographed. And of course our wonderful editor Sarah James for her advice, support and enthusiasm.

Foreword

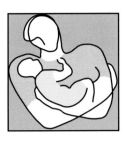

It was a great pleasure to be invited to write the Foreword to this timely and important book. Timely, because of the recent media and Government attention given to choice and care for childbearing women and timely because of the recent publication by the UKCC of the 1994 Edition of the Midwife's Code of Practice. This Edition includes sections on complementary therapies, the administration of homeopathic medicines, and also addresses issues of accountability for the midwife in her practice.

This book provides, as is the authors' stated intention, an introduction and overview to complementary therapies for pregnancy and childbearing and their application in midwifery, rather than a detailed 'how to' guide. This in turn provides a useful introductory 'menu' to what is available and what may be the choices for an increasing number of women. There is much food for thought in the text and whilst I may not necessarily agree with all the views stated, I know that this book will contribute very positively to the wider debate, the questions, the knowledge, the need for further research and the issues of accountability.

In my role as the Professional Officer for Midwifery in the statutory body which regulates the nursing, midwifery and health visiting professions in the United Kingdom, I meet with and hear from many practitioners who are wanting to become informed, skilled and accountable in their provision of complementary therapies in practice. I believe that the reader will in this book find the questions and answers to the initial consideration of at least eight different complementary therapies as well as useful references to addresses of institutions providing education and training, lists of books containing more detailed information and available research data.

The author in the introduction refers to the 'growth industry' of complementary medicine within the healthcare field for both consumers and professionals. I welcome this book in its response to the identified need for information on this 'growth industry' and for providing such information against the backdrop of the midwives' legislation and codes of practice. It is worth reminding midwives that their legislation is about actively enabling rather than limiting practice, and allows, in common with this book, for the development of the profession in the interests of safety of mothers and babies.

Jane Winship RGN RM MTD DipN(Lond)
Professional Officer, Midwifery
United Kingdom Central Council for Nursing,
Midwifery and Health Visiting
September 1994

Denise Tiran

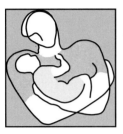

Chapter 1 **Introduction**

Complementary or alternative medicine is a growth industry within the healthcare field, for both consumers and professionals. Many nurses and midwives are beginning to use therapies such as massage and reflexology as an adjunct to their work (Martin, 1990), and the National Health Service reforms are encouraging general practitioners to offer additional services such as hypnotherapy and acupuncture (Fulder, 1989).

Holistic health centres abound particularly in the south-east of England. London's largest centre, the Hale Clinic, offers 60 different practitioners, while therapists elsewhere offer a peripatetic service (Martin, 1989; Wheater, 1990). Health food shops are employing consultants within their stores to offer advice on the wide range of self-help nutritional and herbal treatments (Wheater, 1990), and one large high street pharmaceutical company has introduced a new range of homeopathic remedies for over-the-counter purchase. The vast array of books and journals in any bookstore is also an indicator of the explosion of interest in the subject amongst the general public.

Why then is complementary medicine enjoying such a renaissance? The boom may be due in part to increasing demands from consumers to be involved actively in their own healthcare and the desire to be treated as individuals. There is also a growing belief that conventional or allopathic medicine may not be appropriate for all illnesses; within the overall term of 'conventional' medicine are diverse forms of treatment such as surgery, chemotherapy and radiotherapy to name but a few. Not all of these would be the best or most appropriate therapy for all conditions, so why should 'alternatives' not be better in some instances?

The Chinese have combined orthodox and alternative medicine such as acupuncture for centuries with great success, and French doctors often use homeopathy in preference to more conventional treatments (Bouchayer, 1991). Many other therapies have developed as a result of questioning of traditional methods and an increasing understanding of the body's innate ability for self-healing, on which they are based.

One of the advantages of complementary medicine is that therapists have more time to talk to their clients than many of their colleagues in the National Health Service, mainly due to workload differences. This period of advice and counselling is central to the philosophy of alternative medicine, providing the client with information from which she can make her own choices about treatment rather than merely accepting prescribed care. Conventional medicine further complicates the issue by divisive boundaries or specialities dealing with separate parts of the body, as if it were an engine to be taken apart, mended and reassembled. Complementary practitioners view the client as a whole distinct individual and treatment is geared to achieving optimum health and well-being throughout the body, mind and spirit.

Allopathic medicine can also be said to be suffering a power struggle, with many doctors still lingering under the previously widespread belief in medical omnipotence, while 'patients' (the word implies passive submission) are satisfied no longer with merely being told what to do. Consumers want access to information about their conditions and the treatment options available. Health care, as never before, has become a consumer-directed business, unlike the health service provision of previous decades. What used to be called 'fringe', then 'alternative' medicine is gradually becoming more complementary to conventional treatments.

There is an interesting distinction here in the terminology used, for while 'alternative' implies that treatment is totally discrete from conventional medicine, 'complementary' presumes a degree of cooperation between the care-givers of different disciplines (Thomas, 1991). This does occur in some areas within the National Health Service but is far from the norm. Many doctors, nurses and midwives remain sceptical about the efficacy and safety of types of treatment which they do not understand. It is beholden on these professionals to develop a wider perspective of what constitutes holistic care, particularly at a time when the aim is to work in partnership with clients. Hillman (1986) urges an open mind about the uses and advantages of alternative therapies while continuing to appraise critically their effectiveness. Newbeck and Rowe (1986) argue that the term 'holistic' is not interchangeable with 'complementary' or 'alternative' because care may be fragmented even when given by non-orthodox practitioners. Holistic care is what all health professionals aim to achieve but this not only requires time, a valuable commodity in today's Health Service, but also a change in training programmes of student nurses, midwives and doctors. Until recently emphasis was put almost entirely on alleviating physical symptoms with little consideration given to psychological, social, spiritual and lifestyle factors, to name a few. Newbeck (1986) suggests that holistic care requires planning, and the ability of the practitioner to listen to – and hear – what the client is saying, verbally and non-verbally. It is unfortunate that complementary therapies are not available widely on the National Health Service for not only would this aid the enlightenment of staff, but it would also eliminate, in part, the abandonment of a course of treatment for financial reasons. Activation of the body's self-healing capacity takes time; often the client feels worse initially as the body rids itself of toxins. Cessation of therapy through lack of funds, with a consequent return to the state system leaves the general practitioner to re-establish the doctor–patient relationship and re-commence treatment with the person in a worse condition than before (Freer, 1985). Wider availability would mean easier accessibility and would give tacit approval and respectability to the alternatives. It is claimed that the government would save money by increasing provision of complementary therapies, especially on drugs, such as night sedation (Passant, 1990).

Many people who have sought the advice of a complementary practitioner have refrained from informing their family doctor, perhaps from a desire not to alienate them, thinking that they would not approve. It may be that the medical profession has given this impression because of their own lack of knowledge and their inability to discuss the situation with any degree of authority. In 1993 the National Association of Health Authorities and Trusts (NAHAT) conducted a survey amongst its members to appraise the situation relating to complementary therapies within the National Health Service (NAHAT, 1993). Although a small percentage of health authorities and trusts did provide complementary therapies on an *ad hoc* basis, this was far from the norm, with the justification for this situation being 'lack of proven effectiveness/cost effectiveness' or 'resource constraints'. The therapies most favoured by the authorities were those which involved comprehensive training programmes and which were supported by a significant body of knowledge, namely acupuncture, chiropractic, osteopathy and homeopathy. In addition certain therapies which could reasonably be incorporated into conventional medical practice, such as hypnotherapy and counselling, were included, although the latter certainly should not be considered anything but an aspect of normal care. Interestingly, those therapies which would enhance nursing or midwifery care, including massage, aromatherapy, therapeutic touch and reflexology, were low on the list of priorities. This is probably because 'practitioners' are defined within complementary medicine circles as those using a system of treatment which is a discrete discipline (homeopathy, chiropractic, acupuncture etc.), whereas 'therapists' are those involved in therapies which are an adjunct to other treatments, such as aromatherapy, reflexology, hypnotherapy and shiatsu (Gaier, 1991). It may also, of course, reflect the hierarchy within the healthcare professions in which doctors' views may take precedence over those of nurses and midwives. On the other hand it may be the perception of conventional health carers that, because the training programmes are more comprehensive for the 'approved' therapies, there exists a greater body of scientific knowledge with which to support advocated treatments. This is not necessarily true, for far more research has been carried out into aromatherapy than into osteopathy, for example.

Complementary therapies and research

However, it remains one of the problems of the relationship between orthodox and complementary practitioners in that there has been little research into the alternatives. The response from doctors when discussing complementary therapies has often been that they are unproven and therefore can be of no use to their patients. (It should be pointed out that some medical practices are also unevaluated; furthermore, the lack of scientific data does not mean that complementary therapies are ineffective or of no value.)

The situation is now slowly changing and, whereas previous small-scale research trials were published in complementary medicine journals, contributions to conventional respected journals such as the *British Medical Journal* and the *Lancet* are increasing. Indeed there is a growing number of doctors who have witnessed at first hand the effects of different therapies on their patients and are themselves becoming involved in clinical trials to increase the body of scientific knowledge.

Exeter University was the first academic institution to pursue the subject of complementary therapies, with the establishment in 1990 of a Bachelor of Philosophy degree course in the subject (Martin, 1991). The department has also developed a database called Extract (Exeter Traditional Medicine, Pharmacology and Chemistry project) to coordinate the results of clinical trials on herbal medicine from all sources, including medical doctors, botanists, pharmaceutical companies and biologists. Facilities exist also to search for results of research into other therapies.

The Research Council for Complementary Medicine began in 1983 with charitable status and promotes research into alternative medicine and the dissemination of the results, with the aim of improving the relationship between practitioners of conventional and complementary medicine. Links with the British Medical Association and the Medical Research Council have been forged and the organisation has earned respect from the World Health Organization.

These reputable organisations are influencing the attitudes of many members of the medical and nursing/midwifery professions; conversely they are impressing upon practitioners of complementary medicine the need for academic rigour and scientific knowledge to support the claims made for the various therapies.

An additional factor which has affected the availability of research findings in Britain is that much of the research which has been carried out is published in foreign language journals. The majority of research into traditional Chinese medicine such as acupuncture, shiatsu and herbal aspects has been conducted in the East. Other therapies such as therapeutic touch have been investigated in the United States or, in the case of homeopathy, in Europe but few of the findings have been ackowledged in the United Kingdom.

In reality, the medical establishment has often scorned any research into complementary therapies in the belief that only randomised double-blind controlled trials have any merit or significance. Obviously it is impossible to conduct double-blind trials into some of the therapies, for example hypnotherapy or reflexology, as the client and therapist would be aware whether or not conventional or complementary treatment was being given, while others, such as aromatherapy and herbal medicine, are more easily investigated with a control group using placebos. It is interesting to note that this system of research is relatively youthful, whilst the empirical evidence for the effectiveness of some complementary therapies can be traced back five thousand years or more. It is also increasingly recognised that multivariable single case reporting can demonstrate statistically significant results and it may be that this is the way forward for research into complementary therapies. Therapists record the efficacy or otherwise of a particular treatment for a specific problem, compiling comprehensive results from a significant number of cases, and identifying any other factors which may have positively or negatively affected treatment outcomes.

However, the number of research trials carried out by doctors, midwives and nurses remains minimal and the research tends to be still in those therapies which lend themselves to accepted randomised controlled trials. There are now trials being carried out in aromatherapy by nurses, in particular those working in areas such as intensive care, geriatrics and learning disabilities (Sanderson and Harrison, 1991; Buckle, 1992; Hewitt and Woolfson, 1992). On the other hand, comparative studies into therapies such as hypnotherapy (Guthrie et al., 1984; Brann and Guzvica 1987) and acupressure (Hyde, 1989) are also being conducted. Therapeutic touch, which is a relatively new phenomenon in Britain, has been used effectively and researched comprehensively in America and Canada, and is another therapy which could be very easily incorporated into midwifery and nursing practice (Heidt 1990; Feltham 1991; Krieger 1990; Thayer 1990; Quinn 1988).

Research into chiropractic, acupuncture, osteopathy and homeopathy is increasing too, perhaps because these are therapies often taken up by medical practitioners (Skelton and Flowerdew, 1985; Dundee et al., 1988; Klougart et al., 1989; Budd, 1992). It is noticeable, however, that reflexology research is almost non-existent, and yet this is a therapy which could so easily be incorporated into midwifery or nursing practice.

Education, training and regulation

Another factor which has been detrimental to the relationship between conventional and complementary practitioners has been the lack of clarity about training courses. In England anyone can set up in private practice as a 'therapist' so long as they do not make claims guaranteeing cure, especially for certain named conditions such as cancer and diabetes, or pose as a medically qualified doctor. English Common Law allows this situation, as anyone can do anything if it is not in direct contravention of the law. There are numerous training colleges in alternative therapies, offering 'diplomas' after lamentably short courses, and even qualifications in 'hands on' techniques following correspondence courses!

This factor has contributed to the scepticism with which the medical establishment has viewed complementary therapies. In the British Medical Association's report into 'non-conventional' therapies there is a recommendation for a single national regulating body for each therapy and suggestions as to how the scientific background of the therapy should be increased (British Medical Association, 1993). Many of the recommendations are valid and are being adopted by a majority of the therapies – there has been a flurry of educational activity in complementary medicine circles partly in response to the BMA report and partly due to increased self-awareness. The three main organisations, the Institute for Complementary Medicine, the British Complementary Medicine Association and the Council for Complementary and Alternative Medicine, are all actively involved in encouraging the development of academically supported training programmes in the various complementary therapies. Some of the leading aromatherapy schools formed the Aromatherapy Organisations Council to improve and standardise training requirements. In January 1994, new regulations for training were established, with a minimum of 180 classroom hours and specifications as to the content of individual training programmes. Within acupuncture, the various colleges have voluntarily set up the British Acupuncture Accreditation Board to determine standards for training and regulation, and it is hoped that this will set an example to other therapies (Shifrin, 1993).

Together with other professional education, complementary therapies are looking to advance knowledge and practice in each speciality by offering undergraduate and postgraduate degrees in an attempt to increase the scientific basis and improve the credibility of the different therapies. This is particularly apparent in those therapies which have longer pre-registration trainings such as osteopathy, acupuncture, chiropractic and homeopathy. The University of Middlesex is to start a Bachelor of Science degree in herbal medicine in October 1994, and the University of Greenwich offers Master of Science degrees in osteopathy and chiropractic, as well as a Diploma in Complementary Therapy for qualified health professionals. Exeter University's Bachelor of Philosophy in complementary medicine has been available since 1990. Another London university is to offer a Master of Art degree in bodywork, and the Universities of Manchester and Liverpool are also involved in alternative therapies education.

In June 1992 the British Complementary Medicine Association, which evolved from the former National Consultative Council for Alternative and Complementary Medicine, was launched as the main umbrella organisation to represent the interests of therapists at a national level. The BCMA maintains registers of practitioners and has a Code of Conduct which all member organisations have endorsed and which, if not complied with, may result in the exclusion of an individual from the organisation. However there remains no statutory mechanism for ensuring that anyone excluded from the BCMA does not practise again.

While it includes many of the organisations for different therapies such as aromatherapy, massage, yoga and reflexology, the BCMA also has as members practitioners from some of the more obscure therapies such as crystal therapy, polarity therapy and dowsing, yet those therapies which are gaining tacit approval from the medical establishment such as acupuncture and homeopathy have not joined the BCMA. Osteopaths, who became an accepted adjunct to normal medical care in the 1993 Parliamentary session, do not view themselves as an 'alternative' and therefore see no need to join the organisation.

Likewise midwives and nurses are under no compunction to join the BCMA if they are using their skills as a complement to normal practice, for they are professionally enabled to do so by the legislation of the United Kingdom Central Council; members of the Royal Colleges of Midwifery or Nursing are also covered for insurance claims and therefore do not require this facility from the BCMA (Trevelyan, 1992)

The effect of the single European market

Since 1992 when Britain became part of the single European market various changes have taken place which have had far-reaching implications for complementary therapists in Britain. The European system of law is based upon Napoleonic law, which states that no one can do anything unless it is approved under the law. One issue which has arisen and, at the time of writing, is not yet resolved, is the use of the word 'therapist' which, in Europe, only medically qualified doctors may use – therefore those practitioners traditionally using this suffix, such as aromatherapists, reflex zone therapists and hypnotherapists will need to seek alternative titles. Additionally anyone qualified in a complementary system of medicine may only practise under the auspices of a doctor. It remains to be seen whether Britain will be required to follow suit on this issue; at present member countries have been left to follow their own policies. Legislation at European Community level is in fact unlikely in the near future, according to the Commission of the European Communities (British Medical Association, 1993).

However one positive factor which has resulted from the move into Europe is that the onus of proof of adequate training is now on the practitioner rather than the client. There are as yet no specifications as to what constitutes 'adequate training' but increased regulation will at least eliminate the unscrupulous and incompetent practitioners. There will also need to be some radical changes made in the training programmes of some therapies to conform to the European Community directive concerning higher education.

Midwives wishing to utilise any of the complementary therapies within their midwifery practice are bound by the codes of practice laid down by the United Kingdom Central Council for Nursing, Midwifery and Health Visiting (UKCC). In the Midwives' Rules, number 40 (UKCC, 1993) states that the midwife should not undertake any practice for which she has not been properly trained. However in the 1992 publication on the Scope of Professional Practice emphasis is not on collecting certificates, but rather places responsibility for professional accountability firmly with the midwife (UKCC, 1992b). For midwives using different forms of complementary medicine, this means that as long as they can justify what they are doing and have had 'adequate and appropriate' training this is within the boundaries of their professional midwifery practice. At present it would, in any case, be extremely difficult for the UKCC to specify particular recommended trainings because of the diversity of courses in the individual therapies.

Midwives must also, of course, abide by any other regulations of their profession, and referral to the UKCC's publications on record keeping (UKCC, 1993), advertising (UKCC, 1985) exercising accountability (UKCC, 1989) and administration of medicines (UKCC, 1992a) is of paramount importance. The 'Guidelines for the Administration of Medicines' (UKCC, 1992a) is one document which mentions complementary and alternative therapies specifically. It highlights the importance of the need for informed consent, the right of the individual to decline, or indeed to receive alternative treatment, and the accountability of the practitioner in acting as an advocate for the client's health, whether this is by supporting their desire to use an alternative, or by questioning the interaction of a therapy with conventional care.

As with all systems of medicine and client care there are potential dangers in using alternative therapies, for 'natural' does not necessarily mean free from side effects, nor does it preclude complications from overdose. Midwives using any form of complementary therapy must be fully informed about its particular misuses, and act cautiously within the constraints of professional accountability (Cresswell, 1993). Well-meaning midwives who have a little knowledge of a complementary therapy could cause major problems for their clients, their clients' babies and their own professional integrity. Examples of the potential misuses of different therapies include aromatherapy oils which can initiate epileptic fits, herbal remedies or shiatsu techniques which cause miscarriage, osteopathic manoeuvres which trap nerves, or reflexology overdose leading to prolonged general malaise.

Policies and guidelines

Where maternity units wish to consider the implementation of complementary therapies into normal practice it is wise to develop policies or guidelines relevant to the local area (Armstrong, 1991). These should ideally be devised in conjunction with midwives, managers and supervisors, educators and students, obstetricians and paediatricians and possibly, representative consumers. Midwives should anticipate demand in order to be well prepared when parents do request the use of complementary therapies (see Chapter 2).

In summary, the following issues are relevant to the use of complementary therapies by midwives:

- midwives should have received some form of training in the therapy they wish to practise, and recognise the limitations of that practice;
- the practice of complementary therapies should be based on sound knowledge and available research findings;
- written records and verbal communications with colleagues must be maintained in order to achieve optimum care for the client;
- the use of complementary therapies should not be at the expense of normal midwifery care nor should it conflict with conventional medical care;
- midwives must seek informed consent from the client and respect the right of the individual to decline treatment on moral or religious grounds;
- employed midwives should gain the approval of their managers and the consultants before embarking on treatment with one of the alternative therapies;
- all midwives are subject to the normal parameters of control by supervisors of midwives.

So what of childbearing women? Pregnancy and birth are normal physiological life events and maternity care in Britain has seen a swing away from the mechanisation of the 1970s and early 1980s, back to allowing nature to take its course, within the bounds of safety. Women have found their voices once again, aided by such proponents for natural birth as Sheila Kitzinger, Janet Balaskas and Caroline Flint. That their active campaigning should never have been necessary is less relevant now, for in their vocalising and rallying of others the philosophy of maternity care has been examined closely and adapted to the needs of the consumers at the end of the century. Women have sought their own alternatives to the conventional care on offer and are able to opt for the type of care they want. A vast selection of options are available (in theory at least) from private consultant 'high-tech' delivery to a homeopathic home birth, from a hospital delivery, perhaps in water, with transfer home after a few hours, to the mother employing an independent midwife at home. Preparation for birth and parenthood may be at the hospital- or community clinic-based classes, or expectant parents may choose a course of massage, shiatsu, yoga or 'aqua-natal' classes. In addition to statutory midwifery care, postnatal follow-up may include home-help services or baby massage sessions.

Mothers and midwives are looking to complementary therapies to avoid the risks of drugs on the unborn child, to provide more natural advice for the relief of common discomforts of pregnancy and the postnatal period, and to seek alternative forms of pain relief in labour. Midwives are qualifying as acupuncturists or reflex zone therapists and utilising massage, aromatherapy and herbal remedies in their work. Labouring women are learning hypnosis or being attended not only by a midwife but also by their homeopath, acupuncturist or reflexologist. Specialist clinics are available for expectant mothers in some areas such as the one at the British School of Osteopathy to which women can refer themselves.

As complementary medicine becomes increasingly popular midwives will need to expand their knowledge and re-evaluate their attitudes in order to provide comprehensive care for pregnant and childbearing women. Expectant parents will wish to consult alternative practitioners and should not be made to feel they are being underhand by so doing.

This book is not intended as a 'how to' guide, although many simple remedies such as the dietary measures can be safely suggested to mothers. There are many excellent texts on each of the therapies discussed, some of which are recommended for further reading at the end of each of the chapters. Additionally, useful addresses are included to enable midwives wishing to pursue training in one of the therapies to find out more. The identification of priorities for midwives involved in using complementary therapies, either directly or indirectly, is essential. The issue of professional accountability is considered to be paramount, and is addressed throughout.

It is not the purpose of the book to denigrate the medical or pharmaceutical professions, both of which have vital but different roles to play in the care of childbearing women and their families. Any perceived disparagement is merely a factor in discussions regarding the current nature and status of complementary therapies in relation to conventional care. Indeed it is hoped that the text may go some way towards improving the relationship between midwives, doctors and complementary therapists in order to extend the range of treatments available to our clients.

It is the intention to offer an introduction for midwives into the potential uses, and abuses, of complementary therapies for childbearing women. An exploration of some of the commoner therapies with which midwives might come into contact is provided. Mothers may request advice about specific therapies or aspects of complementary medicine and midwives should be equipped to furnish them with adequate information to make a decision about their uses. Interested midwives may wish to undertake training in a certain therapy to enhance their care of women throughout pregnancy, labour and the puerperium. Clients may be receiving treatment from therapists outside the conventional system and maternity staff should have an understanding of the interrelationship between all carers.

All professionals need to learn to work in harmony in order to provide the best quality and most appropriate care for pregnant, labouring and newly delivered mothers and their families. Mothers have a right to choose whatever they perceive as best for their individual situation, and this has been emphasised in the 'Changing Childbirth' report (Department of Health, 1993). Only by increasing our understanding of the different therapies currently termed 'alternative' will they become truly complementary to our normal care.

References

Armstrong F. (1991) A complementary strategy. *Nursing Times*, **87(11)**, 34–36

Bouchayer F. (1991) Alternative medicines a general approach to the French situation. In: *Complementary medicine and the European Community*, pp. 45–60 C.W. Daniel.

Brann L. and Guzvica S. (1987) Comparison of hypnosis with conventional relaxation for antenatal and intrapartum use: a feasibility study in general practice. Journal of the Royal College of General Practitioners **37(303)**, 437–440

British Medical Association (1993) *Complementary medicine – new approaches to good practice*. Oxford University Press, Oxford.

Buckle J. (1992) Which lavender oil? *Nursing Times*, **88(32)**, 54–55.

Budd S. (1992) Traditional Chinese medicine in obstetrics. *Midwives Chronicle*, June, 140–143.

Cresswell J. (1993) Handle with care. *Nursing Times*, **89(1)**, 18–19.

Department of Health (1993) *Changing Childbirth*. HMSO, London.

Dundee J.W., Sourial F.B.R., Ghaly R.G. *et al.*, (1988) P6 acupuncture reduces morning sickness. *Journal of the Royal Society of Medicine*, **81(8)**, 456–457

Feltham E. (1991) Therapeutic touch and massage. *Nursing Standard*, **5(45)**, 26–28

Freer C. (1985) What kind of alternative is alternative medicine? *Journal of the Royal College of General Practitioners*, October, 459–460

Fulder S. (1989) A complementary NHS? *Here's Health*, February, 46–47

Gaier H. (1991) Reveille for biocentric medicine. In: *Complementary medicine and the European Community*, pp. 9–34, C.W. Daniel.

Guthrie K. *et al.* (1984) Maternal hypnosis induced by husbands during childbirth. *Journal of Obstetrics and Gynaecology*, **4(5)**, 93–95

Heidt P. (1990) Openness: a qualitative analysis of nurses' and patients' experiences of therapeutic touch. *Journal of Nursing Scholarship*, **22(3)**, 180–186.

Hewitt D. and Woolfson A. (1992) Intensive Aromacare. *International Journal of Aromatherapy*, **4(2)**, 12–14.

Hillman A. (1986) Alternative medicine – an introduction. *Nursing*, January, 26–28.

Hyde E. (1987) Acupressure therapy for morning sickness. A controlled clinical trial. *Journal of Nurse-Midwifery*, **43(4)**, 171–178.

Klougart N. *et al.* (1989) Infantile colic treated by chiropractors: a prospective study of 316 cases. *Journal of Manipulative and Physiological Therapeutics*, **12(3)**, 281–288.

Krieger D. (1990) Therapeutic touch: two decades of research, teaching and clinical practice. *NSNA/IMPRINT*, September/October, p83–88.

Martin S. (1989) Hale health. *Here's Health*, August, 44–45.

Martin S. (1990) Nurses take in alternatives. *Here's Health*, February, 18–20.

Martin S. (1991) Where's the proof? *Here's Health*, December, 36–38.

NAHAT (1993) Complementary therapies in the NHS. National Association of Health Authorities and Trusts.

Newbeck I. (1986) The whole works. *Nursing Times*, **82(30)**, 48–49.

Newbeck I. and Rowe (1986) Going the whole way. *Nursing Times*, **82(8)**, 24–25.

Passant H. (1990) Complementary therapies – a holistic approach on the ward. *Nursing Times*, **86(4)**, 26–28.

Quinn J. (1988) Building a body of knowledge: research on therapeutic touch 1974–1986. *Journal of Holistic Nursing*, **6(1)**, 37–45.

Sanderson H. and Harrison J. (1991) *Aromatherapy and Massage for People with Learning Difficulties*. Hands On Publishing.

Shifrin K. (1993) Setting standards for acupuncture training – a model for complementary medicine. *Complementary Therapies in Medicine*, **1(2)**, 91–95.

Skelton I. and Flowerdew M. (1985) Midwives and acupuncture. *Midwives Chronicle*, May, 125–129.

Thayer M. (1990) Touching with intent: using therapeutic touch. *Pediatric Nursing (Canada)*, **16(1)**, 70–72.

Thomas K. (1991) Non-orthodox healthcare in the UK. In: *Complementary Medicine and the European Community*, pp. 125–133, C.W. Daniel.

Trevelyan J. (1992) Complementary care. *Nursing Times*, **8(29)**, 23.

UKCC (1985) *Advertising by Registered Nurses, Midwives and Health Visitors*.

UKCC (1989) *Exercising Accountability*.

UKCC (1993) *Midwives' Rules*.

UKCC (1992a) *Guidelines for the Administration of Medicines*.

UKCC (1992b) *Scope of Professional Practice*.

UKCC (1993) *Standards for Records and Record Keeping*.

Wheater C. (1990) In-house help for health. *Here's Health*, June, 50.

Denise Tiran

Chapter 2

An Overview of Complementary Therapies for Pregnancy and Childbirth

Many physiological changes occur in the body during pregnancy resulting in a variety of troublesome discomforts. The medical profession refers to these as 'minor' disorders for they are not normally of a pathological nature – but they may be major inconveniences for the expectant mother. Additionally, because they are naturally occurring manifestations of the pregnancy, there may be very little to offer in the form of treatment. The pregnant woman is prescribed medication only when absolutely necessary, to avoid risk to the unborn child, but this may lead to an implicit medical attitude that she should 'put up' with the complaint as it is only temporary.

In labour the mother may wish to use a form of pain relief not normally offered within mainstream maternity care, and in response midwives could expand the selection from which the mother may choose. Postnatally 'alternative' therapies are often gentler for mothers and their infants at a time when they are feeling vulnerable.

Perhaps more than anything women want to be in control of their own bodies; they want to make informed choices about what they consider to be the best treatment available, or to be able to try several methods of dealing with the physical and psychological upheaval which is facing them at this time. However, midwives need to be aware of their professional responsibilities when advising the women in their care about the alternatives available. It is sometimes difficult to know where to 'draw the line' when discussing complementary therapies, so as not to exceed accepted professional boundaries (see Chapter 1). It can also be confusing knowing which therapy to suggest for different problems, although some are more clearly defined than others, for example the first choice for women with back problems is likely to be an osteopath. Deciding which therapies a midwife can use or recommend may depend upon local availability; if there are midwives qualified in specific therapies it is preferable that they should utilise their skills in conjunction with their midwifery practice. If no midwives within a particular area have developed the relevant skills, undertaking training in a therapy may be influenced by financial or time constraints. If a mother wishes to be referred to a therapist outside her normal antenatal care system, this will also be affected by the proximity of reputable therapists, and perhaps their availability on the National Health Service e.g. homeopathy, or through private medical insurance schemes, some of which will now allow claims for osteopathy, chiropractic, acupuncture and homeopathy and occasionally aromatherapy.

This chapter aims to provide midwives with an overview of the various uses of complementary therapies for childbearing women and to expand on the discussion from Chapter 1 about what exactly the midwife is allowed to do. Each of the conditions is dealt with in more detail by the specialist contributors in the chapters relating to the specific therapies, but this overview is intended to highlight the possible, though not exhaustive, range of alternatives for any one condition.

Let us then explore some of the commoner conditions of the childbearing year, with which midwives may have to deal, and analyse the ways in which complementary therapies can be of use. It is assumed that the reader will already be familiar with the conventional management of most of the disorders and this has been omitted.

Infertility Secondary infertility or subfertility, while not normally the province of the midwife, may occur in women already known to them. The usual advice about diet, lifestyle, sexual activity etc. can be discussed but some women may wish to pursue other means of dealing with the condition.

Complementary therapies such as homeopathy, acupuncture, osteopathy, shiatsu, herbal medicine and chiropractic all have a part to play, particularly as the therapists will take a much more comprehensive, or perhaps one should say a more broadly focused, case history than some conventional medical practitioners. Many of the therapists will attempt to find and treat the cause whilst others aim to alleviate the psychological upset which often accompanies infertility. Acupuncture may be able to treat causative factors, such as pelvic inflammatory disease (Robinson, 1988). Homeopaths would search for all possible related signs and symptoms, and may prescribe the appropriate constitutional remedy in the first instance or others such as silicea, phosphorous or natrum mur. according to the symptoms. Treatment with medical herbalism may include St John's wort to improve circulation or chasteberry to regulate the menstrual cycle. Realignment of the musculos-keletal system with osteopathy, chiropractic or the Alexander technique can facilitate a return to normal of the endocrine and reproductive systems.

Jenny was receiving osteopathic treatment for a back problem. Coincidentally, or so she thought, a long-term menstrual disorder, which had resulted in an inability to conceive, seemed to improve. On questioning the osteopath she explained that Jenny had had a problem in the upper cervical vertebrae which in turn had caused tension on the pituitary gland in the brain. Release of this tension with osteopathic techniques had facilitated a return to normal of Jenny's menstrual cycle and indeed she was proud to report that she was pregnant within 6 weeks of the treatment.

Drama therapy has also been used with success to treat infertile couples by engendering an outpouring of stress and anxiety. Other therapies which assist in relaxing the potential parents can be useful, such as aromatherapy, reflexology, relaxation exercises, meditation, t'ai chi, yoga, art, music or even humour therapy, hypnotherapy or therapeutic touch.

The examination of the nutritional status of both partners may elicit deficiencies in zinc, manganese, essential fatty acids or vitamin E, particularly in women who suffer recurrent miscarriages (Davies and Stewart, 1987, p. 327). Research into male infertility has shown that the nutrients which may be lacking include zinc, chromium, selenium and arginine (Piesse, 1983; Davies and Stewart, 1987, p. 328).

Once pregnant, the majority of women will experience a variety of symptoms related to the altered physiology, and it is in the management of these that complementary therapies can be of such value.

Sickness Sickness in pregnancy, thought to be caused by the hormones oestrogen and human chorionic gonadotrophin, but exacerbated by low blood sugar, affects about 50% of mothers. Traditional advice has been to drink a cup of tea and eat a piece of dry toast before rising, but this will not suit everyone, and in fact tea and coffee intake should be reduced because of the effects of caffeine which may cause headaches. Dietary modifications may be of use – eating small, frequent meals, avoiding fatty and spicy foods and drinking plenty of (pure) water. Nutritional therapists suggest eliminating dairy produce from the diet and taking daily supplements of vitamin B6 and zinc (50 mg of each). Many women in early pregnancy, particularly those who were previously taking the oral contraceptive pill, may be deficient in these elements, and preconception administration may even prevent gestational nausea and vomiting (Davies and Stewart, 1987, p. 341).

The use of ginger is helpful and can be used either in cooking, or as ginger root tea or capsules, or crystallised ginger can be advised (Roach, 1985; Stewart, 1987; McIntyre, 1988, p. 79). Yoghurt has been found to be of benefit also (Butler, 1985). Midwives could advise any of these dietary adaptations within their normal sphere of practice.

Acupuncture from a suitably experienced practitioner has been well documented as an effective treatment (Skelton and Flowerdew, 1986; Dundee *et al.*, 1988; Budd, 1992). There has also been interest recently in the use of bands worn around the wrists which apply pressure over the appropriate acupuncture points (via acupressure). Research has shown that the bands are very effective both during pregnancy and for cancer patients receiving chemotherapy (Stannard, 1989; Hyde, 1989; Sadler, 1989), and it is now possible to purchase them in large health stores and pharmacies. Midwives would need to refer mothers for acupuncture treatment to a qualified practitioner, but could suggest the wristbands within their own accountability. It would not be expensive for antenatal clinics to keep a supply of acupressure wristbands for loan to mothers suffering sickness.

Herbalists would suggest teas of lemon balm, camomile, lavender, red raspberry leaf or black horehound, but the mother should again seek qualified help in unresponsive cases (Fulder, 1991). Midwives could recommend that mothers try camomile tea, as this is available from health food stores and supermarkets.

There are several over-the-counter homeopathic remedies available such as ipecachuana, sepia or nux vomica (Castro, 1992, p. 95), but it is advisable to discuss the precise symptoms with a qualified homeopath to find the most appropriate solution for the individual. Although it is often thought that no harm can be done by taking homeopathic remedies which have no effect, this may not be so, and indeed the symptom intended to be treated may be exacerbated. However the increased demand from both mothers and midwives has led to plans at the Faculty of Homeopathy of the Royal London Homeopathic Hospital to develop a short course for midwives to enable them to learn the principles of homeopathy and for limited homeopathic prescribing in pregnancy and childbirth.

Reflexology may be beneficial in alleviating nausea and vomiting, especially if it is related to stress and tension, and midwives who have received the relevant training may perform the technique. This must still be within professional boundaries and in accordance with local policy.

Referring the mother to a hypnotherapist can be useful but midwives should assure themselves that the practitioners they suggest are adequately trained and have a reputable practice. It may be useful for staff in local maternity services to identify certain complementary practitioners to whom mothers could be referred and to keep an 'approved' list, according to locally defined criteria.

Occasionally yoga can be of help in mild cases, but unless they have practised yoga previously mothers may not feel inclined to learn the positions at a time when they are feeling unwell.

Heartburn Heartburn plagues many women especially in the latter part of pregnancy, due to hormonal and weight changes. It can be relieved by common sense dietary adjustments such as avoiding acid or fatty foods, but may be helped additionally by taking garlic, either as capsules or used in cooking. Unpeeled cloves soften when cooked and the pulp can be squeezed out; in this way more garlic can be used without overwhelming the tastebuds or the breath. It should be noted however that herbalists recommend the ingestion of a whole raw garlic clove daily as the active ingredients may be destroyed to a certain extent by heat. Care must be taken when buying garlic capsules to ensure that they contain the active ingredients – allicin and various sulphur-containing compounds. It is these which give garlic its characteristic smell, but while some 'odourless' capsules release the allicin slowly after ingestion, others contain very little of the active ingredients.

Although milk and milk products have traditionlly been thought to be effective in treating heartburn by reducing acidity, nutritional therapists believe that this is not necessarily so and that they may even exacerbate symptoms. Excessive use of antacids is to be avoided, especially those which contain aluminium as this is absorbed by the mother and may be toxic to the fetus. It is recommended that women with heartburn avoid tea, coffee, sugar, alcohol and smoking, all of which aggravate the condition, and avoiding food additives in the E220–276 range may reduce the intensity (Davies and Stewart, 1987, p. 342).

Shiatsu techniques can be taught to mothers to perform on themselves, without the risk of any adverse effects. They should be shown how to find the point four fingers breadth above the umbilicus, in the midline, and to press intermittently with two fingers for 10 seconds at a time over a period of about 5 minutes (Fig. 1).

A homeopath may suggest the use of capsicum or other appropriate remedies. Mothers are perfectly at liberty to purchase homeopathic remedies for themselves, and may receive expert assistance in some health food stores, but midwives should refrain from making suggestions about possible treatments unless they are familiar with the system of homeopathic medicine. If a mother mentions that she is taking self-prescribed remedies the midwife can help by ensuring that she is aware of the correct way of taking them. Homeopathic medicines should be handled as little as possible, and dispensed into the lid of the bottle rather than a spoon; if a spoon is used it should be made of plastic not metal. The mother should refrain from using mint-flavoured toothpaste and other strongly aromatic substances such as coffee for the duration of the treatment, and her mouth should be free of food and drink for an hour before taking the tablets. These rules need to be followed as homeopathic remedies may be antidoted by coming in contact with

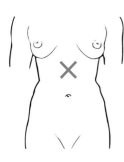

Fig. 1. To show the shiatsu point to press for the relief of heartburn – intermittent two-fingered pressure on the midline point four fingers breadth above umbilicus.

strong flavours. For the same reason they should be stored away from essential oils, particularly peppermint, preferably in a separate cupboard.

Likewise, women wishing to use herbal medicine would best be advised to consult a qualified practitioner who may recommend slippery elm, dandelion root, ginger or camomile tea. It is possible for women to purchase for themselves slippery elm lozenges, so midwives may want to suggest these while stating that they are not familiar with their use so are unable to give further information. Alternatively midwives could suggest that mothers make a tea from infusing a piece of ginger root in a pot of camomile tea, and sipping this, either hot or iced.

Aromatherapists also utilise camomile, either as a tea or for abdominal massage, perhaps combined with lavender. Here again midwives could advise mothers to buy some of the camomile tea bags for themselves but should be cautious about recommending camomile oil unless they are familiar enough to advise on blending, dosage, storage and application.

Osteopathy has been shown to be invaluable in treating heartburn (Montague, 1985), and mothers could refer themselves to an appropriately qualified and experienced osteopath in their area. Yoga classes may also enable the mother to learn various poses to alleviate the heartburn, and some areas organise sessions specifically for pregnant women.

Constipation Constipation during pregnancy occurs normally as a result of the hormone progesterone which dilates the smooth muscle of the intestines and slows down intestinal action, but the condition is aggravated by the consumption of tea as tannin 'clogs' the gut (Davies and Stewart, 1987, p. 206; Sharon, 1992, p. 109). One only has to see the inside of a teapot to imagine what happens within the intestines! Replacing early morning tea with hot water and lemon and drinking herbal and fruit teas during the day will alleviate the problem. Senna is a well-known aperient but may be too purgative for some in pregnancy; mallow capsules or adding artichoke to soups and casseroles may be gentler (McIntyre, 1988, p. 70). Eating plenty of fibrous and vitamin C-containing foods such as citrus fruits, especially blackcurrants, and wholegrain foods is conventionally recommended, but supplements of vitamin C and magnesium may be necessary occasionally. Midwives can also recommend that the mother eats plenty of raw garlic, onions, parsley and nettles in salads, and some authorities suggest starting every meal with raw food (Kenton, 1986).

Medical herbalists also prescribe dandelion root tea for its laxative properties, while homeopaths may select nux vomica, bryonia, natrum mur. or another appropriate remedy according to the symptoms.

Abdominal massage in a clockwise direction, particularly if enhanced by the use of essential oils of mandarin or orange, is one of the cheapest and most effective means of dealing with constipation and may be applied ante- and postnatally, as well as on babies. Midwives could quite easily perform the abdominal massage but should only incorporate the essential oils if they have had some training in their use (see Chapter 3).

The mother can follow up the massage with a shiatsu technique by locating the point halfway between the pubic bone and the umbilicus, in the midline, and (as with heartburn) applying intermittent two fingered pressure for 10 seconds at a time (Fig. 2).

Additionally, midwives could utilise an aspect of reflexology without applying the specific technique. In reflexology the arches of the feet correspond to the intestines and gentle clockwise massage of this area would also help to stimulate peristalsis; in fact the mother could ask her partner to do this for her at home. However for postnatal constipation following Caesarean section this is contraindicated by midwives not qualified in reflex zone therapy as the zone on the foot relating to the incision may be over-stimulated and could cause pain (see Chapter 4).

Ensuring time, warmth and privacy when using the toilet is important to avoid reflex inhibition, and indeed postnatal mothers may be treated best by early transfer home.

Once again yoga poses can be beneficial, as can acupuncture and osteopathy if the mother is already consulting one of these professionals, but the simpler and cheaper manual techniques described should be the first means of tackling the condition, and are usually just as effective.

Anaemia Constipation may be worsened by the routine administration of iron, still prescribed by many obstetricians and general practitioners, despite research indicating that the practice is not only futile and contrary to normal physiology, but also undesirable and economically non-viable (Hemminski and Starfield, 1978; Sheldon *et al.*, 1985). Some authorities believe now that zinc supplements would be far more beneficial as this is required for cell formation and fetal development, and many women are deficient through poor dietary intake, stress (zinc is lost in the urine at times of stress), drinking alcohol or smoking (Davies and Stewart, 1987, p. 65; Bryce-Smith, 1986). Iron supplements should be avoided if the woman is taking zinc, as iron interferes with absorption of zinc through the intestines. Women whose haemoglobin level is pathologically lowered should increase their vitamin C intake to assist with absorption of dietary iron, and consider taking a herbal iron-rich preparation such as Floradix, available from health food stores. Blackcurrants are a particularly rich source of vitamin C; carotene, found in raw carrots, and thyme assist in binding iron and facilitating absorption. Other herbs which could be added to the diet include parsley, mint, fennel, rosemary, savory; watercress and horseradish are also good sources of iron. (For a comprehensive list of iron-rich foods see Chapter 8.)

Homeopaths may prescribe China for women who are anaemic due to preconceptional or antenatal haemorrhage, or remedies such as ferrum met., arsenicum, pulsatilla or natrum mur., depending on the individual.

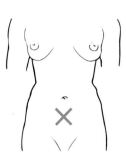

Fig. 2. To show the shiatsu point to press to ease constipation – intermittent two-fingered pressure in the midline, halfway between the umbilicus and the symphysis pubis.

Varicosities Varicosities sometimes occur in later pregnancy due to extra weight and pressure and should disappear within 6–8 weeks of delivery as hormone levels return to normal. Direct massage of varicosed areas of the legs is contraindicated, as this can not only be painful but may also precipitate the release of thrombin into the circulation. However a witch hazel compress or bathing in warm water to which has been added the essential oil of lemon (in a 3% blend, see Chapter 3) may ease the aching which accompanies the condition. Whirlpool baths can be soothing but jacuzzis should be avoided because of the addition of chemicals. Sitting in a bowl of warm water containing oil of cypress is useful in late pregnancy for haemorrhoids but midwives should be wary of recommending this as cypress is one of the oils contraindicated in pregnancy. It is possible to use it in very low dilutions for local application in late pregnancy but this should only be advised by a qualified aromatherapist. This example demonstrates the potential minefield for midwives in that 'a little knowledge is a dangerous thing'.

Garlic helps to tone the circulatory system and can be taken throughout pregnancy, and other dietary recommendations are aimed at generally improving the circulation. Herbal remedies include yarrow, golden seal, horse chestnut and hawthorn for varicose veins of the legs and lesser celandine for haemorrhoids, but these are best prescribed by qualified herbalists. However midwives could advise the direct application to haemorrhoids of grated raw potato to reduce swelling and discomfort. Homeopaths may suggest pulsatilla or hamamelis virginica.

Yoga poses can be taught which will ease the discomfort but it is unlikely that the varicosities will be resolved until the reduction in hormone levels occurs postnatally.

Oedema Oedema of the lower legs, whether of physioloical or pathological origin, can be eased by firm bimanual massage in an upwards wringing motion, which could be performed for just 2 or 3 minutes by the midwife conducting antenatal care. If the mother is wearing tights no oil needs to be used for the material will prevent friction occurring; alternatively if the mother's legs are bare a small amount of talcum powder, which could be kept in each clinic cubicle, would serve the same purpose (see Fig. 7 in Chapter 3,). Once the mother is aware of the movement and pressure required she could ask her partner to perform this for her. Essential oils of geranium and rosemary will complement the massage but care must be taken with rosemary due to its hypertensive action, so again, unless this has been advised by an aromatherapist, it is best avoided.

Yoga may be effective if the mother is referred to an approriate class. Likewise leg cramps will respond to massage and gentle extension of the muscles. The application of an olive leaf compress is recommended by herbalists, or the inclusion of parsley, onion and garlic in the diet, while reflexology will tone and relax the body and act as a preventive measure in women susceptible to cramps.

Cabbage, geranium or rhubarb leaves applied to the oedematous area provide a simple and inexpensive means of relieving the discomfort. The treatment is also effective for engorged breasts in the early postnatal days (see Chapters 3 and 8).

Backache Backache can be a serious discomfort in pregnancy due to the hormonal effects of progesterone and relaxin as well as the increased maternal weight. Lumbosacral pain in labour is common whilst postnatally pain may be felt in the neck and upper back, particularly if breastfeeding without adequate support.

Osteopathy is usually acknowledged as the most appropriate form of treatment, but acupuncture or shiatsu from a qualified therapist can be successful, or yoga can be taught and practised. Tutorials in the Alexander technique will also improve posture and alleviate back pain, although this demands a degree of commitment from the mother which she may not feel able to fulfil at this time.

In the last month of pregnancy or in labour, transcutaneous electrical nerve stimulation (TENS) is beneficial, especially when there is sciatic pain, but it should be avoided before 37 weeks as anecdotal reports suggest that it may prematurely induce labour. TENS is now available in many maternity units and has become part of the repertoire of analgesia which the midwife can offer, although it is certainly not the norm in all units (see Chapter 12). The United Kingdom Central Council (UKCC) has approved the use of TENS by midwives when caring for labouring women (see p. 27).

Mustard capsules have been used to good effect by phytotherapists, or a warm mustard compress can be self-administered by dissolving mustard powder in warm water, soaking a cloth in it and applying it to the affected area. Back and leg massage with essential oils of geranium, marjoram and lavender is a relaxing means of treating the problem and can be performed before, during and after labour as necessary. The safest oil for midwives to suggest is lavender, although this is contraindicated in the first trimester of pregnancy (see Chapter 3). Reflexology, particularly along the inner edge of the feet may provide temporary relief in acute cases but is not the treatment of choice for gestational backache which results from the lumbar lordosis (see Chapter 4).

Various homeopathic medicines are suitable, including arnica if the cause is trauma or sepia or nux vomica when the back pain coincides with constipation.

Headache Headache can be soothed by massage of the scalp in a firm 'hairwashing' action or the application of two drops of neat lavender oil to the temples, similar to the use of lavender water so beloved of elderly ladies earlier in the century. Lavender is one of the few essential oils which can be used neat for certain conditions, but it is important to buy a good quality brand and not rely on that which is available from popular high street stores unless they can guarantee its authenticity.

Reflexology around the big toes can help also as these are the zones for the head, and midwives could apply simple firm massage to the toes (see Chapter 4). Dietary measures include the elimination of caffeine – in tea, coffee, cola and chocolate, and avoiding the E200s range of food additives. Headache is common in early pregnancy due to progesterone dilating the cerebral blood vessels. However any complementary therapies can only be used symptomatically if there is pregnancy-induced hypertension accompanied by oedema and/or proteinuria. In cases of impending eclampsia, gentle massage may relieve anxiety, improve circulation and facilitate excretion of urine, but the midwife must always work within the constraints of medical direction.

Osteopathy, especially craniosacral therapy, or chiropractic manipulations will release musculoskeletal tension if this is found to be the cause of physiological rather than pathological headache. A simple shiatsu technique involves pressure with two fingers underneath the occiput which works on one of the meridians to rebalance the energy flow. One-to-one tuition in the Alexander technique may help in this situation as well as with backache.

Insomnia Insomnia may become a problem as pregnancy progresses due to the inability to find a comfortable position, as well as heartburn, nocturnal fetal activity and a need to pass urine frequently during the night. The mother-to-be should avoid all stimulants (caffeine, alcohol, cheese etc,) and try to 'wind down' for 2 hours before retiring.

A warm camomile bath and a cup of camomile or valerian tea will aid relaxation and induce sleep, and a massage with camomile and marjoram will enhance the feeling of well-being. The use of pillows to support the back, legs and abdomen will facilitate a more comfortable position and some women find relief from resting their heads on a herb- or hop-filled pillow from which they can inhale the aromas. Any of these could be suggested by midwives and it may be possible to offer blended aromatherapy oils for women to add to their baths while in the ante- or postnatal wards, or for them to take home. These would need to be accurately blended, either by the pharmacy staff or a midwife aromatherapist, and permission of the obstetrician obtained. Shiatsu, performed before retiring by a qualified practitioner, can be relaxing too.

Hypnotherapy training can help to calm an overactive mind which could be the cause of an inability to fall asleep, or the use of spoken or instrumental relaxation tapes may help. Midwives could maintain a selection of the cassette tapes for loan or hire to women for use in their own homes and may wish to consider their value in both ante- and postnatal wards, as well as for relaxation in labour.

Various homeopathic remedies may be suitable, according to the precise symptoms, such as coffea when the brain seems overstimulated (as when someone has drunk too much coffee). Herbal medicines such as valerian are best prescribed by a qualified therapist.

Mood swings Mood swings and mild depression can be a normal aspect of pregnancy when there are physical, emotional, social and financial concerns. Massage or using room vaporisers with geranium, lavender or camomile oils soothes the nerves and, in the case of massage, eases muscle tensions, while practising yoga combined with daily meditation or other relaxation exercises may help some (see Chapter 5). Herbalists may suggest valerian or lavender taken as a decoction but the commoner anti-tension remedy of passiflora is to be avoided during pregnancy as it may have a stimulating action on the uterus.

Regular reflexology can also help to relieve tension but unless this is a service offered within the maternity unit women would have to pay a practitioner outside the National Health Service.

Bach (pronounced 'batch') flower remedies can be self-administered, the remedy chosen according to the precise nature of the mood. Women who become very anxious, perhaps even suffering panic attacks, may find the Rescue Remedy of particular value. This is an inexpensive Bach remedy which contains a combination of five of the Bach flower remedies, in homeopathic (i.e. minimal) doses and is excellent for reducing panic, anxiety, hysteria or shock. Four drops applied neat to the tongue is the optimum means of administering to an adult, or added to a small glass of water and sipped. Children should have a half dose and health visitors may wish to investigate its benefit as a remedy for toddler temper tantrums. Other remedies may be chosen according to the cause of the problem, for example, mimulus if the mother is afraid of possible fetal abnormalities or of the approaching labour, olive for tiredness and weariness, or crab apple as a cleanser for the woman who dislikes her changing shape or has a general feeling of unpleasantness (Howard, 1992). Bach remedies are available in many health stores with accompanying directions for use so that the mother can select the most appropriate one for herself, but midwives who are unfamiliar with them should not recommend them to the women in their care. Midwives should state only that they have heard that the remedies can be effective but that they are not in a position to comment further; the conversation should be recorded in the notes.

Hypnotherapy may be a valuable tool for those women who are anxious about the forthcoming labour, but midwives should ensure that any recommendations they give are for reputable practitioners; hypnotherapy in particular is a field in which a poorly trained or unqualified therapist can do untold harm to the mother.

Encouraging the mother to increase her exercise and physical activity may facilitate a reduction in tension and it may be that for some women conventional parent education classes and exercises to prepare for labour and the postnatal period could be replaced by t'ai chi, pregnancy aerobics or 'aquanatal' (see Chapter 6), under the direction of appropriately qualified exercise teachers or physiotherapists.

Natrum mur. would seem to be the homeopathic remedy of first choice for prenatal depression although others such as phosphorous may be more appropriate for some mothers.

Thrush Irritating common infections such as thrush, caused by changes in vaginal acidity, can be treated with dietary measures, for example by avoiding all yeast products (including vinegar), sugar (beware 'hidden' sugars in savoury processed foods), and antibiotics if possible (including those used in the deep freezing of meat). Garlic is a natural antibacterial agent and can be taken in food or as capsules. More direct use of garlic involves wrapping a raw, peeled and oiled clove in muslin for insertion in the vagina (see Chapter 8). Other herbal remedies include marigold or thyme. Dipping a tampon in live natural yoghurt and inserting this vaginally may combat the thrush as may a tampon dipped in diluted tea tree oil. However while the yoghurt remedy can be safely recommended by midwives, the tampon-in-tea-tree solution should only be sugested by midwives who are familiar with its use. Pessaries containing tea tree oil are now available in health stores which the mother could buy without the risks of mixing an incorrect blend of the essential oil. Tea tree is antibacterial, antiviral and antifungal so if the diagnosis is not candidiasis, the condition may still be treated effectively. However, midwives should again record any conversation with the mother about the vaginal discharge and irritation as it is outside the limits of the midwife's practice to diagnose and prescribe treatment for an abnormality – medical opinion should be sought. Midwives could produce scientific evidence from complementary and conventional medical journals to demonstrate to the consultants the effectiveness of tea tree in an attempt to convince them of the value of stocking the pessaries on standing order (see Chapter 3).

If a mother chooses to consult a homeopath she may be prescribed a compound such as candida acidophilus or sepia, according to her symptoms and her own remedy classification. Eating a daily portion of live active yoghurt containing acidophilus may act as a preventative measure for women susceptible to candidiasis.

Cystitis Cystitis may be treated with homeopathic, herbal or aromatherapy preparations such as camomile, and reflexology can aid excretion of urine and a consequent flushing of the urinary tract. Even osteopathy can be effective in easing frequency of micturition of a non-infective origin through manipulation of the musculoskeletal system and indirectly of all its appendages. Any woman who is susceptible to cystitis and urinary tract infections may benefit from drinking a small glass of cranberry juice daily as a preventative measure, and copious amounts of camomile tea and homemade pearl barley water to neutralise acidity if the condition does arise. Nettle or marigold tea can also be beneficial.

Many women are worried about the onset, course and duration of labour as well as their ability to cope with the contractions, but there is much that midwives can suggest to help women.

Onset of labour The use of raspberry leaf tea or tablets could be commenced at about 28 weeks of pregnancy, gradually increasing from one cup of tea or one tablet a day to four of either by term. Raspberry leaf tones the uterine muscle and makes labour contractions more efficient and possibly less painful. It serves to assist in 'ripening' of the cervix prior to labour and can be drunk throughout the first stage (hot or iced) to stimulate contractions. It has long been recommended by herbalists (McIntyre, 1988, pp. 48-49; Peterson, 1989, p. 67) but midwives who are unfamiliar with it may only advise that they are aware of its benefits but are not sufficiently cognisant with it to offer more comprehensive information. If a mother asks about drinking it in labour midwives can be reassured that it is safe to use and will have no adverse effects on any medically prescribed drugs.

Herbalists seem to disagree amongst themselves about when the raspberry leaf should be commenced in pregnancy; McIntyre (1988, p. 54) advises it in cases of threatened miscarriage, and from mid-pregnancy, whilst Peterson (1989, p.67) states that it is contraindicated until late in the third trimester because of its contractile effects on the uterus. Most authorities however encourage its use in the puerperium to facilitate involution.

Suitable essential oils added to a base massage oil include bergamot (uplifting), camomile (relaxing, good for cramping pains), geranium (relieves anxiety), lavender, marjoram (alleviates stress), rose (soothing) and ylang ylang (creates a sense of well-being). For women whose labour is not yet established simple sacral massage with a blend of lavender and mandarin essential oils can be much more pleasant, have less side effects than the ubiquitous oral analgesia and sedation, and may in fact enhance and coordinate uterine action.

Nipple stimulation can be suggested to some mothers who appear receptive, to aid cervical ripening and initiate uterine contractions through the natural release of oxytocin from the pituitary gland. Only one nipple at a time should be massaged by rolling between finger and thumb as oxytocin release may be excessive and cause hypertonia if both breasts are stimulated together. Midwives could advise this method of cervical ripening and 'DIY' induction within the limits of their own practice for it is based on a normal knowledge of physiology. The usual accountability issues pertain here, i.e. adequate information about the pros and cons of the technique must be given to the mother to enable her to make an informed choice and the advice given must be recorded in the notes.

Sexual intercourse near term may help also in triggering labour because of the prostaglandins in semen and the local release of maternal prostaglandins from the cervix. Many midwives have suggested this to women over the years, especially those anxious to avoid a hospital induction when they have booked a home birth. Clitoral stimulation could also be advised to selected mothers. Clitoral stimulation causes the release of endorphins from the brain which create a sense of euphoria and ease discomfort in labour, so it can be an additional means of analgesia for some women. If it also results in orgasm during which the uterus contracts it may initiate contractions in the mother whose cervix is ripe, or aid the ripening process in others.

Women who are already receiving help from a qualified therapist such as an acupuncturist, herbalist or homeopath may be facilitated towards the onset of labour by their practitioners. This may be acceptable for mothers who are supposedly 'overdue' and who may have been advised to have labour induced in hospital for this reason alone.

Reflex zone therapy, performed by a midwife qualified in the therapy, with medical approval, may be effective in stimulating the body's own mechanisms to initiate labour, particularly when the therapist works on the zones to the uterus and the pituitary gland (see Chapter 4). However if midwives are made aware that a mother is receiving alternative assistance to increase uterine action, they should record this knowledge in the notes. It is of course preferable that any treatment intended to initiate contractions, by whatever means, is undertaken in the full knowledge of all concerned, including the parents and both conventional and complementary practitioners. Likewise if midwives become aware that a mother is taking action to induce labour herself, this should be recorded. Some cultures encourage the use of a variety of natural methods of self-help, most of which are traditionally handed down from mother to daughter and have been found to be effective. For example West Indian women may eat okra in order to stimulate labour, but of course the midwife would not, on her own accountability, recommend this to women without further information with which to support the claim.

Pain control Pain control in labour is a controversial subject but some maternity units now 'permit' mothers to be accompanied by their alternative practitioners. Midwives too are gaining qualifications in different therapies to enhance their work and provide additional choices for mothers. The presence of a homeopath, acupuncturist, herbalist or other therapist should not cause conflict if planned in advance in cooperation with the midwives and doctors. However with the increasing involvement of alternative therapists in the care of childbearing women, maternity unit staff would be well advised to develop appropriate policies relating to visiting practitioners.

These should address issues of accountability, overall supervision of the mothers' care, insurance and the role of the alternative practitioner within the maternity unit. It is preferable to anticipate that some women may wish to be accompanied by their therapists, even in units where this has not occurred before, and to consider the multidisciplinary development of a policy, rather than be caught unawares. Potential antagonism from any staff can be worked through and a positive reception to mothers' requests to bring in their therapists should result in far greater collaboration between all carers, whether conventional or complementary, and the parents (see Chapter 1).

If a midwife feels unable to care for a mother using complementary thera-pies, she should endeavour to deploy a different midwife who is sympathetic to the mother's wishes. However, it should be highlighted that, following a meeting on 'appropriate technologies for birth', the World Health Organization recommended that natural birth without the routine adminis-tration of analgesia should be advocated (Wagner, 1993). This has implications for those midwives who seek to 'control' women by quietening them with analgesia, effectively to reduce the 'midwives' distress syndrome'. Midwives should make every effort to learn about and begin to use the alter-natives which are available so that they can offer a wider range of pain relieving methods to women in labour.

Hypnosis can be self-administered in labour, having been learned and practised in pregnancy. Trials in various units have shown that hypnotherapy can be a valuable aid in labour by reducing stress and anxiety and facilitating the mother's ability to cope with the pain of the contractions (Gartside, 1982; Guthrie *et al.*, 1984; Brann and Guzvica, 1987; Conway, 1987; Boot, 1987; Fitzgerald, 1987; Woods, 1989; Wine, 1989; Steven, 1990; Jenkins and Pritchard, 1993).

Self-help in the form of yoga positions learnt and practised during preg-nancy will enhance relaxation and indeed may be effective in correcting an abnormal position of the fetus (Balaskas, 1990). Midwives may be able to recommend suitable classes or plan to invite a yoga teacher to run classes in the maternity unit. The person involved would need to be assessed as being the most appropriate according to locally defined needs. Yoga as a discipline has several schools of thought, some of which are more esoteric or related to Eastern philosophies than others, and midwives should identify a type which best seems to suit the local clientele.

Transcutaneous electrical nerve stimulation (TENS) is a relatively new means of pain relief in labour and is being offered increasingly by midwives who wish to provide a wider choice for their clients. TENS works by inter-rupting the pain impulses travelling to the brain and thereby decreasing the intensity of pain perceived by the mother. It is gaining popularity amongst parents because it is controlled by the mother and is non-invasive. The UKCC has approved the use of TENS by midwives as an additional means of pain relief in labour but they should, of course, have been trained in its use within the limits of professional accountability.

Massage is comforting for some women in labour although it must be remembered that others dislike being touched at this time. However if touch is used positively, from a psychological viewpoint its physiological benefits are undoubted. Regular massage (effleurage or circular stroking) of the abdomen and back and other areas of tension helps to relax the mother prior to and during labour and this can be performed by midwives or the mother's partner. Many midwives spontaneously apply pressure to the sacral area during the first stage of labour and a simple shiatsu technique to relieve pain can also be carried out by the midwife. By pressing intermittently during each contraction with the thumb tips in the 'dimples' either side of the spine from the coccyx to the waist, the nerve pathways which serve the uterus will be affected and contraction pain will be eased (see Chapter 7 and Fig. 5 in Chapter 3).

Aromatherapists suggest the application of a warm compress of clary sage oil just above the pubic bone and on the lower back to ease the aches often experienced in early labour, while lavender can enhance contractions and relieve the pain of established labour.

Reflexology can be useful in stimulating the pituitary gland to release oxytocin, with direct work on the parts of the feet which relate to the uterus. It is also soothing and relaxing and will reduce stress and tension which can hinder the progress of labour. Bach remedies such as the Rescue Remedy for panic and anxiety, especially around the transition stage, or aspen for non-specific fears of the unknown are effective in calming some women.

The idea of labouring and even delivering in water has become fashionable recently but this is no new phenomenon. Hydrotherapists have advocated the use of a whirlpool or spa bath to alleviate many discomforts and contemporary mothers have grasped the notion as another means of retaining control over their own bodies as well as facilitating the birth process (Burns and Greenish, 1993). Herbs such as rosemary and red raspberry leaf could be added to the bath water by hanging a bunch of the dried herbs under the tap while the hot water is running.

In units where mothers are 'allowed' to bring a complementary therapist with them midwives may observe relief of labour pain from acupuncture (Ledergerber, 1976; Skelton and Flowerdew, 1985, 1986; Meiyu, 1985; Budd, 1993), herbal remedies such as squaw vine, birth root, raspberry leaf, echinacea or ginseng (Bunce, 1987; Maus 1989; Singingtree, 1989), or homeopathic substances, for example, caulophyllum, arnica, natrum muriatricum (Farrent, 1985; Priestman, 1988; Holt 1988).

The concept of pain relief in labour has caused consternation for many years amongst both professionals and consumers, for the traditional selection has been limited and each carries certain fetal or maternal risks. The utilisation of the many alternatives offered by practitioners of non-allopathic therapies increases the choices available to mothers and has no known detrimental effects on the fetus if used appropriately. It allows women to reclaim their bodies and to work in partnership with their carers, resulting in satisfying and fulfilling experiences for all concerned. Midwives could develop their knowledge and skills in the use of several of the above-mentioned methods of pain relief within the limits of their practice, and so enhance their care of the mothers.

Other problems Other problems which occur in labour can be treated with alternative remedies. For example inefficient uterine action can be improved by herbal cures such as black and blue cohosh or raspberry leaf; mild disproportion may be eased by reflexology to the zones corresponding to the pelvic girdle; overactivity of the uterus can be calmed by acupuncture; and a retained placenta may be encouraged to separate by reflex zone therapy, homeopathic treatment such as pulsatilla, acupuncture, herbs (myrrh or feverfew) or aromatherapy (jasmine oil).

Much can be done through the use of complementary therapies to ease the transition into motherhood, for women may suffer a variety of discomforts as they did in pregnancy, due to the changing physiology as the body readapts to the non-pregnant state.

Breast tenderness Breast and nipple tenderness is not uncommon, whether the mother breastfeeds her baby or not. Lactation can be stimulated by the use of reflex zone therapy around the distal dorsum of each foot (see Chapter 4), and drinking fennel or other herbal teas may help. Of course there is no substitute for frequent demand feeding and correct fixing of the baby to the breast, but despite this some mothers have initial problems with the milk supply and with soreness of the nipples.

If milk engorgement of the breast causes discomfort cabbage leaves can be used to good effect (see Chapter 3). Venous engorgement responds dramatically to reflex zone therapy (see Chapter 4). Soreness of the nipples can be prevented or alleviated by smearing a few drops of colostrum around the areola after each feed and allowing this to dry. Calendula or camomile both have soothing effects and can be bought as proprietary creams or the essential oils may be mixed into a base cream. However the latter should be wiped off before the baby is put to the breast as essential oils should not be taken internally. Alternatively, Bach Rescue Remedy cream is very soothing, rubbed into the nipples, but again should be removed before the baby starts sucking (Howard, 1992). The mother could also steep two camomile tea bags in boiled water, let them cool and then place the two tea bags inside the bra over the nipples. Geranium leaves applied over the nipples will also help to combat soreness.

The flow of milk can be encouraged by massage from the axillae towards the nipples, and by hydrotherapy; suppression of lactation may be aided by the application of a cold compress of essential oil of peppermint, and jasmine has been found to be useful in these cases (Shrivastav *et al.*, 1988).

Perineum The perineum can be particularly uncomfortable following vaginal delivery irrespective of whether the mother has required sutures. There may be severe bruising of the perineum, vulva and buttocks to which arnica cream in a homeopathic concentration could be applied, although not directly over the wound. Oral arnica tablets should help if there is an open wound or bruising and should be commenced immediately following delivery. However unless the midwife is fully cognisant with the use of arnica the mother will have to administer this for herself or have them prescribed by her homeopath. Certain independent midwives recommend arnica to their clients, but unless they have had some homeopathic training or can justify that they have sufficient knowledge for safe and accountable use, they are putting their professional registration in jeopardy. While it is highly unlikely that any adverse effects would arise from administering arnica, the midwife could find herself in a difficult legal position if complications arose which led to a court case, particularly if she was unable to discuss the subject authoritatively.

Sitting in a bath of warm water to which has been added a small amount of witch hazel can be soothing, and is readily available from chemists. Adding a few drops of Bach Rescue Remedy and crab apple to the bath or bidet will help to combat shock and act as a cleanser, respectively. Essential oils of cypress and lavender as a sitz bath will aid healing, as will marigold tincture, from a herbalist. Nutritional therapists promote healing from within by ensuring that the body has adequate levels of zinc and vitamins B_6 and C, and midwives could make suggestions about suitable foods (see Davies and Stewart (1987) for food items containing different vitamins and minerals).

Postnatal depression The severity of postnatal depression may be lessened in susceptible women, by regular use of jasmine in the days following delivery, either in a tea (which the midwife could recommend) or as a massage or bath with essential oil (which will also have the effects of increasing the mother's confidence and incidentally improving the flow of vaginal blood loss). Herbalists may recommend agnus-castus, and nutrition therapists suggest supplements of zinc and vitamin B6 as in pregnancy. Various homeopathic remedies are beneficial, for example sepia, but would be prescribed according to individual symptoms. Bach remedies which are suitable include mustard, gentian or Star of Bethlehem, depending on the type of depression.

A trend in the early 1980s for eating the placenta for its high hormone and vitamin levels seems to have lost its popularity, for various reasons.

Urinary retention Urinary retention responds well to reflex zone therapy, and is the subject of current research by the author. Homeopathic and herbal substances could also be used.

Constipation Constipation, as in pregnancy, can be treated with massage, aromatherapy, reflexology, dietary, herbal or homeopathic methods.

The newborn baby For the neonate, complementary therapies offer a natural gentle means to ease the transition into extrauterine life. Some examples include the use of craniosacral therapy to reduce distress and trauma in babies delivered by forceps or to treat an infant who has become hyperactive; massage and aromatherapy to treat constipation and colic; and herbal preparations or homeopathic remedies for the baby whose skin is eczematous. However it is not within the scope of this book to discuss the myriad uses of alternative therapies for babies and children, and midwives are referred to the lists of further reading to find out more.

It can therefore be seen that alternative remedies can truly be used as a complement to orthodox treatment at a time when women are most receptive to suggestions which encompass safety and self-control. Many remedies are becoming increasingly popular amongst midwives who see the tremendous value in being able to offer non-medical and non-pharmaceutical treatment. Many of the treatments suggested throughout this book can be used by midwives, or self-administered by the mother. Others require the assistance of qualified therapists, whether they are a normal part of the maternity services or selected practitioners from outside the National Health Service. At all times midwives must be aware of the accountability issues, but with greater understanding of how the different therapies can be of use, they may be able to refer to an appropriate therapist without jeopardising their professional situation. The benefits far outweigh the perceived problems of the sceptics, and midwives and mothers need to continue to promote the inclusion of complementary therapies and therapists within the maternity services in order to enhance the choices for care.

Useful Addresses

British Complementary Medicine Association
Harold Gillies Ward, St Charles' Hospital, Exmoor Street, London W6, UK
Tel: 081 964 1205
This organisation acts as a resource on all matters relating to complementary medicine, including maintenance of registers of member groups from the different therapies. It is pressing for greater recognition of the therapies within conventional healthcare through Parliamentary liaison.

Institute for Complementary Medicine
PO Box 194, London SE16 1QZ, UK
Tel: 071 237 5165
Another organisation which acts as a resource, the ICM has registers of practitioners, and is working for improved standards of training in complementary

therapies. It intends to establish an international college of complementary medicine by 1997.

Research Council for Complementary Medicine
60 Great Ormond Street, London WC1N 3JF, UK

Tel: 071 833 8897
The RCCM is concerned with rigorous examination of complementary and alternative therapies in order to increase credibility and the scientific basis on which their incorporation into mainstream healthcare may stand or fall.

References

Balaskas J. (1990) *Natural Pregnancy* Sidgwick and Jackson.

Boot M. (1987) Hypnosis in pregnancy, labour and the puerperium. *Journal of the Association of Chartered Physiotherapists in Obstetrics and Gynaecology*, **60**, 30–31.

Brann L. and Guzvica S. (1987) Comparison of hypnosis with conventional relaxation for antenatal and intrapartum use – a feasibility study in general practice. *Journal of Royal College of General Practitioners*, **37(303)**, 437–440.

Bryce-Smith D. (1986) Prenatal zinc deficiency. *Nursing Times*, **82(10)**, 44–46.

Budd S. (1992) Traditional Chinese medicine in obstetrics. *Midwives Chronicle*, **105** (June), 140–143.

Bunce K. (1987) The use of herbs in midwifery. *Journal of Nurse-Midwifery*, **32(4)**, 255–259.

Burns E. and Greenish K. (1993) Pooling information. *Nursing Times*, **89(8)**, 47–49.

Butler K. (1985) Nausea in pregnancy. *Women Wise*, **8(1)**.

Castro M. (1992) *Homeopathy for Mother and Baby*. Macmillan.

Conway A. (1987) Hypnotherapy. *Health Visitor*, **60**, 83.

Davies S. and Stewart A. (1987) *Nutritional Medicine*. Pan.

Dundee J.W. Sourial F.B.R. and Ghaly R.G. (1988) P6 acupuncture reduces morning sickness. *Journal of the Royal Society of Medicine*, **81(8)**, 456–7.

Farrent F. (1985) Homeopathy for mother and baby. *Association of Radical Midwives Magazine*, **25**, 26–28.

Fitzgerald A. (1987) Hypnosis helping ease childbirth. *Essex Chronicle*, 6.2.87.

Fulder S. (1991) Help yourself to superherbs. *Here's Health*, February, 101–105.

Gartside G. (1982) Easy labour – personal experience of childbirth under hypnosis. *Nursing Times*, **51(78)**, 2187–2188.

Guthrie K. *et al.* (1984) Maternal hypnosis induced by husbands during childbirth. *Journal of Obstetrics and Gynaecology*, **4(5)**, 93–95.

Hemminski E. and Starfield B. (1985) Routine administration of iron and vitamins during pregnancy – review of controlled clinical trials. *British Journal of Obstetrics and Gynaecology*, **85**, 404–410.

Holt M. (1988) Homeopathy in childbearing. *Midwives Chronicle*, **1206(101)**, 225–226.

Howard J. (1992) *Bach Flower Remedies for Women*. C.W. Daniel.

Hyde E. (1989) Acupressure therapy for morning sickness – a controlled clinical trial. *Journal of Nurse-Midwifery*, **43(4)**, 171–8.

Jenkins M. W, and Pritchard M. H. (1993) Hypnosis: practical applications and theoretical considerations in normal labour. *British Journal of Obstetrics and Gynaecology*, **100(3)**, 221–226.

Kenton L. (1986) Raw Energy – *Eat Yourself to Radiant Health*. Century Arrow.

Ledergerber C. (1976) Electroacupuncture in obstetrics. *Acupuncture and Electrotherapeutics Research International Journal*, **2**, 105–118.

Maus C. (1987) An herbal. *Texas Midwifery*, **4(3)**, 18–19.

McIntyre A. (1988) *Herbs for Pregnancy and Childbirth*. Sheldon Press.

Meiyu C. (1985) Acupuncture anaesthesia for Caesarean section. *Midwives Chronicle*, **1168(98)**, 107.

Montague K. (1985) Osteopathy during pregnancy. *Nursing Mirror*, **161(5)**, 26–28.

Peterson N. (1989) *Herbs and Health*. Bloomsbury.

Piesse J. (1983) Zinc and human male infertility. *International Clinical Nutrition Reviews*, **3(2)**, 4–6.

Priestman K. (1988) A few useful remedies in pregnancy, labour and the first few days of the babies' life. *British Homeopathic Journal*, **77(3)**, 172–173.

Roach B. (1985) Ginger root (*Zingibar officinale*). *California Association of Midwives Newsletter*, **1**, 2.

Robinson N. (1988) Infertility and subfertility. *Nursing Times*, **84(44)**, 42–43.

Sadler C. (1989) Can acupressure relieve nausea? *Nursing Times*, 85(51), 32–34.

Sharon M. (1992) *Optimum Nutrition*. Prion,

Sheldon W. *et al.* (1985) Effects of oral iron supplements on zinc and magnesium levels. *British Journal of Obstetrics and Gynaecology*, September, 892–898.

Shrivastav P. George K. and Balasubramaniam N. (1988) Suppression of puerperal lactation using jasmine flowers. *Australia and New Zealand Journal Obstetrics and Gynaecology*, **1(28)**, 68–71.

Singingtree D. (1989) Managing postpartum haemorrhage. *Midwifery Today*, **10**, 14–15.

Skelton I. and Flowerdew M. (1985) Midwifery and acupuncture. *Midwives Chronicle*, **1168(98)**, 125–129.

Skelton I. and Flowerdew M. (1986) Is there a place for acupuncture on labour wards? *Midwife, Health Visitor and Community Nurse*, **12(22)**, 423–426.

Stannard D. (1989) Pressure prevents nausea. *Nursing Times*, **4(85)**, 33–34.

Steven C. (1990) Labour smoothed by hypnosis. *The Independent*, 23.1.90.

Stewart N. (1987) New ways to beat sickness. *Mother Magazine*.

Wagner M. (1993) *The Birth Machine*. Temple University Press, Philadelphia.

Wine P. (1989) Superficial hypnosis – an aid to midwifery. *Midwife, Health Visitor and Community Nurse*, 25(12), 518.

Woods M. (1989) Pain control and hypnosis. *Nursing Times*, **7(85)**, 38–40.

Further Reading

Maher G. (1992) *Start a Career in Complementary Medicine*. Tackmart Publishing.

Rankin-Box D. (1988) *Complementary Health Therapies – a Guide for Nurses and the Caring Professions*. Croom Helm.

Wells R. and Tschudin V. (Eds) (1994)

Wells' Supportive Therapies in Health Care. Baillière, Tindall, London.

Denise Tiran

Chapter 3

Massage and Aromatherapy

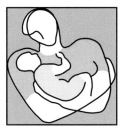

Aromatherapy is the very ancient art and, more recently, the science of using highly concentrated essential oils or essences distilled from plants in order to utilise their therapeutic properties. It is the combination of various chemical compounds which give each oil its own particular properties and indeed different parts from the same plant may produce several different oils, e.g. the orange tree provides orange oil from the peel, neroli from the orange blossom, and petit grain from the leaves and twigs.

The term 'aromatherapie' was first used in the 1920s by Rene Maurice Gattefossé, a chemical perfumier. During his laboratory experiments he burnt his hand and plunged it into the nearest available liquid which happened to be essential oil of lavender. He was astounded to find that his hand healed rapidly with no pain, blistering, infection or scarring, a fact which led him to research extensively into essential oils for medicinal purposes.

However, in Britain aromatherapy has developed not from the medical perspective but from the beauty therapy angle. This has resulted in both public and medical opinions that massage and aromatherapy are merely a luxury with which to pamper oneself and that essential oils are harmless, pleasant-smelling substances to assist in the process. This is not so, and in the last 10–15 years health professionals have begun to take an interest in their uses for treatment.

The effects of Common Market changes

The establishment of the single European market is altering the position for all complementary therapies, particularly in Britain. One of the issues under discussion is the use of the word 'aromatherapy' as in France, Germany and Switzerland only medically qualified doctors can practise 'therapy' where the word implies diagnosis and prescription of appropriate treatment. A meeting in Zurich in 1992 was attended by leading aromatherapists, perfumiers and essential oil manufacturers to discuss the issue, and eventually the term 'aromatology' was agreed – 'aroma' meaning 'smell' and 'ology' meaning 'study of' (Price, 1992).

Unlike England's current Common Law which allows one to do anything as long as it is not against the law, Europe uses Napoleonic law which means that no one can do anything unless it is approved by the law. If Britain is forced to change to the European legal system the implication for aromatherapists in the United Kingdom is that unless they possess a medical qualification they will be required to practise under the delegation of a doctor. For midwives who work as independent practitioners this may prove restrictive in that many of the physiological symptoms of pregnancy can be treated with essential oils and at present midwife-aromatherapists can do this on their own accountability. It remains to be seen whether the British legal system will need to conform to the European system.

The history of aromatherapy

Essential oils or the chemical properties of plants have been used since ancient times and have even been found in fossilised pollen from archaeological exploration of primitive burial sites. The Chinese are thought to have used the medicinal properties of plants as early as 4500 BC, including opium, pomegranate and rhubarb; the mummification of the dead incorporating essential oils not only for their fragrances but also for their antibacterial properties is well documented (Davis, 1988, p.2; Worwood, 1990, p.9; Lawless, 1992, p.120; Arcier, 1992, p.8). The Greeks are thought to have used many plants including myrrh for the treatment of wounds sustained in battle, and fennel seeds were chewed to suppress appetite during marches. Even Hippocrates acknowledged the benefits of plant substances.

However the 'father of aromatherapy' was the Arab physician Avicenna, who documented the effects on the body of over 800 plants and is credited with discovering the method of extraction of essential oils. Sadly the European Dark Ages of the tenth century, during which many written records were destroyed, deprived future generations of much of the contemporary and abundant knowledge of plant medicine. By the sixteenth century herbs and other plants were once again being used for their therapeutic characteristics and many herbalists compiled relevant texts – some such as Culpepper's Herbal are still in use today.

Unfortunately for herbalists, the growing science of chemistry in the seventeenth century elicited new substances for use in medicine and this seems to have coincided with the practice of burning witches at the stake, who were often merely women who had been found collecting plants to treat illnesses.

Although essential oils remained in limited use, synthetic production of drugs with their attendant side effects has increased up to the present day. It is perhaps due to public challenge of these drugs that we are now seeing a return to natural plant remedies and that the medical and allied professions are beginning to examine the scientific basis of the essential oils.

As previously mentioned, Gattefossé was instrumental in reviving interest in essential oils in the early twentieth century, and other French physicians and scientists have continued his research. Doctor Jean Valnet used the oils during the First World War to treat burns and injuries, to good effect. He is still considered one of the world's leading authorities on the therapeutic uses of essential oils, and his book *The Practice of Aromatherapy* (Valnet, 1980) is considered one of the definitive texts on the subject.

How do essential oils work?

Essential oils are highly concentrated substances containing a variety of chemical compounds which give them their therapeutic properties. It is the scientific analysis and the acknowledgement that the compounds have various medical qualities which will convince sceptical doctors, midwives, nurses and others that there truly are clinical benefits to their use. Indeed, essential oils have been used in French medicine for many years and much of the research that has been performed was carried out in France.

All of the constituents in essential oils are organic, their molecular structures being based on carbon atoms bonded to one another and to hydrogen atoms. Some essential oils contain oxygen atoms, sometimes with nitrogen and/or sulphur atoms. Essential oils typically contain several hundred different constituents, although when one sees an analysis of an individual oil it is the major components which have been classified.

The chemical components, grouped into hydrocarbons and oxygenated compounds, have been known since 1818 when the first analysis was carried out. The hydrocarbons contain hydrogen and carbon atoms only, and the oxygenated compounds contain hydrogen, carbon and oxygen atoms in their molecules.

Hydrocarbons Hydrocarbons take the form of terpines which are broken down into monoterpines, diterpines and sesquiterpines, each of which can be further subdivided. Terpines are found in all essential oils in varying amounts. Gattefossé stated that the highest proportion of terpines is found in oils distilled from wood, then those extracted from leaves, with the smallest quantities in oils produced from flowers (Tisserand, 1993, p. 40), although Tisserand, a contemporary leading authority, disputes this (p 141).

Terpines can have irritant and toxic effects if used incorrectly, which led Gattefossé to produce terpineless oils, although Tisserand (1993, p. 142) states that this does not necessarily make them any safer to use. Pinene, one form of terpine, has antiseptic properties and is found in oils such as eucalyptus, while limonene, in lemon oil, is antiviral. The sesquiterpine, chamazulene, a major constituent of camomile oil, has recently been found to possess anti-inflammatory and antibacterial properties (Lawless, 1992, p. 34).

Oxygenated compounds Oxygenated compounds are divided into esters, aldehydes, phenols, ketones, alcohols and oxides.

Esters Esters are acidic compounds which Gattefossé states can produce epileptiform fits (Tisserand, 1993, p. 45) and while Tisserand agrees in part, it is generally felt that ketones are more toxic than esters (p. 142) (see below). Massive doses have also been found to produce fatal cardiac failure (Tisserand, 1993, p. 45). Linalyl acetate (in lavender, clary sage and bergamot) and geranyl acetate (in marjoram) are antifungal and sedative while benzyl benzoate (in ylang ylang) is antispasmodic.

Aldehydes The antiseptic properties of aldehydes are considered to be much safer than those of phenols (Tisserand, 1993, p. 45). All essential oils have some degree of antiseptic property although certain oils are more readily used as such, e.g. lavender, eucalyptus and lemon, while others have antiseptic effects on specific systems of the body, such as bergamot, camomile, sandalwood, and lavender for the urinary tract, eucalyptus, tea tree, basil and myrrh for the respiratory tract, and marjoram, lemon, camomile and juniper for the gastrointestinal system. This is due in the main to the presence of the aldehyde citral, which can be found in the citrus oils such as lemon, lemongrass, verbena and some eucalyptus. Aldehydes are also sedative, particularly camomile, lavender, clary sage, sandalwood and ylang ylang.

Phenols Phenols are extremely effective antibacterial compounds and also act as stimulants. The degree to which they can cause skin irritation is disputed between Gattefossé and Tisserand (Tisserand, 1993, pp. 48 and 143), although Lawless (1992, p. 35) seems to agree with the latter. Thymol found in thyme oil can be an extreme irritant to mucous membrane, yet in small doses can be effective in treating infections of the upper respiratory tract. Thymol is, in addition, a particularly good disinfectant and vermifuge and although Gattefossé (Tisserand, 1993, p. 48) found another phenol, carvacrol, to be equally effective but less toxic than thymol, new research confirms the effectiveness of thymol.

Ketones Ketones are considered to be the most toxic of all substances found in essential oils, especially thujone which is present in sage, mugwort and tansy. Gattefossé's observations that fenchone in fennel oil can 'turn livers brown' (Tisserand, 1993. p. 47) was after 'repeated ingestion' of fennel solution and neither Tisserand (1993, p. 142) nor Lawless (1992, p. 35) consider fenchone to be toxic. Ketones can in fact be useful in respiratory infections, serving to ease congestion and aid the flow of mucus – hyssop and sage are particularly noted for these purposes. Other similarly useful ketones include camphor, menthone and pinocamphone, all of which are present in oils such as eucalyptus. The ketone pulegone, found in peppermint and in pennyroyal, the latter being known for its abortifacient properties, is useful for its calming effects on the digestive system. Peppermint, in fact, is the only essential oil currently licensed as a medicine in Britain, but the presence of pulegone makes it suspect for use in pregnancy. (Balacs, 1992a).

For midwives therefore one of the most significant toxic effects of ketones is the abortifacient action they may have on the pregnant woman, especially oils such as sage, a powerful emmenagogue.

Alcohols Alcohols comprise the greatest quantity and strength of any of the chemical compounds found in essential oils, even more so than terpines. They are antiseptic and antiviral and are also uplifting. Generally too they are not toxic. Types of alcohols include linalol (in lavender and rosewood), citronellol (in lemon, rose, geranium and eucalyptus), geraniol (in geranium), borneol, menthol and others.

Oxides Oxides such as cineol, a principal constituent of eucalyptus, tea tree, cajeput and rosemary are those with a noticeably camphorous odour. Recent trials in France have concluded that eucalyptus is safe to use in pregnancy, contrary to previous thinking (Pages *et al.*, 1990).

Toxicity of essential oils

Many essential oils can cause a variety of adverse effects ranging from skin irritations to death. Some, such as sage, rosemary, fennel and hyssop, may initiate epilepsy in someone who has never had a fit before. Certain oils are hypertensive, especially rosemary, sage, hyssop and black pepper; others lower the blood pressure, including lavender, clary sage and ylang ylang. Clary sage can potentiate the effects of alcohol; some oils are stimulating, for example basil, peppermint, black pepper and rosemary. Still more increase photosensitivity and should be avoided if the skin is to be directly exposed to the sun, particularly bergamot. If the therapist wishes to achieve one of these effects, then judicious use of appropriate essential oils can be valuable aids to treatment, but it can be seen that misuse through lack of knowledge could produce disastrous consequences.

There are many oils which should not be used for babies and children. Davies (1988, p. 86) suggests that the safest oils for children are camomile, lavender, mandarin and rose. However it is important to note that in no case, child or adult, should any one oil be used continuously for more than 3 weeks as skin sensitivity may occur. The safest route of administration for children and babies is via the skin in massages or in the bath water.

Pregnancy and childbirth

Many essential oils are to be avoided in pregnancy as they are thought to be emmenagogue (i.e. they produce uterine bleeding), such as sage, basil, clary sage, juniper, hyssop, lavender, marjoram, myrrh, rosemary and rose (Davies, 1988, p. 366). However a recent article by Tony Balacs in the *International Journal of Aromatherapy* (Balacs, 1992a) disputes the possibility that emmenagogue oils are actually abortifacient. He adds camphor, cypress, jasmine, nutmeg and peppermint to the list of emmenagogue oils. Balacs also classifies others by their oestrogen-stimulating action (aniseed and fennel), mild carcinogenicity (basil, sassafras and tarragon), general toxicity (boldo, horseradish, mustard and wormseed) and abortifacient tendency (pennyroyal, rue, savin, mugwort, sage, tansy, thuja, plecanthrus and wormwood). Other oils which are considered to be moderately toxic include bitter almond, clove, hyssop, myrrh, parsleyseed, oregano, savory, thyme and wintergreen (Table 1).

Table 1. Essential oils which should not be used in pregnancy

Emmenagogue
Basil Camphor Clary sage Cypress Juniper Jasmine Hyssop Lavender Marjoram Myrrh Nutmeg Peppermint Rose Rosemary Sage

Abortifacient
Mugwort Pennyroyal Plecanthrus Rue Savin Sage Tansy Thuja Wormwood

Oestrogen-stimulating
Aniseed Fennel

Carcinogenic
Basil Sassafras Tarragon

Toxic
Boldo Horseradish Mustard Wormseed

Moderately toxic
Bitter almond Clove Hyssop Myrrh Parsleyseed Oregano Savory Thyme Wintergreen

In addition Balacs clarifies the confusion over juniper communis and juniper savin (more commonly known as savin oil), the latter being definitely contraindicated in pregnancy, but the former – juniper oil – being acceptable in small doses (Balacs, 1992a).

Midwives may be concerned here about mothers' use of herbs in the diet, but it should be remembered that the amount of essential oil in a single plant is miniscule. It is therefore safe for mothers to use herbs in their cooking or for teas, to obtain some of the positive effects of the contraindicated oils, although none should be used to excess. Similarly, the mugwort sticks used by acupuncturists to turn a breech to a cephalic presentation (see Chapter 10) will cause no harm to the mother or fetus as it is not the concentrated essential oil being absorbed by the woman.

In addition to those essential oils which are emmenagogue, abortifacient, carcinogenic or toxic, certain other oils may affect fetal development, although this has not been proven, and some may interfere with the mother's health, for example by raising the blood pressure.

On the other hand, Daniele Ryman, in her controversial book *Aromatherapy*, suggests that all essential oils are to be avoided in pregnancy (Ryman, 1991, p. 28). Most other authorities disagree with her but the issue of using essential oils for expectant mothers needs urgent research, a fact which is to be addressed by the Scientific and Research Committee of the Aromatherapy Organisations Council (Sapsford, 1993).

It should be stressed that the benefits to be gained from the use of essential oils during the childbearing year are enormous if they are used with care. Midwives wishing to enhance their care of women should therefore be fully informed about the oils they are using. Professional accountability as a midwife is the first priority, for pregnant women are in a vulnerable position and deserve to have the midwife act as their advocate. Midwives should refer to the UKCC's publications on the Scope of Practice (1992b), Guidelines for the Administration of Medicines (1992a) and the Midwives' Rules (1991).

Blending oils

Essential oils should principally be chosen to elicit the desired therapeutic effect in the client. A maximum of five oils can be blended together and it is in the blending that the art of aromatherapy is seen. Using more than five oils may overpower the person's olfactory sense, and the versatility of many oils makes it unlikely that more than five oils will be needed to obtain the required effects. It is perfectly acceptable to use a single oil for a specific purpose but the combined effects of more than one oil will be greater than if each oil was used separately – this is called the synergistic effect. Additionally the end product needs to have an aroma which is pleasing to the recipient and therapists should always be guided by their client's choice; some aromatherapists believe that clients will automatically choose the oil which is not only the most pleasing but also the most appropriate therapeutically.

There are several different means by which therapists will choose oils to blend. Some aromatherapists use the perfumery system of 'notes' to achieve a balanced blend. The therapeutic oils are ususally the middle notes; those which 'fix' the blend and have a long-lasting effect are the base notes; and the presenting aroma of the blend will be the top notes. Oils derived from roots and wood are the base notes, those which are from leaves, particularly the culinary herbs, are the middle notes and oils produced from flowers constitute the top notes.

Whichever method the therapist uses to decide on a blend, the rules in relation to therapeutic use of essential oils are exactly the same as for conventional medicines, i.e. the blend chosen must be the correct dose of the correct oils given to the correct person by the correct route and at the correct time.

As a general rule a 3% blend would be used for massage of an adult, although in pregnancy this may be reduced to 1.5–2%; for debilitated perhaps elderly adults and for children the strength would also be diluted to between 1% and 2%. A similar amount would be used for facial massage. If using essential oils in the bath a mix of between 4% and 10% could be used but it is always best to err on the side of caution in pregnancy and use a 4% blend as maximum. This strength is also suitable for inhalations.

To calculate the correct number of drops of essential oil to be added to the base or carrier oil the following formula is used:

To every 5 ml of base oil add the same number of drops as the percentage required

ie.   for a 1% blend – 5 ml of base oil + 1 drop of essential oil
       for a 3% blend – 5 ml of base oil + 3 drops of essential oil
       for a 6% blend – 5 ml of base oil + 6 drops of essential oil

Obviously for a 1.5% blend it is impossible to add one and a half drops of essential oil therefore the amount is doubled:

i.e.   for a 1.5% blend – 10 ml of base oil + 3 drops of essential oil

If more than one essential oil is used the number of drops is the total amount:

e.g.   for a 3% blend using lavender and camomile - 5 ml of base oil + 2 drops of lavender + 1 drop of camomile, or
        5 ml of base oil + 2 drops of camomile + 1 drop of lavender

Base or carrier oils

The oil used as a base into which essential oils are blended will vary according to the purpose for which it is required in addition to being merely a lubricant. For example a nourishing oil such as avocado may be used for very dry skin, while wheatgerm is rich in vitamin E and good for scar tissue, but as it is thick it usually needs diluting with another thinner oil. The most commonly used carrier oils in aromatherapy (and the most economical) are grapeseed and sweet almond, although Davis (1988, p. 76) states that sesame seed oil has the advantage of washing out of towels more easily than the others.

Buying and storing oils

It is very true in aromatherapy that 'you get what you pay for'. Many essential oils are extremely expensive due to the complicated process of extracting them from the plant. Orange oil, for example, is relatively cheap to produce

– even peeling an orange will sometimes produce a spurt of the essence from the rind. Jasmine, on the other hand, requires a vast number of flowers to produce a small quantity of oil because of the delicate nature of the flowers; in addition they are collected by hand at night when the fragrance is at its strongest, and the process of extraction (enfleurage) is costly in terms of skill and time.

All of these factors combine to price essential oil of jasmine in the region of £90–96 for 10 ml, a fact which may lead some producers to use a cheaper system yielding an oil which does not have the same therapeutic properties.

It is interesting to note that Daniele Ryman (1991) states that production costs for oils such as jasmine became prohibitive in the late 1980s and that the subsequent change in the production process yields an absolute which is not for medicinal purposes. More alarmingly she believes that 'it is likely that any jasmine labelled as an essential oil is really the absolute and is only suitable for use as a fragrance' (Ryman, 1991, p. 116). This has implications for midwives using jasmine oil, for example for postnatal depression, as the oil could have been adulterated. Rose oil too could be diluted by the addition of geranium, bois de rose or palmarosa to avoid the huge costs of true rose oil, for which about 5 tonnes of rose petals are required to produce 1 kg of essential oil! (Ryman, 1991, p. 181). It is therefore vital when buying esential oils that the retailer can confirm what you are buying by using the Latin name of the plant.

There are several reputable essential oil producers including Natural by Nature, Neal's Yard, Culpepper's, De Fraine, Shirley Price, Tisserand and Gerard. There are also other brands obtained from organically grown plants, in consideration for the ecological effects of the greatly increased consumption of essential oils (Henglein, 1992). At the other end of the spectrum are several popular high street stores which offer pleasant smelling but therapeutically inadequate oils and which are to be avoided by anyone seriously wishing to use aromatherapy within their professional practice.

Midwives are advised to buy a limited number of versatile oils which will be used up relatively quickly. Once opened, most essential oils will retain their therapeutic properties for up to 2 years but some, particularly the citrus oils, will only last about 6 months. Additionally it is professionally more expedient to keep a limited selection and to know their uses thoroughly than to acquire such a large number of oils that it is impossible to be fully cognisant of their uses and dangers.

Essential oils should be stored in dark blue or brown bottles in a cool place with the lids securely on, as light, heat and air cause them to deteriorate more quickly. Certain oils such as jasmine and the citrus oils are probably best kept in the refrigerator. If this is in a maternity unit the normal health and safety rules regarding storage of medicines must be adhered to. Essential oils should not be stored near homeopathic remedies as the strong odours may inactivate the remedies, even when the bottle tops are on.

Peppermint is a particularly strong aroma which will antidote homeopathic medicines, and anyone using homeopathy should avoid the use of peppermint oil for the duration of their treatment.

Methods of administration of the oils

Essential oils can be administered either through the skin, by inhalation or orally, although the latter should only be used by medically qualified aromatherapists as in France.

Massage Massage is perhaps the most usual and certainly the most relaxing means of administration via the skin, and one which provides its own additional benefits, i.e. massage is de-stressing, it relaxes muscles, aids circulation, excretion and digestion, and facilitates communication between giver and recipient.

Although there are many different forms of masssage there is nothing especially difficult about intuitive massage – if it feels right to the recipient it is right! Simple stroking will often suffice in the absence of knowledge or confidence to attempt more specific techniques.

Due to lack of time midwives wishing to administer essential oils to mothers will probably not perform a full body massage, although this can be wonderfully relaxing in cases where the woman is stressed, anxious or depressed. It is far more likely that midwives would choose to massage a particular part of the body for a specific reason, for example, the feet in labour to warm them, an aching back in pregnancy or labour, oedematous ankles, or the scalp to relieve headache.

Midwives and nurses occasionally question the cost of the time involved in performing massage on clients or patients, for it is true that it costs more in the short term to massage them, for instance to aid sleep, rather than to give them night sedation, but it is more difficult to count the long-term cost. Penny Fromant (1991), while discussing intensive care nursing, nevertheless feels that some of the nurturing of nursing (and likewise midwifery) has been lost in the effort to attain cost-effectiveness and efficiency. The very act of touching the women for whom we care has become 'functional' rather than nurturing, perhaps due to excessive workloads and staff shortages, but perhaps also because of the trend towards the promotion of self-help, almost in a 'do it yourself' way. Additionally for some health carers, not touching clients/patients facilitates a professional 'distance' which avoids the need to become too emotionally involved. Obviously these are generalised statements and there are many midwives who provide excellent nurturing for the mothers in their care, but often this is related to the personality of the individual midwife as to how close she becomes to them, either physically or emotionally.

There are numerous accounts of massage, with or without essential oils, being used in nursing – for oncology and other terminally ill patients (Horrigan, 1991), in intensive care (Martin, 1990; Fromant, 1991), in cardiology units (Maxwell, Hudson 1990), for physically handicapped children and children with learning disabilities (Cohen, 1987; Maxwell Hudson, 1990; Sanderson, 1992; Payne, 1993), for HIV and AIDS patients (Hagan, 1992) and in bereavement work by health visitors (Armstrong, 1991). In midwifery some midwives are teaching mothers to massage their own babies, particularly in the neonatal intensive care unit (Paterson, 1990), using essential oils in the labour ward (Reed and Norfolk, 1993) or easing some of the physiological discomforts of pregnancy with aromatherapy (Guenier, 1992).

In addition, the benefits of massage as a means of relieving occupational stress have only recently been recognised, and some institutions, both commercial and the public sector, are introducing it for staff (Redding, 1991).

Performing a massage Before beginning any massage adequate preparation is necessary. Both the mother and the midwife should be comfortable in a warm, quiet room where they will not be disturbed. (Remember to disconnect the telephone if at home, or give ward keys to a colleague if in the maternity unit.) Towels should be used to cover the mother for dignity, and for warmth after the massage has finished; this is particularly important as it is thought that occlusion of the skin may facilitate absorption of the essential oils into the bloodstream. The midwife should remove rings and wrist watch to avoid scratching the mother and should warm her hands before commencing.

The oil is poured into the hands, never directly onto the recipient and, if used without therapeutic essential oils, acts merely as a lubricant to prevent friction of skin to skin rubbing. It is preferable to start with a little oil, about 5 ml, as it is easier to apply more than it is to remove excess. If this occurs, wiping the hands on a towel will leave sufficient oil on the mother to continue the massage. Occasionally women with very dry skin will require more oil to be applied.

Massage should be rhythmical but varied using different pressures, speeds, parts of the hands and techniques. As a general rule slow deep massage will calm and relax whilst brisker movements will stimulate and act as a 'pick me up'. The one exception to performing a deep slow, soporific massage would be in a woman who is pathologically (clinically) depressed, for this could deepen her sense of introversion and introspection; this woman would benefit from a much more stimulating massage with refreshing oils.

Figure 1 shows a pregnant woman receiving abdominal massage.

The movements There are several simple massage movements which can be used in any sequence to make the massage a pleasurable experience.

• Stroking – using the flat of the hands, fingertips or thumbs, stroking enables the oil to be spread over the body surface and creates a flow between other more specific movements. It is important to be creative and imagine you are 'performing a ballet' on the skin, which will enhance the feeling of nurturing. Stroking has the physical effect of relaxing

Fig. 1. Pregnant mother receiving abdominal massage. (Courtesy of Nursing Times).

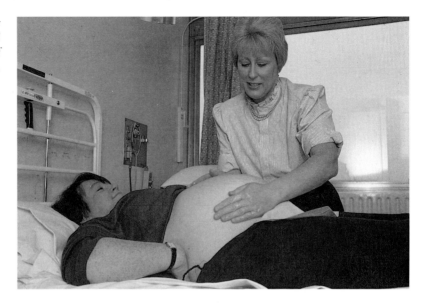

Fig. 2. To show direction of stroking movements on the face.

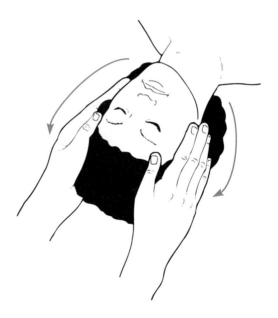

muscles and improving circulation and a calming effect upon the emotions. The massage is more pleasurable if a variety of strokes are used, with a combination of straight, circular, small, large, deep, light, brisk and slow movements. Stroking should normally be in the direction of venous return, towards the heart, although on the legs, stroking down from the thigh to the feet will give the sensation of removing tension. On the face movements are performed upwards ('in a smile') taking the tension out of the top of the head (Fig. 2).

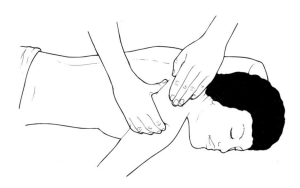

*Fig. 3. To show kneading
movements.*

- Kneading – grasping the flesh beween thumbs and fingers in a flowing motion alternating from one hand to the other is particularly effective on the shoulders, hips and thighs. Kneading can also be used on other fleshy parts of the body to relax muscles, aid circulation and excretion and to work more directly on certain areas. Where muscles are very tense, for example the shoulders, kneading may be uncomfortable, but by working briefly, moving elsewhere and then returning to the area the desired effect can be obtained (Fig. 3).
- Pressure – using fingertips and thumbs to work directly on specific muscles, sometimes with small circular movements, can be very pleasurable, especially either side of the spine during a back massage (Fig. 4). The knuckles can also be used to produce a different sensation.
- Percussion – cupping, hacking and pummelling, as in Swedish massage, can be used on fleshy muscular areas for stimulation and to improve circulation, although it may be omitted during a very relaxing massage. This is one of the techniques used by physiotherapists when treating postoperative patients.

Massage in pregnancy Abdominal and sacral massage is to be avoided during the first trimester of pregnancy for although there is no conclusive proof that any problems have occurred as a result, any woman who miscarries may search for a reason and implicate the massage as a cause.

Regular massage during pregnancy can be extremely beneficial, calming both mother and fetus.

Melanie was a particularly anxious woman for whom weekly massage was performed from about 10 weeks' gestation, commencing initially with just upper back, shoulders, neck, face and head. Back, abdominal and leg massage was added in the second trimester. Melanie always slept exceptionally well following the session which was usually in the evening at her own home, and the

*Fig. 4. To show pressure
movements.*

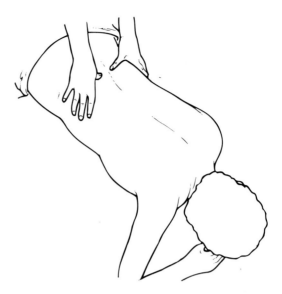

*fetus seemed calmer without its usual burst of evening activity. She
was so enthusiastic about her weekly 'fix' that on one occasion the
massage was continued in total darkness throughout a power cut! In
fact the lack of visual stimuli seemed to enhance the effects so much
that she felt this was the best massage of any she received during her
pregnancy.*

This example serves to raise the issue of the environment. Obviously one
would not normally perform a massage in total darkness although dimmed
lighting can be calming; the masseuse however needs to observe the client
for non-verbal signs that she is relaxing or alternatively perhaps uncomfortable or ill at ease.

Auditory stimuli is also questionable. A full body massage will take longer
to perform than a foot massage and the degree of relaxation achieved will be
greater. Therefore it may be preferable not to initiate conversation with a
mother who may opt to be silent. Other women may choose to talk and
indeed the sense of being cared for can trigger emotional responses which
may otherwise have remained hidden. In a few cases it may be necessary to
cease tactile contact and resort to a counselling session if appropriate. Many
massage therapists believe that counselling skills are a vital prerequisite for
good practice, and midwives using massage in their work must be confident
and competent enough to deal with this scenario if it arises.

The use of music is also debatable as some therapists feel it may detract
from focusing on the sensations of touch, while others believe that carefully
selected music can enhance the relaxation; however only specific relaxation

music, of which there is a good selection at most health shops, should be used. With repeated listening the music itself will have a Pavlovian effect and trigger relaxation.

Positioning the mother for massage requires the midwife to be flexible. For example back massage can be performed with the mother lying on her front in early pregnancy if she is comfortable, then on her side, changing to the other side as appropriate, or sitting leaning over a chair as the pregnancy progresses.

If the mother has varicose veins of the legs deep localised massage is contraindicated as this may not only be painful but also precipitate release of clots into the circulation. However simple light stroking over the affected area can be incorporated. Foot massage is an excellent means of offering therapeutic touch to the woman and in reflexology terms she is receiving the equivalent of a full body massage (see Chapter 4). However in the first trimester it is important to avoid vigorous movements around the heels as these are the reflex zones for the pelvis and this type of massage could potentially disrupt the pregnancy.

The midwife should also be comfortable, paying particular attention to her back through good posture, for there is no point in achieving relaxation for the mother if the midwife ends up needing a massage herself!

Use of essential oils in baths The addition of a few drops of essential oil to the bath water can be relaxing and therapeutic. Midwives could advocate this method in the postnatal wards as it does not require the midwife's presence and is therefore more cost effective. (Dispensing by appropriately trained personnel and the usual issues of professional accountability apply – see Chapter 1.) However as with massage the dose used is important and the essential oils are normally diluted in base oil to disperse them. This is because oil floats on water, and skin contact with undiluted oils can cause dermatitis in women with sensitive skin.

The essential and base oil mix is added to a warm bath under running water and thoroughly blended. A 4% blend is sufficient in pregnancy and this can be increased to a 6% blend postnatally, i.e. 4 or 6 drops of essential oil respectively to 5 ml of base oil. For neonates only a 1% blend should be used, i.e. one drop of essential oil to 5 ml of base oil thoroughly dispersed in the bath water. Doors and windows should be closed to contain the vapours which are inhaled and add to the benefits obtained through skin absorption. If the bath is not enamelled the surface should be cleaned immediately after use to avoid permanent stains from some of the darker oils. For more localised treatment the mother could use a foot bath or a bidet.

Inhalation Inhalation of essential oils is particularly valuable for respiratory tract infections but may be the preferred method of administration for other conditions. Daniele Ryman (1991, p. viii) states that this is her most often used method and that because the oils penetrate the mucous membrane the treatment becomes systemic. Facial saunas are also useful. A number of proprietary tools are available to facilitate vaporisation of the volatile essential oils which can then be inhaled. These are ideal to give a room a pleasant but also therapeutic odour. Indeed, the concept of the 'fragrant hospital' is promoted in some states of America (Steele, 1992), although the ethical issue of administering the oil to everyone in the room should be resolved.

Compresses Compresses act more locally than an all-over massage or bathing and are useful for inflamed or infected areas of the body, for example the perineum following delivery. A cloth soaked in either hot or cold water to which has been added the required essential oil is wrung out to remove excess liquid and then applied direct to the affected area. Compresses containing an appropriate essential oil applied to the sacral and suprapubic area in labour can ease the intensity of pain during contractions.

Ingestion Oral administration of essential oils is recommended by medically qualified doctors in France and is very successful in the treatment of many conditions. However this is only suggested under strict control and it is to be totally avoided by anyone without the relevant knowledge. Inappropriate use may lead to damage to the gastrointestinal tract and other problems. The therapeutic properties of the oils can still be ingested by using the whole plant in cooking or as herbal teas. Certain United Kingdom insurance policies specific to aromatherapy would be invalidated if the therapist was found to have been prescribing essential oils for internal use.

Essential oils for use by Midwives

Midwives need to become totally familiar with a few versatile essential oils. Micheline Arcier (1992, p. 86) recommends the use of mandarin (tangerine) as one of the gentlest oils for relaxation in pregnancy, except for anyone who is allergic to citrus fruit. Perhaps the most universal oil is lavender, and camomile is beneficial in small amounts. Neroli, sandalwood, tea tree, geranium and rose are also of value for specific conditions. In labour jasmine and clary sage can be added, and of course once the mother is puerperal, any of these and many other oils can be utilised. For babies mandarin and camomile can serve a multitude of purposes.

Let us then examine in detail the characteristics and properties of this small but flexible selection of essential oils.

Mandarin (tangerine) – *Citrus reticulata* (Rutacea family) Essential oil of mandarin is derived from the rind of the fruit and has a light, refreshing aroma reminiscent of the actual fruit. Most authorities are of the opinion that mandarin is safe to use in pregnancy (Davis, 1988, p. 214; Arcier, 1992, p. 44; Lawless, 1992, p. 125; Metcalfe, 1992, p. 42; Sellar, 1992, p. 100) although the danger of phototoxicity has been questioned but not proved conclusively. Ryman (1991, p. 137) suggests that it may be adulterated by the cheaper orange or even lemon. This is important particularly with the latter as lemon is even more phototoxic than mandarin is claimed to be, so it is important to ask specifically for the oil by its Latin name of *Citrus reticulata*.

Mandarin, in common with other citrus oils, deteriorates quickly so it is best to buy it in small quantities, store it in the refrigerator and only blend the amount required. It blends particularly well with lavender and neroli, but can also be mixed with camomile, sandalwood, geranium and jasmine to produce a pleasant aroma. The oils chosen will of course depend on the desired therapeutic effects.

The chemical constituents include limonene (terpene), methyl methylan-thranilate (ester), geraniol (alcohol), citral and citronellal (aldehydes) and other lesser compounds.

Mandarin is antispasmodic, antiseptic, sedative, tonic and digestive.

Lavender – *Lavandula augustifolia/officinalis* (Labiatae family)

Lavender oil is obtained from the leaves or the flowers and that produced from Alpine lavender is considered to be the best. Inexpensive lavender oil may have been adulterated by lavandin (spike lavender) which has a different balance of chemical constituents and will therefore have different therapeutic properties.

Lavender has a high proportion of phenols which give it a very strong antiseptic and antibacterial action. It contains the alcohols borneol, geraniol, linalool and lavandulol, together with esters (geranyl acetate, lavandulyl acetate, linalyl acetate), terpenes (limonene, pinene, caryophyllene) and the ketone cineole.

Due to its emmenagogic action lavender should be avoided during the first trimester, but is safe to use in small doses towards the end of pregnancy.

Lavender is analgesic, antiseptic, antidepressant, antibacterial, antispasmodic, antiviral, carminative, decongestant, deodorant, diuretic, emmenagogic, sedative and hypotensive. It aids wound healing and is an excellent treatment for burns and scalds, relieving pain and preventing blistering and infection. Lavender is one of the few oils which can be applied neat to the skin in this instance and should be poured liberally over burns. The analgesic property makes it useful for headaches, and in labour.

It can be seen that lavender has many different uses, but as with all other oils it should not be administered for more than 3 weeks without a break. Arcier (1992, p. 32) states that it may overstimulate the nervous system if used in excess; and this author personally finds that it can cause irritation of the eyes if inhaled for a prolonged period of time.

In general healthcare lavender is effective in treating eczema and other skin rashes, is antipyretic and antispasmodic. Holmes (1992) identifies the cardiotonic, cell and biliary stimulant, immunostimulant and antiemetic properties amongst others.

Lavender blends well with most of the oils in the selection outlined but especially with mandarin, camomile, jasmine and geranium.

Neroli (orange blossom) – *Citrus bigaradia/aurantium* (Rutaceae family) Neroli oil is obtained by an intricate process of enfleurage (see Glossary) from the delicate petals of the bitter or Seville orange tree and is therefore one of the most expensive oils and something of a luxury. However the price is worth paying as a very few drops can be extremely effective in a variety of conditions.

The chemical compounds include phenylacetic acid, linalyl acetate, neryl acetate, methyl anthranilate (esters), nerolidol, linalool, geraniol, terpineol (alcohols), camphene and limonene (terpenes) and jasmone, a ketone, in small amounts.

Neroli is an excellent antidepressant and is effective in alleviating nervousness, tension and anxiety. It can be invaluable in times of hormonal upheaval such as premenstrual tension, postnatal depression and again at the menopause. In addition the sedative action of neroli has recently been demonstrated in research on mice (Jaeger *et al.*, 1992) and its relaxing and calming effects were evaluated in research carried out in the intensive care unit at the Middlesex Hospital, London on patients who had had cardiac surgery (Stevenson, 1992).

As with all essential oils it is antiseptic and antibacterial and could be used in a room spray to ward off infections, such as colds in the winter months, whilst also making use of its deodorising effects It is carminative and regulates the digestive system, being useful for constipation, flatulence, diarrhoea and sickness. Combined with mandarin as an abdominal massage it can be extremely effective for any of these conditions, but in particular for constipation. Neroli also has a toning effect and could be beneficial to aid circulation in the legs with massage or in a foot bath.

Camomile – *Matricaria chamomilla* (German)/*Anthemis nobilis* (Roman) – Compositae family Camomile essential oil is another oil with many uses and is so gentle that Davis (1988, p. 86) refers to it as 'the children's oil'. It is distilled from the flowers of the camomile plant and, depending on its geographic origin and the consequent amount of azulene (see below) within it, may be any colour from a pale to deep blue or yellow to green. The quality will also of course affect the price, with some camomiles being extremely costly.

The most important constituent is not present in the flower but is formed during the process of extracting the oil from the plant. This is a fatty aromatic substance called azulene which has strong anti-inflammatory properties and aids wound healing and other skin problems. German camomile contains a higher proportion of azulene than Roman or Moroccan but otherwise the properties of the different camomiles are very similar to one another.

Other constituents include coumarin, the esters of angelic and tiglic acids, pinene (terpine), farnesol and nerolidol (alcohols) and pinocarvone (ketone), plus others in smaller amounts.

Camomile can be used in any situation where there is inflammation and infection for its anti-inflammatory and antibacterial characteristics come into their own. Menstrual or labour pain may be eased by the use of camomile im massages, baths or as a tea, and hormonal tensions and depressions can also be alleviated – premenstrually or postnatally. Use in pregnancy should however be delayed until the last trimester as it is thought to have some emmenagogic properties.

The soothing and calming nature of camomile is helpful in promoting rest and sleep, and could be of use throughout the childbearing period and for children and babies. Its action on the digestive tract will ease colic and diarrhoea in children, and a 1% blend rubbed into a teething infant's cheeks reduces fretfulness at these times.

Camomile has an affinity with the urinary tract and can act as a urinary antiseptic. A compress over the kidneys may ease discomfort during an infection. It may also be useful to put camomile tea bags, which have been soaked in boiling water and cooled, over the eyes in cases of conjunctivitis, or on the neck over the Eustachian tube when there is an ear infection. Influenza responds well to an inhalation using camomile oil and this will also relieve blocked sinuses.

Tea/ti tree – *Melaleuca alternifolia* (Myrtaceae family) Tea tree oil is a wonderfully versatile oil derived from the leaves of an Australian bush, and which has been used by the Aborigines for centuries. Indeed its fame grew in the middle of the twentieth century but later declined due to its relative inaccessibility (it grows in snake-infested marshes in New South Wales) and due to new drugs being manufactured. However it is enjoying a resurgence of popularity and the many purported benefits of tea tree oil are now being scientifically investigated.

Tea tree oil contains a massive 60% of terpines as well as various alcohols and sesquiterpenic alcohols. It is the large proportion of terpines which make tea tree such a useful oil for it is antiseptic, antibacterial, antiviral, antifungal and immunostimulant, a fact which has led to investigation of its use in HIV and AIDS, and for various skin infections (Wheater, 1991).

Tea tree products are now widely available from health food stores, including the essential oil, creams and pessaries. It is effective in treating candidal and other vaginal infections, including those in which causative organisms cannot be found, as reported by Blackwell (1991).

Although it has a rather pungent medicinal smell this can be subdued by blending it with other oils such as lavender which will enhance the therapeutic properties of each oil. Tea tree could be used as a room purifier where there is generalised infection, as an inhalation for respiratory infections, as a douche for infections of the reproductive tract (although this is not to be advised by midwives unless qualified aromatherapists), or applied neat to spots, verrucae or other localised inflammations and infections. Mixed into an appropriate cream in a regulated dose it could be applied to the buttocks of babies who develop infected nappy rash.

A massage with dilute tea tree oil over the kidneys and suprapubic area can also be effective in cases of cystitis.

Sandalwood – *Santalum album* (Santalaceae family) This is a rich exotic-smelling oil which has popularly been known for its aphrodisiac properties. Due to its price, as a result of near-extinction of the trees, sandalwood is another oil subject to adulteration, so it is best to purchase from a reputable supplier, in small quantities.

Sandalwood's chemical constituents include the alcohol santalol, santalene, a sesquiterpine and various aldehydes. Therapeutically sandalwood is antiseptic, antispasmodic, aphrodisiac, astringent, carminative, diuretic, expectorant, sedative and tonic. It blends well with lavender, rose, jasmine, geranium, neroli and ylang ylang.

Geranium – *Pelargonium odorantissimum* (Geraniaceae family) The essential oil of geranium is derived from the flowers and leaves of the plant and has a heavy but sweet smell, sometimes thought to be similar to rose, a fact of which unscrupulous suppliers take advantage by adulterating rose oil with geranium.

Geranium contains a high proportion of alcohols such as terpineol, geraniol, citronellol and linalool, plus the phenol eugenol, citral, an aldehyde, sabinene, a terpine and methone, a ketone. It is best avoided in large amounts during pregnancy, particularly around the abdominal and sacral areas for it is known as a hormone regulator. It can however be used for specific massage such as ankle oedema and is useful for other hormonally related periods such as premenstrually, at the menopause and postnatally. Alternatively the application of geranium leaves to the legs should reduce oedema.

Geranium is analgesic, antidepressant, antiseptic, astringent, diuretic, haemostatic, vasoconstrictive, insecticidal and tonic. It blends well with bergamot, clary sage, jasmine, lavender, neroli, orange, rose and sandalwood.

Rose – *Rosa centifolia/damascena* (Rosacea family) Rose is one of the most luxurious oils for, like jasmine and neroli, the delicate nature of the petals make extraction of the essential oil an expensive process. However it has a wonderful aroma which is particularly feminine and lends itself to use in midwifery and gynaecology. The cost can sometimes result in adulteration with cheaper oils so it is important to ask for the oil by its Latin name; *Rosa damascena*, produced mainly in Bulgaria may be called rose otto or attar of roses, while the French *Rosa centifolia* produces a rose absolute which is by far the most expensive.

The principal constituents include geranic acid, alcohols of citronellol, geraniol, nerol and farnesol, the phenol, eugenol and the terpine, myrcene. These chemicals result in rose being an especially effective antidepressant, but also antiseptic, antispasmodic, diuretic, emmenagogue, haemostatic, laxative, sedative and tonic. Its use is contraindicated in pregnancy as it may initiate uterine bleeding but it can be used with caution in the last 2–3 weeks and is good to use in labour.

Massage with essential oil of rose in labour will not only calm and cheer the mother but enhances uterine contractions; this same property can be harnessed in the premenstrual phase for non-pregnant women, and again postnatally to aid involution and prevent postnatal 'blues'. It is thought to be of use for nausea and vomiting but as it is contraindicated in the first and second trimester it is not appropriate for gestational sickness.

Rose is also recommended for sexual difficulties including frigidity and impotence and could be helpful in the early weeks of the puerperium to facilitate the resumption of sexual activity.

Rose blends well with mandarin, camomile, neroli, jasmine, lavender, sandalwood, clary sage and geranium; if mixed with tea tree oil it is effective for respiratory tract infections.

Jasmine – *Jasminum officinale* (Oleaceae family) This is another costly oil which has a truly exotic aroma but which can be quite oppressive for some women so care should be taken in the amount used.

There is a variety of alcohols in the oil such as geraniol, terpineol and nerol, as well as esters, linalyl acetate and methyl anthranilate, and the ketone jasmone. It is this latter with its adverse effect on the fetus which makes jasmine contraindicated in pregnancy, but it is perhaps the best essential oil to use in labour. Jasmine can enhance uterine action, accelerating or regulating contractions and easing pain and discomfort.

Jasmine is also antidepressant, and is therefore a valuable addition to a massage or the bath in the puerperium and is noted for its beneficial effects in severe depression. Its galactogogic action helps to stimulate lactation, so adding a few drops to a bath will treat or prevent several postnatal disorders. Premenstrual tension and menstrual pain also respond well to jasmine, and it can be valuable in cases of infertility as is it said to increase spermatozoa production.

Jasmine blends well with mandarin, rose, sandalwood, neroli and geranium.

Clary sage – *Salvia sclarea* (Labiatae family) Clary sage is a member of the same family as sage (*Salvia officinalis*) but because it contains a far lower proportion of the ketone thujone it is much safer to use in women of reproductive years. Menstruating women have suffered menorrhagia after using sage oil, and although it can be useful in certain circumstances such as sports injuries, sage oil is best avoided by the novice.

Clary sage contains other ketones such as cineole, as well as the sesquiterpine caryophyllene and various esters and alcohols. It is anticonvulsive, antidepressant, antiseptic, antispasmodic, aphrodisiac, digestive, hypotensive, sedative and tonic. However overdosing can result in headaches or loss of concentration so clients should be advised not to drive immediately after use. It is also known to potentiate the effects of alcohol – but is not a cheap means of becoming inebriated! Indeed it is thought that clary sage was sometimes added to cheap wines in the eighteenth century as it gave them a taste rather like Muscatel.

Clary sage can be very relaxing for women who are stressed and anxious and can be safely used in labour to ease pain and create a sense of euphoria. Its emmenagogic action precludes its use in pregnancy but it comes into its own in early labour and the postnatal period. Like rose and jasmine oils, clary sage also reduces abdominal and sacral pain during menstruation, labour and involution.

Digestive and kidney problems may respond to the use of clary sage, especially if blended with an oil such as mandarin for constipation.

Clary sage blends well with geranium, grapefruit, orange, mandarin, jasmine, lavender and sandalwood.

It can be seen that our selection is extremely versatile and that all the oils blend with at least three of the others. Let us then consider how these oils could practically be utilised in midwifery.

Utilising essential oils for pregnancy, labour, the puerperium and neonates

Anxiety Periods of anxiety or worry are a common occurrence in pregnancy and essential oils are invaluable in these situations. There are many oils which are safe to use either for massage, in the bath, in room vaporisers or as teas.

For women in the first trimester camomile tea is one of the safest means of providing the effective ingredients, without the potential problems of massage or concentrated oils directly on the skin. Room vaporisers are useful and it is possible to purchase traditional joss sticks of sandalwood, which is one of the most suitable oils. Later in pregnancy, massage (foot, back, face or the luxury of a full body massage) or oils added to the bath can be used, taking into account the correct blending as discussed previously.

Essential oils which can be beneficial in cases of anxiety include bergamot, camomile, lavender, neroli, mandarin, sandalwood and rose. In labour jasmine, clary sage and ylang ylang may also be used.

During her sixth pregnancy Mary was seen in the hospital antenatal clinic for her 32 week examination. The midwife spent a long time with Mary who seemed particularly anxious. From discussion it transpired that, although all previous labours had been normal, as each had approached Mary had become increasingly agitated and convinced of her own impending mortality. In her mind she knew this was illogical but the feelings had worsened with successive pregnancies so that by now she was emotionally drained and her concerns were affecting the rest of the family.

Mary had no knowledge or experience of complementary therapies but was 'willing to try anything'. At that appointment she was given a simple foot and leg massage, ostensibly to reduce ankle oedema, and she found this very pleasurable and relaxing. No essential oils were available at that time but the effect of the massage was very positive and it was suggested to Mary that someone at home could perform a similar massage for her. Mary was also recommended to drink camomile tea, and to purchase a small bottle of Rescue Remedy to take (see Chapter 2) when the feelings of panic were overwhelming.

About 7 weeks later the same midwife met Mary leaving the clinic after a subsequent appointment. Mary reported that she had followed the suggestions and used the Rescue Remedy in addition to the camomile tea and that this had been the best pregnancy of all. The following day she was to have labour induced due to mild cephalopelvic disproportion but with the help of her 'anti-anxiety remedies' she felt ready for labour and for the process of induction.

Backache The effects of progesterone and relaxin can cause chronic backache throughout pregnancy, labour and the puerperium which is very wearing for the mother. A gentle massage over the sacral area (except in the first trimester) can ease the discomfort, and if essential oils of lavender and/or camomile are added to the base oil the effects will be even more dramatic. These oils can also be added to a deep warm bath. Some aromatherapy books advise the use of rosemary for relieving backache in pregnancy but this is better avoided because of its tendency to raise the blood pressure.

Backache in labour, due to occipitoposterior position of the fetus, can best be relieved by sacral massage with lavender which will also facilitate effective uterine contractions and possibly anterior rotation of the fetal head. The massage can be performed by the midwife or by the birth companion and carried out between contractions. Firm circular movements with the heel of the hand around the sacral area can be very soothing as can small circular movements with the thumbs up either side of the spine.

In addition a simple shiatsu technique is useful in relieving the intensity of backache during labour and can be performed by the midwife or the mother's partner (Fig. 5).

Breast feeding Lactation can be stimulated by encouraging the mother to drink herbal teas such as fennel, dill or aniseed, or by using one of these

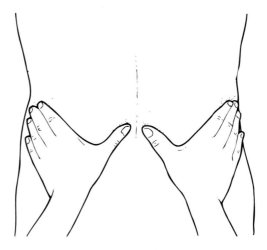

Fig. 5. To show shiatsu technique for relief of backache in labour (see also Fig. 15 in Chapter 7).

plants in cooking, especially fennel. Sore and cracked nipples may be relieved by the use of calendula and there are several proprietary calendula creams available to recommend to mothers.

Relief of milk engorgement can be achieved by using cabbage leaves and recently geranium leaves, have been used with similar but not quite such dramatic effects. Rhubarb leaves can also be used although the breasts should be wiped before feeding as rhubarb leaves are poisonous if ingested; it is probably advisable, therefore, not to recommend them to mothers for use at home. If the mother uses cabbage it should be very dark green as it is thought to be a substance in the chlorophyll which is the active ingredient. The leaves are wiped clean and cooled in the refrigerator, then applied to the breasts, left in place until wet, and then replaced with two more. This process is repeated until relief is obtained; in some cases the leaves become wet in seconds as the osmotic pressure takes effect.

Essential oil of peppermint can be used in a cold compress for the same reason but this must be wiped off before the baby goes to the breast to avoid ingestion, and for both practical and professional reasons cabbage leaves are the treatment of choice here.

Colic Neonatal colic can be as distressing for the parents as it is for the newborn baby. Simple abdominal massage with a base oil such as sweet almond is all that is required in most cases. If the 'wind' appears to be near the beginning of the intestines, anticlockwise abdominal massage will cause the air bubble to move and be expelled upwards, whereas air lower in the intestines should be encouraged to be expelled via the rectum by performing clockwise massage. If in doubt it is best to carry out clockwise massage which will stimulate peristalsis in the direction of the rectum (see Fig. 7).

Community midwives could employ this simple remedy if they are called

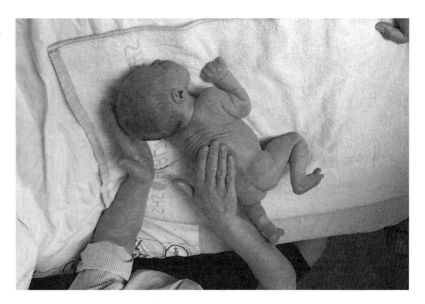

Fig. 6. A baby being massaged. (Courtesy of Nursing Times).

out by distraught parents in the middle of the night. Not only will the massage calm the baby but the manner in which it is performed, of necessity, will help to relax the parents. It may be even more beneficial if after a few minutes the mother or father is encouraged to carry out the massage themselves.

Constipation By far the most effective treatment for constipation in pregnant or postnatal women or their babies is to use abdominal massage in conjunction with essential oils. The massage should be in a clockwise direction across the whole abdomen, following the direction of the large intestine (Fig. 7).

The oils most appropriate for constipation are mandarin, orange and grapefruit, especially if used in combination.

Fig. 7. To show abdominal massage for ante- and postnatal constipation and neonatal colic.

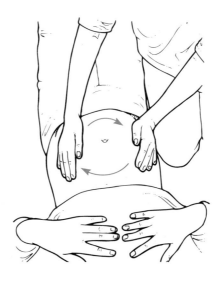

Ruth was a 30-year-old lady expecting her fifth baby. She had always had a tendency towards constipation, particularly in pregnancy which, on this occasion, was exacerbated by painful haemorrhoids which prolapsed following defecation.

Ruth was seen by the midwife at 30 weeks' gestation when the problem was causing her great distress. The midwife, an aromatherapist, performed clockwise abdominal massage for about 10 minutes, using a 2% blend of mandarin and orange oils. Normal advice about dietary and fluid requirements was reiterated.

Ruth was given a small amount of the blended oil to take home with her to perform abdominal self-massage. In addition she was given essential oil of lemon and juniper in a 1% blend to use in the bidet or a small bowl for her haemorrhoids. She was visited at home 2 weeks later and reported that she had used the oils as suggested with great relief to both her constipation and her haemorrhoids. She asked her husband to perform the abdominal massage which he normally did just before she went to bed, and the calming effect of the massage had improved her quality of sleep as well.

Postnatally Ruth again had problems, particularly with the haemorrhoids, and she used a combination of cypress and juniper oils in the bidet for local relief, and took homeopathic pulsatilla as the appropriate remedy which eased the haemorrhoids quickly and effectively.

Cystitis It is obvious that in some women the symptom of cystitis indicates a more serious urinary tract complication which requires medical consultation. However for those women who experience mild cystitis essential oils may reduce the symptoms, and can be an additional means of treating infection in conjunction with antibiotics.

The essential oils which have a particular affinity for the urinary tract include camomile, sandalwood, bergamot and lavender, all of which could be used for suprapubic massage, in compresses or in the bath, and garlic which could be added to the diet.

Bhupinder had a long history of cystitis. Although she was delighted at being pregnant she was nevertheless worried about the effects it would have on the urinary tract. Bhupinder's mother was instrumental in encouraging her to use complementary therapies, for cultural traditions at home involved the use of essential oils and other plant products.

The first episode of cystitis occurred at 9 weeks' gestation when mild burning sensations were felt during micturition. Bhupinder was advised to drink copious amounts of camomile tea which acts as a urinary antiseptic. She also increased the amount of garlic in her diet. This can be done by using greater numbers of cloves of garlic but without cutting or crushing them. If used whole in cooking the taste and odour will not be overpowering but the active ingredients will be present in larger quantities.

Sandalwood sticks were used regularly around the home so that Bhupinder would inhale the vapours. This combination of remedies seemed to be effective and the symptoms subsided.

However the cystitis returned with a vengeance at 34 weeks of pregnancy. The previously used regime was implemented and in addition Bhupinder was advised to wash the vulval area following micturition with a strong solution of warm camomile tea to cleanse the area and reduce stinging. She also prepared compresses to apply suprapubically when the discomfort was at its worst – she soaked a cloth in a solution of warm water (half a litre) to which had been added the essential oils of bergamot and camomile in a 2% blend. She asked her mother to use the same blend as a massage around the sacral area and this combination served to reduce the symptoms considerably.

The general practitioner was amenable to Bhupinder's self-treatment but following laboratory analysis of a midstream specimen of urine antibiotics were also prescribed. It poses a difficult ethical dilemma to withhold conventional treatment in order to await the results of 'alternatives' but it would have been interesting to observe the effects of the essential oils alone rather than to pursue the 'just in case' philosophy which can be so much a part of both medicine and midwifery. In Bhupinder's case the use of the essential oils truly was complementary to the orthodox care and caused no problems either for mother or fetus.

Haemorrhoids The pain of severe haemorrhoids, especially when they prolapse, can be relieved by sitting in a bowl of warm water to which has been added the essential oil of cypress and/or juniper in a 2% blend (i.e. to 5 ml of base oil add one drop each of cypress and juniper). These are both astringent and will reduce the throbbing sensation which often accompanies 'piles'. In addition lemon has a toning effect on the circulatory system and lavender can be beneficial as it will reduce pain and act as an antiseptic agent to cleanse the area. The mother could be given a bottle of the blended oils to use in the bidet or a bowl of water after each bowel action. This would need to be prescribed on 'standing orders' in agreement with medical staff.

Headache The headaches of early pregnancy which are a result of the action of progesterone on the cerebral blood vessels do not normally herald a more serious problem but those occurring in the third trimester may obviously require further investigation. However some symptomatic relief can be obtained by using lavender oil. This is one of the few exceptions to the rule of never using essential oils neat on the skin, for two drops on the forefingers of each hand rubbed gently into the temples can work wonders for a mild headache. Alternatively an ice cold compress made by soaking a cloth in iced water with a 2% blend of lavender may be welcomed by some women.

In someone who is not pregnant the synergistic effect of using lavender and peppermint together is even better, but as mentioned previously, peppermint oil is contraindicated in pregnancy.

Hypertension Massage alone can be extremely beneficial for the hypertensive woman, and for those admitted antenatally a simple back or foot massage could be effective in lowering the blood pressure. Its cumulative nature means that its optimum effects are obtained when the massage is repeated regularly and midwives could teach partners to perform massage, perhaps during visiting hours for inpatients or prior to bedtime in the home.

Lavender and camomile essential oils both have hypotensive and sedative properties and these could be alternated or combined for their synergistic effect (in which the combined effects are greater than the oils used singly).

Mandarin and neroli are also useful for their indirect hypotensive effects through their anxiety-relieving action on the mother.

McCardle describes her care of a woman with impending eclampsia who was not responding to intravenous therapy. Essential oils of rosewood and ylang ylang were massaged into the mother's back and legs for half an hour until the blood pressure decreased to within relatively normal limits. She poses the question 'was it due to the continuous infusion of drugs, was it due to the essential oils or was it due to the massage?' (McCardle, 1992) – a question which repeatedly presents problems for those attempting to carry out research.

Indigestion Many women suffer heartburn in later pregnancy to such an extent that it interferes with their appetite, sleep pattern and mood. Camomile and ginger are useful oils, and the mother could prepare a tea from grated ginger root or use one of the proprietary camomile teas. A gentle abdominal massage using camomile oil would be very relaxing, or a compress with camomile placed over the upper abdomen may help.

Insomnia Women nearing the end of pregnancy often experience difficulty in sleeping due to a variety of discomforts. The midwife can advise the ubiquitous camomile tea to be drunk just before retiring. Camomile or lavender oil added to a bath in a 3–4% blend could also be tried by the mother at home or in the antenatal ward. Massage could be even more relaxing, but for women in hospital it may be a less practical suggestion due to lack of time or other resources.

It may be possible in both ante- and postnatal wards to use electric vaporisers to dispense relaxing and calming oils into the air – ylang ylang is perhaps the most effective but as some people find its aroma rather cloying it could be blended with neroli or lavender. Staff would however need to obtain permission from all women in the ward/bay as everyone in the room would be receiving the vaporised oils.

Nausea and vomiting One of the difficulties in using essential oils to treat nausea and vomiting in pregnancy is that the symptom occurs usually in the first trimester when the woman is seen less often by the midwife, and at a time when many essential oils are contraindicated.

The safest method of utilising the therapeutic properties of appropriate plants is to make a tea, and camomile is the optimum choice. It is a gentle oil which will also relieve the anxiety which can occur and assist in promoting sleep. Women can buy this for themselves and it is acceptable for midwives to recommend it as an adjunct to any other treatment for sickness. Ginger is also very effective in relieving nausea and vomiting and drinking ginger tea will utilise the therapeutic properties of the plant without too high a proportion of essential oil. Alternatively the mother could chew on crystallised ginger pieces (Stewart, 1987).

Sickness in labour, which sometimes occurs, could also be relieved by sipping camomile tea, either hot, perhaps with the addition of honey, or iced. Midwives conducting parent education classes could suggest that the women bring in their own flask of camomile tea. If the partner drinks it as well it could serve to calm him down!

For neonates who posset frequently or for those who suffer vomiting caused by swallowing mucus during delivery, an abdominal massage with a 1% mix of camomile would be helpful. Encouraging the mother to perform this massage will have the additional benefit of relieving her anxiety at seeing her baby in distress.

Oedema Geranium and rosemary work well in reducing ankle and leg oedema if combined with bimanual upwards massage of the legs (Fig. 8). Midwives can demonstrate this to mothers in the antenatal clinic or parent education classes and the women could then perform it on themselves or ask their partners to do it, even without the essential oils. However care should be taken with the use of rosemary oil in pregnancy as it has hypertensive properties. Geranium, too, requires caution as, in a similar way to alcohol, it may exacerbate the mood of the mother, so that if she is depressed it can worsen the condition. Wrapping geranium leaves around the mother's ankles and legs should have the desired effect without exposing her to excessive quantities of the essential oil.

Fig. 8. To show leg massage for oedema.

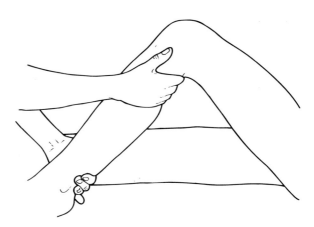

Pain relief in labour Aromatherapy has a very real part to play in the care of labouring women and can truly be used as an adjunct to any other conventional means of pain relief. It is the time when midwives often feel at a loss to offer sufficient choice to the mothers, particularly as many of the traditional methods have associated side effects or possible complications.

It is important to recognise that some women do not like to be touched during labour, but in fact if the midwife gently perseveres with a massage the mother often accepts it and then enjoys it. The most effective essential oils in labour include clary sage, lavender, mandarin and jasmine. For women who are coping with contractions but seem anxious, a foot massage with mandarin and rose can be very comforting – women in labour quite literally experience cold feet for their energy is focused elsewhere. Gentle but firm massage of the heel and sole in particular will also stimulate the appropriate reflex zones to enhance uterine action.

Margaret was a 33 year old primigravida, booked for a home birth with two midwives and a consultant obstetrician, all of whom were personal friends. She had performed nipple massage daily from the 37th week of pregnancy, had been taking raspberry leaf tablets since 30 weeks and went into labour on exactly her due date. During the early hours Margaret used a combination of transcutaneous nerve stimulation alternated with periods in the bath to which had been added essential oil of clary sage and lavender. It was unfortunate that after the second episode in the bath she returned to using the TENS machine only to find that the batteries were inactive. The delay in obtaining new batteries resulted in labour having progressed too far for the TENS to have any real effect so Margaret turned to the clary sage again. She made a compress from a clean sanitary pad and immersed it in a solution of warm water and clary sage (2% blend) – this was pressed against the suprapubic area with considerable relief.

The fetal position was found to be occipitoposterior and the first stage lasted 23 hours, including what appeared to be a 3 hour transition period between first and second stages. Margaret continued to use the clary sage for most of this time in conjunction with inhalational analgesia, relaxation and distraction techniques and accompanied throughout by one or both of her midwives.

Eventually the obstetrician joined the midwives and after a short period of spontaneous pushing everyone decided that a forceps delivery was needed. Twenty-four hours after the onset of labour (still at home), Margaret was delivered of a healthy baby boy weighing 4.6 kg (10 lb 4 oz)!

Perineal care Some mothers can be advised to perform daily perineal massage in the last 6 weeks of pregnancy to stretch and lubricate the area in preparation for the delivery. Using a few drops of base oil they should massage both outside and inside the perineal area, paying special attention to previous scars, and stretching the tissue by inserting their two thumbs inside the introitus and pressing downwards in the direction of the rectum. This should facilitate stretching of the perineum during delivery and can make the difference between needing an episiotomy or not.

Following delivery, trauma to the perineum, either due to episiotomy or lacerations, can be encouraged to heal more quickly by using lavender oil in the bath or bidet. Recent research by Sheila Cornwell and Ailsa Dale at Hinchinbrook Hospital in Huntingdon, Cambridgeshire, has shown that, while there was no statistically significant difference in wound healing, the use of lavender oil as a bath additive resulted in less perineal discomfort between the third and fifth days post-delivery (Dale and Cornwell, 1994).

Postmaturity In the absence of any fetal or maternal contraindications, aromatherapy could be used to initiate labour in a mother whose pregnancy is postmature – 42 weeks' gestation or more. A daily gentle abdominal massage with a 3% blend of lavender, jasmine and clary sage (i.e. one drop of each in 5 ml of base oil) should stimulate uterine action. This same mix can be used in labour which has commenced spontaneously but in which the contractions are either irregular or ineffective. However it is important to remember that induction is normally the province of medical staff and midwives must therefore consult with them prior to using essential oils likely to trigger contractions.

Postnatal 'blues' In the early days when many new mothers react tearfully to minor upsets, essential oils can again be of benefit. Room vaporisers with uplifting oils such as orange, mandarin and neroli or bergamot, geranium and rose will help to cheer everyone including the staff, if in hospital, or the rest of the family, if at home. The oils can also be added to the mother's bath in a 6% blend.

For a mother who becomes clinically depressed jasmine, sandalwood and ylang ylang are valuable in the bath or as a massage although the latter should be lighter and brisker than the normal deep slow relaxing massage, to avoid the mother becoming even more introspective. On the other hand the woman who has developed puerperal psychosis could benefit from a short but relaxing massage with rose essential oil, together with intermittent oral administration of the Bach Rescue Remedy, in conjunction with medically prescribed treatment.

Retained placenta Delay in separation and delivery of the placenta need not become a medical emergency which may result in a manual removal under anaesthetic. There is an expectation amongst many midwives that the placenta should be delivered within 10–15 minutes of the birth of the baby and that any delay is abnormal. Midwives need to relearn patience in their work, particularly at this stage of labour. However if after allowing for nature to take its course there still appears to be no separation and descent of the placenta and membranes natural methods to encourage it to do so can be employed.

Nipple stimulation, either by putting the baby to the breast or by manual stimulation will obviously increase the pituitary release of oxytocin. In addition a compress of lavender and jasmine against the suprapubic and fundal areas should initiate further uterine contractions.

This treatment was employed for Prudence, a para three with a history of previous retained placentae. Fifty minutes had elapsed since the baby's birth and the midwife applied a compress of lavender and jasmine to the abdominal area. She also performed reflexology (see Chapter 4) to stimulate contractions. Ten minutes later the placenta was seen at the introitus to the vagina and delivered complete with membranes. One could question whether the outcome was the result of the natural course of events, or due to the aromatherapy or the reflexology – but does it really matter? For the purposes of research it would be important to isolate the causative factors, but on its own merit this case illustrates the virtue of patience.

Striae gravidarum Daily abdominal massage throughout the second and third trimesters of pregnancy with a rich base oil such as jojoba, avocado or peach kernel with added wheatgerm can be enhanced by the addition of a gentle essential oil such as mandarin. Whether this actually prevents stretch marks appearing is questionable, as they may not have manifested in the first place, or if none appear this may be due to the rich base oil rather than the essential oil. However it is certainly pleasurable for an expectant mother to receive a daily massage (she can do this for herself) and many mothers report that their fetuses seem to respond with a perceived calmness in their movements.

Vaginal infections Leuccorrhoea which indicates an infection such as thrush can be treated with a local wash of boiled water and 2% tea tree oil which is antibacterial, antiviral and antifungal. There are now proprietary preparations of tea tree creams and pessaries in regulated doses which midwives may prefer to recommend.

Blackwell, writing in the *Lancet* in 1991, describes the case of a woman who presented with anaerobic vaginosis but who declined the conventional treatment of metronidazole. She treated herself with tea tree pessaries which proved to be effective in resolving the problem which did not recur.

Pruritis without confirmed infection can be eased by using a vulval wash of lavender or camomile, or adding this to the bath or bidet. Once again, those midwives unsure in their usage of essential oils could suggest a strong solution of camomile tea for the vulval wash, and mothers could of course prepare this for themselves.

Conclusion

Aromatherapy provides a wonderful array of pleasant-smelling aids to the midwife's normal practice if used cautiously and responsibly. Of all the complementary therapies enjoying a resurgence of popularity aromatherapy is perhaps the one in which midwives and nurses are most interested. The use of touch enables a return to the nurturing which has, to a certain extent, been lost in the last decade in an attempt to justify the increased use of technology.

Aromatherapy should in no way be considered an alternative to conventional treatment, but as a complement, as an additional tool for symptom relief, to resolve so many of the conditions which midwives already treat.

Midwives have much to offer women in their care and must be mindful not to abuse their privileged position. As with any other innovation it is the overenthusiastic midwife, trying to force through aromatherapy, perhaps with inadequate knowledge, poor quality oils or liberal doses who will meet resistance from colleagues. Judicious introduction of 'safe' essential oils, in consultation with medical staff, will enable midwives to demonstrate their effectiveness and gain their acceptance alongside other therapeutic substances. Perhaps in the not too distant future we shall see aromatherapy as an integral component of midwifery practice. It certainly merits consideration. In the mean time this chapter may have served to interest and enthuse readers sufficiently to learn more so that they can be the innovators we need. Good luck!

Training to be an aromatherapist

There is a great number of courses in aromatherapy, of variable quality. Midwives wishing to pursue an aromatherapy qualification should investigate carefully to find the training programme which suits them best.

Although there is no nationally prescribed standard for aromatherapy training, some centres are approved by one of the self-regulating bodies which belong to the Aromatherapy Organisations Council. New directives for training in line with European regulations came into force in 1994, which resulted in some institutions having to upgrade the courses they offered. Those which offer a recognised 'kitemark' such as the International Federation of Aromatherapists (IFA) or the International Society of Professional Aromatherapists (ISPA) are recommended, although midwives should still ascertain if a particular course is appropriate to their needs.

There is also a move towards improving the academic level of many of the courses to diploma standard. One such programme is the Diploma of Higher Education in Complementary Therapy (Aromatherapy) offered to qualified healthcare professionals by the University of Greenwich in south-east London.

It should also be stressed that, while a 10 week evening class in aromatherapy will provide sufficient background for the safe treatment of family and friends, it is not adequate preparation for professional use. The dangers to clients, and to the midwife's professional registration, of 'dabbling' in aromatherapy cannot be emphasised enough.

Useful addresses

The Aromatherapy Organisations Council
3 Latymer Close, Braybrooke, Market Harborough
Leicester LE16 8LN, UK
Tel: 0455 615466

The International Federation of Aromatherapists
Dept. of Continuing Education, Royal Masonic Hospital, Ravenscourt Park, London W6 0TN, UK
Tel: 081 846 8066

The International Society of professional Aromatherapists
Hinckley and District Hospital & Health Centre, The Annex, Mount Road, Hinckley, Leicestershire LE10 1AG, UK
Tel: 0455 890956

The University of Greenwich, Faculty of Health
Elizabeth Raybould Centre, Stonehouse Hospital
Bow Arrow Lane, Dartford, Kent DA2 6PG, UK
Tel: 081 316 9231

References

Arcier M. (1992) *Aromatherapy*. Hamlyn.

Armstrong F. (1991) Scenting relief. *Nursing Times*, **87(10)**, 52–54.

Balacs T. (1992a) Safety in pregnancy. *International Journal of Aromatherapy*, **4(1)**, 12–15.

Balacs T. (1992b) Peppermint pharmacology. *International Journal of Aromatherapy*, Spring, 22–25.

Blackwell A.L. (1991) Letters – anaerobic vaginosis. *Lancet*, **337** (February), 2.

Cohen N. (1987) Massage is the message. *Nursing Times*, **83(19)**, 19–20.

Dale A. and Cornwell S. (1994) The role of lavender oil in relieving perineal discomfort following childbirth: a blind randomised clinical trial. *Journal of Advanced Nursing*, **19(1)**, 89–96.

Davis P. (1988) *Aromatherapy: An A – Z*. C.W. Daniel.

Fromant P. (1991) Let me rub it better. *Nursing*, **4(46)**, 18–19.

Guenier J. (1992) Essential obstetrics. *International Journal of Aromatherapy*, **4(1)**, 6–8.

Hagan S. (1992) Aromatherapy and its benefits to people who are HIV positive. *Aromatherapy World*, Summer, 20–21, 8.

Henglein M. (1992) Essential oil presentation. *Aromatherapy World*, Summer, 29.

Holmes P. (1992) Lavender oil. *International Journal of Aromatherapy*, **4(2)**, 20–22.

Horrigan C. (1991) Complementing cancer care. *International Journal of Aromatherapy*, **3(4)**, 15–17.

Jaeger W. *et al.* (1992) Evidence of the sedative effect of neroli oil, citronellal and phenylethyl acetate on mice. *Journal of Essential Oil Research*, **4**, 387–394.

Lawless J. (1992) *Encyclopaedia of Essential Oils*. Element Books.

Martin S. (1990) Nurses take in alternatives. *Here's Health*, February, 18–20.

Maxwell Hudson. (1990) A licence to touch. *Here's Health*, September, 30–33.

McArdle M. (1992) Letter – Rosewood in pre-eclampsia *International Journal of Aromatherapy*, **4(1)**, 33.

Metcalfe J. (1992) *Herbs and Aromatherapy*. Bloomsbury Books, London.

Pages N. *et al.* (1990) Essential oils and their teratogenic potential: Essential oil of Eucalyptus globulus – a preliminary study. *Plantes Medicinales et Phytotherapie*, **24(1)**, 21–26.

Paterson L. (1990) Baby massage in the neonatal unit. *Nursing*, **4(23)**, 19–21.

Payne B. (1993) Learninig disabilities course. *Aromatherapy World*, Summer 16–17.

Price S. (1992) The position of aromatherapy in European countries other than Britain. *Aromatherapy World*, Summer, 16–17.

Redding D. (1991) When massage is just the job. *Independent on Sunday*, 10.2.91.

Reed L. and Norfolk L. (1993) Aromatherapy in midwifery. *Aromatherapy World*, Summer, 12–15.

Ryman D. (1991) *Aromatherapy – The Encyclopaedia of Plants and Essential Oils and How They help You.* Piatkus,

Sanderson H. (1992) Introducing people with learning difficulties to aromatherapy. Aromatherapy World, Summer, 4–6.

Sapsford C. (1993) Committee communication – research. *Aromatherapy World*, Summer, 6.

Sellar W. (1992) *The Directory of Essential Oils.* C.W. Daniel.

Steele J. (1992) Environmental fragrancing. *International Journal of Aromatherapy*, **4(2)**, 8–11.

Stevenson C. (1992) Orange blossom evalua-tion. *International Journal of Aromatherapy*, **4(3)**, 22–24.

Stewart N. (1987) New ways to beat sickness. *Mother*, May.

Tisserand R. (Ed.) (1993) *Gattefossé's Aromatherapy.* C.W. Daniel.

UKCC (1991) *Midwives' Rules.*

UKCC (1992a) *Guidelines for Administration of Medicines.*

UKCC (1992b) *Scope of Professional Practice.*

Valnet J. (1980) *The Practice of Aromatherapy.* English translation by Tisserand R. (1982). C.W. Daniel.

Wheater C. (1991) First aid in a bottle. *Here's Health*, September, 24–25.

Worwood V. (1990) *The Fragrant Pharmacy.* Bantam Books,

Further reading

Lavabre M. (1990) *Aromatherapy Workbook.* Healing Arts Press, Rochester,.USA

Maxwell Hudson C. (1988) *The Complete Book of Massage.* Dorling Kindersley,

Westwood C. (1991) *Aromatherapy: A Guide to Home Use.* Amberwood.

Denise Tiran

Chapter 4 Reflexology in Midwifery Practice

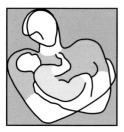

Reflexology or reflex zone therapy involves a sophisticated form of foot massage or manipulation in which the feet represent a map of the whole body. Working on the feet, or the hands which correspond accordingly, parts of the body distal to the feet can be treated. Although reflexology is not a diagnostic tool it is possible to detect areas of disorder or disease which may be present in the body, or to have an indication of previous and even potential problems which may arise in a given area.

The history of reflexology

Reflexology, reflex zone therapy and the metamorphic technique all evolved from the ancient Chinese system of medicine used thousands of years ago. In acupuncture, needles are inserted into a point on the body distal to the source of a particular health problem, in the belief that they are linked by energy lines called meridians. So too, in reflexology, is there the theory of energy pathways linking the feet and hands to the rest of the body. While many Western reflexology authorities feel that these are not the same as the meridians of acupuncture, some believe they are identical.

Other therapists support the theory that reflex points in the feet act as nerve receptors for all the organs of the body, in an attempt to explain in more Westernised terms how reflexology works.

In practice the right foot relates to the right side of the body and the left foot relates to the left side; the dorsum represents the front of the body including the musculature, and the soles of the feet represent the back of the body and the internal organs. Kevin and Barbara Kunz (1984, p. 10) state that the exception to this rule is the cerebral and central nervous systems which are controlled by the opposite side of the brain and thus the reflex areas on the feet for these parts of the body should be on the opposite foot. This concept may support the nerve receptor theory but no mention of it is made by other writers (Marquardt, 1983; Wagner, 1987; Goodwin, 1988; Hall, 1991).

Egyptian tomb paintings have depicted scenes of what appears to be foot massage and it is also thought that primitive tribes elsewhere in the world used similar techniques. Very little is documented about reflexology after this time until its resurgence at the end of the nineteenth century. The four main protagonists of the twentieth century were William Fitzgerald, Eunice Ingham, Hanne Marquardt and Doreen Bayly.

Fitzgerald, an American doctor at the turn of the century, was an ear, nose and throat specialist who observed that patients' perceptions of pain could be affected by pressing elsewhere on their bodies. He had discovered Red Indian tribes practising zone therapy and explored the principle further, developing and refining it into a system of treatment which he used within his medical practice, to great scepticism from his colleagues.

His research led him to divide the body into ten longitudinal zones running from head to toes and fingers (Fig. 1). It is interesting to note that at this time the feet were not singled out for any special significance but that effective treatment could be given through pressure on the hands, feet, tongue and lips. It is the theory of the ten longitudinal zones which enables the therapist to treat any disorder within a specific zone by working on either the hand or the foot in the same zone. This is of particular relevance when it is not possible to work on a client's feet, due to infection or perhaps an amputation, and the therapist would then work on the hands in the same zones as she would have treated on the feet.

Another doctor, J. S. Riley, also used reflex zone therapy extensively but his main claim to fame is as the teacher of Eunice Ingham. In the 1930s Mrs Ingham, an American masseuse, was the first person to use reflexology as it is used today. She devised the special 'grip' technique and refined the therapy to one in which almost all treatment can be carried out on the feet or the hands. Her compression massage was thought to be a way of working on crystalline deposits under the skin which result from excess calcium and uric acid when the metabolism is disrupted. The reflexology technique aimed to disperse these crystals and facilitate their excretion through the blood and lymphatic processes.

A pupil of Eunice Ingham's was Hanne Marquardt, a German, who added the concept of transverse body zones to the existing theory of longitudinal zones. These transverse zones correspond to the shoulder girdle, the waist and the pelvic floor and related transverse zones can be described in the feet (Fig. 2).

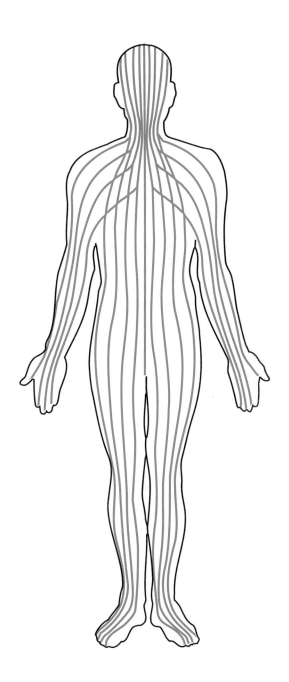

The person credited with bringing reflexology to Britain is Doreen Bayly, who persevered against her critics to demonstrate the many benefits of the treatment and established the first British reflexology training institution.

Another reflexologist, working in the 1960s, Robert St. John, discovered that the inner edge of the foot, which represents the spinal zone, also

Fig. 2. To show the transverse zones of the body and feet.

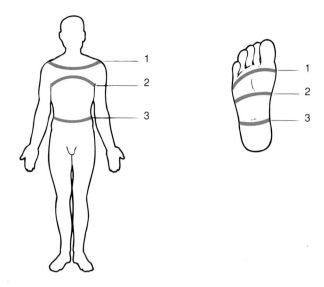

Fig. 3. To show the spinal zones of the feet which relate to the prenatal period in the Metamorphic Technique.

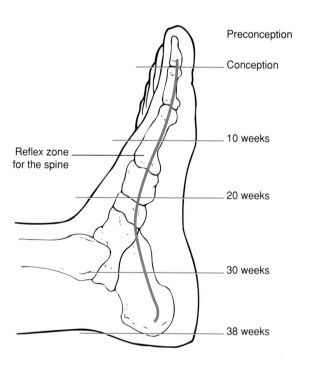

corresponds to the prenatal period. He thus surmised that by working on this part of the feet energy blockages which occurred during fetal life could be released – this became known as prenatal therapy or the Metamorphic Technique (Fig. 3).

Therapists do not aim to treat illness but rather to stimulate the innate capacity of the body to rebalance itself towards optimum health. St. John's most famous pupil, Gaston St. Pierre, investigated the technique further and is considered one of the leading authorities on the subject today (Cohen, 1987; Lambert, 1988).

It is not the aim of this chapter to consider in detail the metamorphic technique but suggestions for further reading are given at the end of the chapter.

How does reflexology/reflex zone therapy work?

Reflexology or reflex zone therapy of the feet can be used to highlight areas of the body in which past, current or potential energy disturbance may be present. This may be identified visually, manually or as a result of the recipient's response to the treatment.

On examination of the feet the therapist may be able to observe discoloration, dryness or rashes on the skin surface or oedema and swelling of certain areas which may or may not be diagnostically significant. Minute tactile examination over the entire surface of both feet may elicit the presence of the crystalline deposits, resistance and tension or pitting oedema. If there is disorder or disease in the body the client may experience a bruised feeling on palpation of the feet, or a pinpricking sensation 'as if the therapist is sticking her nail into the foot' while working on those areas which relate to the affected organs. Either of these responses may indicate energy disturbance but is not a diagnosis of disease in itself. Occasionally when visual evidence is present but the client feels no discomfort at all in that part of the foot, this may be more indicative of disease than a bruised or pinpricking sensation. However as a general rule, the sharp sensation highlights possible acute or current disorder while the bruised feeling identifies previous or chronic problems.

Reflexology can also be performed regularly for stress relief and relaxation and for maintenance of optimum health. It is with this in mind that it becomes such a useful adjunct to normal midwifery or nursing practice, as it can truly be used as a complement to any other orthodox treatment.

Reflexology is performed using the special 'grip' sequence devised by Eunice Ingham in which the therapist's thumbs or fingers move across the feet covering every minute point. This is sometimes called 'thumb walking' (Kunz and Kunz, 1984, p. 23), 'massage' (Hall, 1991, p. 103) or perhaps the most descriptive, 'caterpillar crawling' (Wagner, 1987, p. 44). The purpose of the technique is to activate the body's self-healing capacity by stimulating the reflex points, or to calm and relax zones which indicate an acute disturbance in the body. The former is achieved by an intermittent pressure of the thumb or, in the case of sedation, by a sustained continuous pressure on the relevant reflex point for up to 2 minutes. An example of the latter can be seen in someone suffering an occipital headache. The large toe on each foot represents the head in miniature, with the occipital zone being on the back

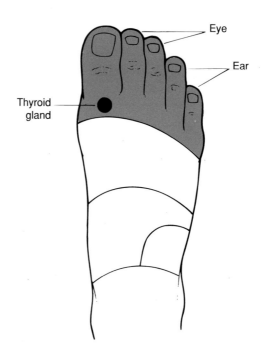

of the big toe at the junction between the toe and the foot (Fig. 4). This point is likely to be painful to touch in someone with an occipital headache, but continuous pressure is sustained until the discomfort in the toes is alleviated – this should be reflected by an easing of the headache.

Logically frontal headache would be relieved by applying the same technique to the relevant part on the dorsum of each toe. There is however one major difference between reflexology and reflex zone therapy, in that whereas the former treats symptomatically, the latter attempts to treat causatively. Therefore a reflex zone therapist treating the same occipital headache would explore both feet and treat any part of the foot which was either painful to touch or which visually demonstrated disorder. This might include, for example, the zones to the kidneys if the cause of the headache was renal hypertension.

Location of specific zones on the feet is easier if the two feet are placed together and a picture of the body is superimposed upon them. However because of the diminutiveness of the feet in relation to the size of the whole body care must be taken that the correct organ zone has been identified. Working one eighth of an inch off the intended zone could mean that an entirely different body organ is being treated. This is especially significant in midwifery when working on the heels, which represent the zones to the reproductive organs (Fig. 5).

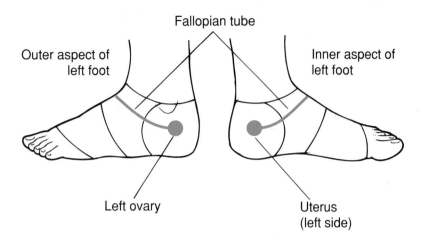

Fallopian tube

Outer aspect of left foot

Inner aspect of left foot

Left ovary

Uterus (left side)

A knowledge of the position of reflex zones is useful when applying simple massage to the feet. It can be seen that the heels represent the pelvic area, and it is this part on which vigorous brisk massage is contraindicated in early pregnancy, to avoid any potential risk of spontaneous abortion (see Chapter 3).

Some reflexologists include the use of 'tools' in their practice, such as elastic bands or clothes pegs, to apply continuous pressure to certain areas of hands or feet, or combs to create friction on specific zones (Hall, 1991, p. 17). However, it is generally considered that the relationship between client and therapist, and the sensitivity of the reflexologist in detecting nuances in the recipient are of paramount importance and result in a more effective treatment. For this reason nothing other than the bare un-encumbered hands of the therapist should be used to perform the treatment – not even oils or creams are required, although some therapists use a small amount of talcum powder to avoid friction of skin to skin con-tact. Other 'gadgets' claiming to stimulate reflexology points are also to be avoided as these may overstimulate and cause pain. In addition the individ-uality of every foot cannot be identified by a standard piece of equipment such as a reflexology sandal, which may put pressure incorrectly on the feet and serve to aggravate existing conditions or even initiate others which are latent.

The theory that pressures on the feet from shoes or specific conditions such as corns, verrucae or athlete's foot may indirectly stimulate disorder elsewhere in the body is often reported anecdotally by therapists, and is wor-thy of further investigation.

Vera, a middle-aged woman who received regular reflexology for relaxation, developed a verruca on the upper surface of her left second toe, which incidentally represents the zone for the left eye. On questioning her it emerged that she had also begun to suffer 'spots' in front of her left eye which had commenced at about the same time as the verruca first appeared.

It is wise to avoid direct reflexology to infected areas so Vera was given essential oil of tea tree to use (one drop neat applied to the centre of the verruca daily and confined by a corn plaster; see Chapter 3). She used the tea tree oil for 5 days when she began to see an improvement in the size of the verruca – and the severity of the visual disturbance lessened. A further 10 days of tea tree application had virtually eliminated the verruca, and the 'spots' before her eyes did not recur after the eighth day.

This does raise the question of whether the situation would have resolved itself spontaneously for no empirical evidence exists to prove otherwise. However many reflexologists recount similar instances, and it would seem to confirm the theory of the interrelationship between the feet and the rest of the body. Franz Wagner (1987, pp. 52–53) identifies several potential problems as a result of common foot complaints, including previous, existing or latent disease, injuries, hyperactive or hypoactive organ functioning, or merely excess exhaustion or tiredness. The theory is supported by Kunz and Kunz (1984, p. 19). Marquardt (1983, p. 74–75) goes further, giving a variety of examples with suggestions as to their specific potential outcomes. These include: hallux valgus causing problems of the cervical spine and thyroid gland; fallen arches/flat feet leading to spinal column disorders; and pelvic and hip conditions arising from injury to or congestion of the malleoli and heels.

In midwifery the supposition that an intravenous cannula inserted into the back of the hand, which is over the zone relating to the breast, may impair the onset of lactation is also worth investigating. Certainly the converse is true in that women with inadequate lactation can be helped by stimulation of these zones on the hands and the feet (Fig. 6).

Contraindications to treatment

It is obviously impractical to attempt to work on someone's feet if there are major problems of the lower limbs, such as severely varicosed veins or ulcers, thrombosis or fungal infections, although unilateral disorders can be treated on the opposite limb. It is also feasible to work on the reflex zones to the hands (see Fig. 1), although deeper manipulation may be necessary as the hands are less sensitive to therapy than the feet.

If a person has an acute infectious disease or is pyrexial it is also advisable to refrain from giving a full treatment, yet simple sedation techniques can be

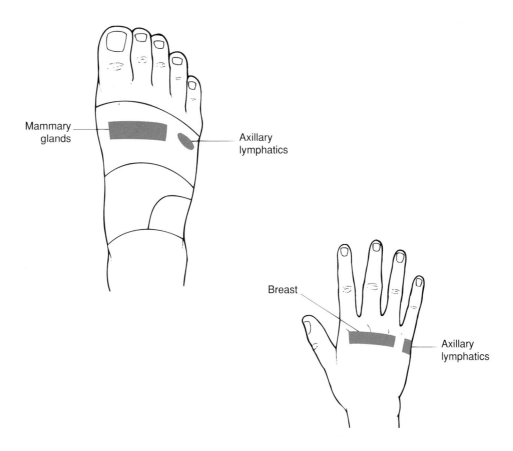

Mammary glands

Axillary lymphatics

Breast

Axillary lymphatics

Fig. 6. To show the zones for the breast in hand and foot.

very soothing to someone emotionally and physically stressed by serious illness. Similarly if the client has carcinoma, multiple sclerosis or a condition requiring surgery reflexology, will not eliminate the cause of the illness. It will however relax and calm the person, activate excretory organs, stimulate the respiratory system and may dramatically reduce pain.

In pregnancy, reflexology or reflex zone therapy is only contraindicated if there is a risk of fetal loss, although Kunz and Kunz (1984, p. 82) dispute this, stating that 'miscarriage is a reaction of the body, NOT a reaction to reflexology'. Great care should be taken however during the first trimester and with the first treatment at any time during pregnancy, but reflexology can be a very pleasurable means of relaxing both the mother and fetus, and enabling the woman's body to find its own equilibrium.

Reactions to reflexology treatment

A variety of positive and negative reactions can occur during, after or between treatments. These arise as a result of the activation of the body's innate self-healing capacity and demonstrate that toxins are being eliminated in an attempt to attain homeostasis. Often there is a healing crisis in which the person appears to get worse before getting better, as the body 'kick starts' itself into action.

All reactions occurring at any time during the course of treatment should be recorded however insignificant or unrelated they may seem.

While administering the reflexology treatment it is important to observe the client for responses to the massage – whether they appear calm and relaxed, agitated, in pain or frightened. Occasionally the person may start to perspire or complain of feeling hot and/or cold – this is often as pressure is applied to reflex zones relating to diseased or disordered organs in the body. However it may be even more significant if the therapist is aware of possible disorder by observation or manipulation of the feet while the client feels nothing and does not respond at all. If reactions do occur during treatment, simple stroking of the feet and 'harmonising' grips can be used until the symptoms subside. For example, the reflex zone for the solar plexus (Fig. 7) can be treated by sustained pressure and will help to calm the client down. This area can also be treated as part of a session for relaxation.

Between treatments, if a client is receiving a course of reflexology, other reactions may occur but are not always recognised as such. These may include improvement in the texture and tone of the skin due to improved

Fig. 7. To show the reflex zones for the solar plexus (left side).

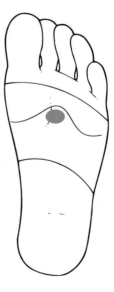

circulation; alternatively skin eruptions in the form of spots and rashes may present as the body attempts to rid itself of toxins (the so-called 'healing crisis'). Most clients report sleeping better although some complain of remembering vivid dreams. Activation of the excretory processes often results in increased diuresis or bowel action, sometimes accompanied by an unusual, somewhat unpleasant odour of either urine or faeces; other secretory processes are stimulated leading to extra mucus production in the respiratory tract or vagina. A few people become feverish, not symptomatic of illness, but rather as a natural defence mechanism, and the fever should not be suppressed by antibiotics. Indeed it has been seen in some clients that latent, perhaps previously suppressed or inadequately treated illness, may surface; completion of a course of reflexology should resolve the problem. Many clients experience mood changes, usually positive, as a response to treatment, and report a sense of relaxation and calm. This is what makes reflexology such a valuable aid to the treatment of stress-related conditions.

Some authorities, such as Wagner (1987, p. 56), suggest that the therapist may also experience reactions due to the energy flow between themself and the client. This may take the form of tiredness and yawning, nausea or headache, and throbbing of the hands and fingers. Wagner recommends that thorough washing of the hands followed by brisk shaking and rubbing of the lower arms should resolve the situation.

The use of reflexology/reflex zone therapy during pregnancy, labour and the puerperium

Reflexology can be extremely beneficial for expectant, labouring or newly delivered women, and for their babies, both to treat a variety of specific conditions and to aid relaxation and induce sleep. Some women enjoy regular sessions throughout their pregnancies which helps to alleviate the adverse effects of physiological changes as they arise, by triggering the body's self-healing and self-regulating capacities.

It is also thought to be useful in cases of infertility or subfertility when treatment of the reflex zones for the pituitary gland and ovaries may stimulate ovulation. This would normally be carried out in conjunction with other treatment such as dietary advice, relaxation exercises and the recommendation to sit in alternate hot and cold baths, with the water level above the waist, in an attempt to improve pelvic lymphatic and nerve supplies.

Identification of the pituitary gland reflex zone (Fig. 8) is vital to the use of reflexology in midwifery as so much of physiology is dependent on pituitary activity.

Throughout pregnancy it is wise to work very gently over the reflex zone to the uterus, although the zone should not be sedated by sustained pressure on the area – this would have the effect of 'sedating' the pregnancy and possibly creating difficulties for maternal and fetal health.

Fig. 8. To show the reflex zone for the pituitary gland.

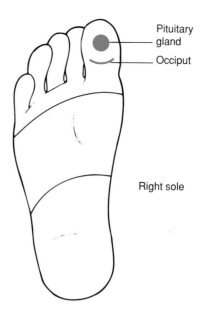

Contraindications Contraindications to reflex zone therapy in pregnancy include major placental disturbance such as placenta praevia or abruption, ectopic pregnancy, threatened abortion, pyrexia or infection and any unstable pregnancy about which the therapist is unsure.

An additional condition which some therapists would avoid treating with reflexology is pre-eclampsia, although gentle harmonising stroking movements may lower the blood pressure sufficiently to prevent eclampsia. Treatment of the kidney zones may also be of use but this should be done with caution to avoid exacerbating renal dysfunction.

Nausea and vomiting Nausea and vomiting of the first trimester may respond to reflexology in conjunction with other treatments as outlined elsewhere in this book. Harmonising massage strokes and sedation of the solar plexus zone may generally relax the mother and treatment of the reflex zones for the endocrine system can relieve severe hyperemesis of hormonal aetiology.

Constipation Constipation responds wonderfully well to reflexology and can be performed antenatally and postnatally as well as on neonates and infants. The arches of the feet correspond to the gastrointestinal tract and clockwise massage of these areas with the thumbs can be very effective (Fig. 9). A qualified therapist would also treat the zone for the liver, but the novice may achieve good results simply by circular massage – it would be acceptable for midwives with limited experience of reflexology to attempt massage of the arches rather than the specific reflexology technique.

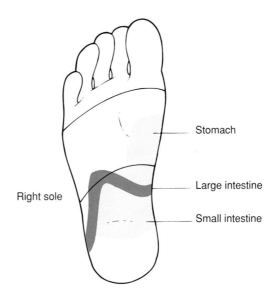

Fig. 9. To show the reflex zones for the intestines – massage in a clockwise direction to stimulate peristalsis (both feet).

Stomach

Large intestine

Small intestine

Right sole

Haemorrhoids Varicosities, particularly Haemorrhoids, can be treated successfully with reflexology, before and after delivery. Sedation of the rectal reflex zone and stimulation of the lymphatic system and intestinal zones will ease discomfort, aid defecation and may reduce swelling of prolapsed haemorrhoids.

Backache Backache due to the effects of relaxin may be relieved by working on the spinal zones along the inner edges of the feet, as well as sedation of the zones for the sacroiliac joint and abdominal musculature. If the problem is exacerbated by laxity of the symphysis pubis, gentle work on the pituitary gland zone should rebalance the hormonal output.

Oedema Physiological ankle oedema can be resolved to a certain extent by working on the reflex zones to the lymphatic system, kidneys, liver and gastrointestinal tract regularly.

Heartburn Heartburn may be alleviated by stimulating the zones for the stomach and intestines and sedating the zones relating to the solar plexus and diaphragm.

Cystitis Most authorities (Kunz and Kunz, 1984, p. 132; Wagner, 1987, p. 139; Hall, 1991, p. 145) suggest that the symptoms of cystitis, pyelitis and nephritis can be treated with reflex zone therapy, but great care must be taken by even the most experienced reflexologist when dealing with this condition in a pregnant woman. The therapist must also be certain to work only in the direction of the urinary tract from the kidneys to the ureters and then the bladder to avoid spreading any infection in the opposite direction. Wagner (1987, p.139) urges discretion in any client in whom renal calculi are suspected for inadvertently enthusiastic treatment may dislodge a loose stone, moving it to a position where it causes a blockage and a subsequent deterioration in renal function.

Frequency of micturition, however, due to pressure from the growing uterus or engaged presenting part, may be improved by gentle reflexology to the urinary tract zones.

Anxiety Anxious or depressed mothers may enjoy receiving regular reflexology from a qualified practitioner throughout pregnancy. This would alleviate insomnia, reduce stress, and may provide an opportunity to discuss in detail their fears and worries. As with other tactile one-to-one therapies, practitioners are advised to be competent in identifying and resolving or referring psychological problems.

Insomnia For those women in whom an active fetus at night prevents sleep, reflexology can help by not only relaxing the mother but also the fetus. Midwives on night duty in an antenatal ward could utilise simple foot massage as a means of facilitating sleep for inpatients. If the mothers are hypertensive, without impending eclampsia, this would help to reduce blood pressure as well.

For midwives, it is in caring for labouring women that reflexology comes into its own.

Induction Technically, labour can be induced by stimulating the zones to the pituitary gland and uterus, but the midwife-reflexologist must not exceed the limits of her practice by attempting this without the express permission of the obstetrician. However, the same treatment could be used in cases where labour needs to be accelerated or when the membranes rupture but spontaneous contractions do not follow.

Pain Pain in labour can be reduced by gentle work all over the feet but paying particular attention to the reflex zones for the uterus, pituitary gland, lymphatic system and other pelvic organs. For the midwife not qualified in reflex zone therapy, simple foot massage will serve to warm the feet, as labouring women quite literally suffer from cold feet as energy is directed elsewhere. Vigorous rubbing of each heel between the midwife's two palms can ease discomfort and enhance uterine action, while encouraging the mother to massage briskly around her wrists for 2 minutes every hour may also be helpful. The wrists and across the top of the ankles correspond to the Fallopian tubes and reproductive lymphatics and this action helps to relieve pelvic congestion. (It is also effective for dysmenorrhoea in menstruating women.)

Contractions Uterine action can be regulated with reflexology, either stimulating or sedating according to whether the contractions are inadequate or excessive. In the event of incoordinate activity, harmonising grips and treatment of the zones to the pituitary and other endocrine glands should help.

Micturition For women unable to pass urine reflexology can initiate micturition and save the mother from the potential complications of catheterisation. This is also an especially effective means of treating retention following delivery or Caesarean section.

Janet, a 25 year old primigravida, went into labour spontaneously at 38 ¹/₂ weeks' gestation and was admitted to the labour suite after 3 hours of regular painful uterine contractions at home. On examination the cervix was found to be 4 centimetres dilated, partially effaced and soft.

She progressed to full dilatation within 2¹/₂ hours. However the relative speed of the first stage had meant that she had only passed urine once, just before leaving home for the maternity unit, and she had continued to drink water throughout her labour. Janet felt a strong urge to push spontaneously but after 1¹/₄ of active pushing the presenting part was still at the level of the ischial spines, and on examinaton per vaginam the bladder was found to be full although Janet was unable to pass urine herself.

The midwife in attendance, a qualified reflexologist, asked if she could treat Janet's feet, to which she readily agreed. Stimulation of the zones to the urinary tract resulted in an almost instantaneous urge to pass urine, and the voiding of 450 ml. Emptying of the bladder facilitated descent of the presenting part, and Janet was delivered of a 3.8 kg boy just 20 minutes later.

Hyperventilation Reflexology can be effective in regulating the breathing of a mother who hyperventilates in labour, particularly in a prolonged second stage, by working on the zones to the solar plexus and respiratory tract.

Cephalopelvic disproportion If mild cephalopelvic disproportion is thought to be the cause of delay in the second stage, treatment of the zones to the pelvic joints and ligaments has been found in practice to create a little extra 'give' in the pelvic canal, sufficient to facilitate a vaginal delivery rather than Caesarean section.

Retained placenta Retained placenta also responds to treatment with reflex zone therapy, with stimulation of the uterine and pituitary gland zones on the feet. Community midwives qualified in reflex zone therapy in the author's area of work have utilised their skills on several occasions to avoid transfer to hospital of a mother who has delivered at home but in whom the placenta is slow to separate. Although these are anecdotal accounts without controls, the subject is worthy of research and could serve as a simple means of dealing with a situation which normally requires medical attention, but with which the midwife is trained to cope in an emergency.

Cynthia, a gravida four, insisted on a home birth despite complications in previous pregnancies – mild hypertension, postmaturity and haemorrhage during the third stage of her last labour. Two midwives were allocated to provide continuity of carer, and the pregnancy progressed normally apart from fluctuating blood pressure readings up to 100 mmHg diastolic towards term.

Labour commenced spontaneously at 42 weeks' gestation and full dilatation was confirmed after 6 hours. An uncomplicated birth of a healthy girl was achieved following 35 minutes of spontaneous pushing. However no further contractions occurred and a period of 40 minutes elapsed with the placenta still in situ. The midwife urged Cynthia to put the baby to the breast but she did not want to suck so nipple stimulation was started in an attempt to make the uterus contract. This had no effect and by now 65 minutes had passed.

The supporting midwife was nearing the end of her training as a reflexologist and asked if she could treat Cynthia's feet. Contractions recommenced after 5 minutes followed by separation and delivery of the placenta 3 minutes later.

In this case reflexology had been used as a last resort before calling medical aid because the midwife was not fully qualified, but she knew enough to justify what she was doing as an accountable midwife. In the future she would attempt to treat a mother's feet earlier to reduce the interval between birth of the baby and separation of the placenta.

It has already been mentioned that reflexology can be useful in initiating micturition, and it is a particularly valuable tool post-delivery, for women who have had a traumatic forceps delivery or a Caesarean section when the bladder and ureters may be bruised. Obstetricians in the author's maternity unit are happy for appropriately trained midwives to use reflex zone therapy on these women. Research to determine the effectiveness of the procedure and evaluate it in terms of cost compared with catheterisation, laboratory urinalysis and antibiotics in the event of iatrogenic infection is due to begin at the time of writing.

Subinvolution If a mother is found to have retained products of conception or subinvolution, reflex zone treatment of the feet can facilitate the physiological process and avoid the need for evacuation of retained products.

Perineal discomfort may be alleviated by working on the zones to the pelvic floor; other discomforts of the postnatal period such as uterine 'after-pains', backache, especially after epidural anaesthesia, headache and shoulder pain from poor positioning during breastfeeding may also be relieved.

Haemorrhoids can be treated to reduce pain and swelling when they have prolapsed by working on the reflex zones to the rectum and the lymphatic system.

For breastfeeding mothers reflex zone therapy is extremely useful in encouraging lactation, relieving engorged breasts, in particular venous engorgement, and stimulating milk flow to prevent stasis in the axillae. As mentioned earlier in this chapter, mothers who have had an intravenous cannula inserted into the back of the hand in labour may be slow to start lactating. Midwives, even those not trained in reflexology, can massage the dorsum of each foot and the back of each hand which should work on the reflex zones to the breasts; a qualified practitioner would also treat the pituitary zone. (see Fig. 6).

Depression The relaxation and de-stressing effects obtained from reflexology are useful in helping women suffering from postnatal 'blues' and may be effective in those with puerperal depression. Any mother would benefit from having a few sessions of reflexology after delivery, for at least it is calming and relaxing, and it may prevent or treat physiological disorders or pathological conditions which arise in the early postnatal period.

Research into reflex zone therapy/ reflexology

While reflexology purports to be a complete discipline in its own right it must be acknowledged that there is not a substantial body of knowledge with which to support it. Much of the discussion in this chapter is of unsubstantiated claims purely from anecdotal evidence. This fact would seem to undermine to some extent the value of reflexology/zone therapy, and without research to underpin theories the situation is unlikely to change. Reflexology is often used as a complement to other therapies, either for diagnosis (although this is not the aim of the therapy) or as an option available to practitioners who are qualified in other therapies.

In preparation for this chapter extensive international searches of relevant literature were made, but they yielded little in the way of specific research into reflex zone therapy/reflexology. Much of what has been written is descriptive without significant reference to other authorities.

It was interesting to note that the few research trials conducted into reflexology were in countries where complementary medicine is more accepted, and the research findings were published in non-English journals (Eriksen, 1992; Ferrer de Diso, 1993; Eichelberger 1993). Much of the English language literature is written by nurses attempting to describe the benefits to nursing/midwifery practice from their personal practice (Barron,

1990; Evans, 1990; Levin, 1992; Lockett, 1992; Tattam 1992). What was fascinating to discover was that the two international searches classified reflexology or reflexotherapy with some aspects of acupuncture. This poses the question of whether reflexology truly is considered to work on the same energy pathways as acupuncture, or whether those who compiled the databases assumed a relationship.

The lack of research is worrying, although the author is aware of several projects in progress around the country. There are many aspects of the use of reflex zone therapy in midwifery which would be well worth evaluating, such as for constipation, retention of urine, inadequate lactation or engorged breasts, induction or acceleration of labour and many more. The difficulty, as always with manual therapies, is the impossibility of carrying out randomised double-blind controlled trials, as it is obvious that the client would know whether or not the treatment was carried out. However randomisation of who receives conventional treatment or reflexology is possible, and this probably has to be the way forward.

International Reflexology

Reflexology around the world seems to be expanding rapidly although there are many differences in status within the various countries. Most countries report an increase in interest amongst consumers and many countries are working hard to develop high standards of educational programmes (Reflexions, 1993). However there does appear to be dissent in certain countries about whether training should be formalised: there seems to be concern that this step would have an adverse effect on the therapy because of the intellectualisation and the perceived loss of intuition in performing the treatment. On the other hand most countries have fought to gain legal recognition within the constraints of the individual country's laws. In some, such as Switzerland, where reflexology is used widely, it is classed with other manual techniques, particularly massage. In America where this is also the case it is hoped that North Dakota will, in 1994, be the first state to pass a reflexology law, in order that therapists can practise without first having to complete a course in full body massage. The Japanese, Israelis and Danish people use reflexology regularly, and in Denmark, the only country in Europe to include complementary therapies in medical training, reflexology institutions have been awarded a substantial budget to commence research. In Australia too, large-scale research, in collaboration with the Global Reflexology Research Institute for Professionals, is in progress (Reflexions, 1993).

In Britain reflexology/reflex zone therapy is also expanding and many health professionals are undertaking training. It is possible to attend evening classes intended to enable people to use the system on friends and family. However there is considerable confusion about reputable training courses for professional use. As with many complementary therapies there is no single regulating body and no national guidelines about standards of training.

From a professional viewpoint it is extremely worrying that nurses and midwives believe they can practise reflexology on clients and patients without attending a reputable and credible course of instruction. Readers are referred to the section on accountability in Chapter 1, and are advised to investigate potential courses thoroughly before joining them.

However the value of reflexology/reflex zone therapy is constantly being demonstrated in practice, and it is certainly a therapy which complements conventional midwifery care well. There is considerable strength of feeling amongst practitioners that the therapy needs further integration into orthodox care, especially within the National Health Service. This must be the optimum means of achieving greater credibility for the therapy. Healthcare practitioners who add it to their current skills will be better placed to provide a more comprehensive range of treatments, supported by their in-depth knowledge of anatomy and physiology, health and disease. Finally the opportunities presented to these practitioners to conduct research into reflexology should work towards developing the theoretical background on which the therapy is based. Only in this way will reflexology be fully accepted as an integral part of British health care.

Fig. 10. Reflexology in the postnatal period. (Courtesy of Nursing Times).

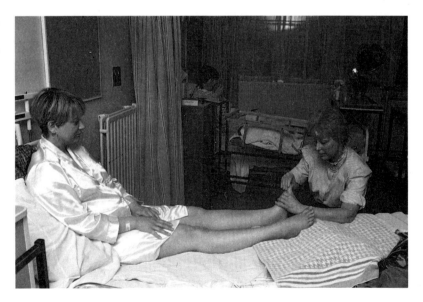

Training in reflex zone therapy/ reflexology

As mentioned previously there are no national standards for reflexology training although many of the reputable schools are moving towards the National Vocational Qualification (NVQ) scheme. Midwives considering the practice of reflexology should thoroughly scrutinise a variety of courses. The following organisations maintain details of training institutions and lists of practitioners.

The British School – Reflex Zone Therapy
87 Oakington Avenue, Wembley Park,
Middlesex HA9 8HY, UK
Tel: 081 908 2201

British Reflexology Association
12 Pond Road, London SE3 9JL, UK
under the auspices of the
Bayly School of Reflexology,
Monks Orchard, Whitbourne,
Worcestershire WR6 5RB, UK
Tel: 0886 21207

Association of Reflexologists
27 Old Gloucester Street,
London WC1N 3XX, UK
Tel: 081 445 0154

Metamorphic Association
67 Ritherdon Road, London SW17 8QE,
UK
Tel: 081 672 5951

References

Barron H. (1990) Towards better health with reflexology. *Nursing Standard.* **4(40)**, 32–33.

Cohen N. (1987) Massage is the message. *Nursing Times*, **83(19)**, 19–20.

Eichelberger G. (1993) Studie uber Fussreflexzonenmassage – Alternative zu Pillen

(Study on foot reflex zone massage – alternative to tablets). *Krankenpfl-Soins Infirm*, **86(5)**, 61–63 (in German).

Eriksen L. (1992) Zoneterapi mod kronisk forstoppelse (Zone therapy in chronic constipation). *Sygeplejersken*, **92(26)**, 7 (in Danish).

Evans M. (1990) Reflex zone therapy for mothers. *Nursing Times*, **86(4)**, 29–31.

Ferrer de Diso M. (1993) Energia y reflexologia como tratamiento holistico (Energy and reflexology as holistic treatment). *Rev Enferm*, **16(174)**, 65–67 (in Spanish).

Goodwin H. (1988) Reflex zone therapy. In Rankin Box D. (ed) *Complementary Health Therapies – a Guide for Nurses and the Caring*

Professions (Ed. D. Rankin Box), pp. 59–84. Croom Helm.

Hall N.M. (1991) *Reflexology: A Way to Better Health*. Gateway Books.

Kunz K. and Kunz B. (1984) *The Complete Guide to Foot Reflexology*. Thorsons.

Lambert M. (1988) *Finding Your Feet (Metamorphic Technique)*. M. & J. Lambert (Publ.).

Levin S. (1992) Why homeopathy, wherefore reflexology? *Nursing (South Africa)*, **7(8)**, 38–39.

Lockett J. (1992) Reflexology – a nursing tool? *Australian Nurse' Journal*, **22(1)**, 14–15.

Marquardt H. (1983) *Reflex Zone Therapy of the Feet*. Thorsons.

Reflexions (1993) Reflexology around the world. *Journal of the International Association of Reflexologists*, **2(1)**, 14–17.

Tattam A. (1992) The gentle touch. *Nursing Times*, **88(32)**, 16–17.

Wagner F. (1987) *Reflex Zone Massage*. Thorsons.

Further reading

Dougans I. and Ellis S. (1991) *Reflexology – Foot Massage for Total Health*. Element Books,

Ingham E.D. (1938, revised 1984). *Stories the Feet can Tell*. Ingham Publishing Inc., Fl.

Sue Mack

Chapter 5

Complementary Therapies for the Relief of Stress

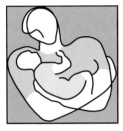

What is stress   There cannot be life without stress. It is the physiological/psychological spur that makes us get up and go and carries us through the day. Positive stress, coped with by the individual, can produce a feeling of satisfaction, happiness or even euphoria. Negative stress, not coped with, can produce illness, fatigue or breakdown. Thus it is both the kind of stress, its origin and intensity, and the coping mechanism of the individual that determines the effect of stress.

The word stress comes from the Old French *destresse*, which means placed under narrowness or oppression. This is exactly how many people would describe the feeling of being stressed.

Stress may be best defined from its effects. We may consider this on a simple cause and effect model, that is stress → strain. Noise may lead to headache, conflict may result in anger. This system while offering a simple explanation takes no account of the individual's response to stress.

We share with all animals a primitive physiological response to stress, the fight/flight mechanism. This is triggered whatever the stressor and is not within our control. Hans Seyle (1956), an endocrinologist, studied the physiological effects of stress and developed a theory he called the General Adaptation Syndrome (GAS) to describe the common human response. The three stages of GAS are first alarm, second resistance, and finally exhaustion. Thus many stimuli result in the same pattern of response. This is in part affected by the interpretation of the stimuli by the individual. The alarm phase provokes a quick response including lowered blood pressure and tachycardia. The resistance phase is the body's fight back. There is increasing production of adrenocorticotrophic hormones, with raised blood pressure and heart rate. If this is prolonged and the adaptation required too great, the body becomes increasingly vulnerable and exhaustion follows. Here it is the adaptation to stress, the coping mechanism, that affects the outcome.

A cognitive model of stress (Lazarus, 1966) includes the importance of thought, experience and the meaning of stress to the individual. Thus stress and adaptation may vary over time and in different situations for the same individual. The career woman who manages a demanding work schedule may find great difficulty in coping with her demanding infant.

To be able to deal adequately with negative stress we need to be able to recognise it, activate our coping skills appropriately and act on them with help and support where available.

Why is stress important?

Stress, or our maladaptive response to stress, has been implicated in many illnesses as well as the damaging attempts we make to relieve it by the use of cigarettes, drugs and alcohol.

The body's response to any stress is to release adrenalin and noradrenalin from the adrenal gland into the bloodstream, thus speeding up reflexes, increasing heart rate and raising blood pressure. This gives an immediate boost to our performance, but if not used as energy has serious implications for cardiovascular disease. Thyroid hormones when released also charge our metabolism but if they continue to be produced can lead to exhaustion and collapse. The cholesterol released from the liver when the body is under stress gives short-term energy but can increase blood cholesterol levels with the risk of arteriosclerosis.

It has been shown that psychological stress does impair the efficiency of the immune system (Jabaaij, 1993). Dutch researchers found that people experiencing stress produce significantly lower titres of antibodies to hepatitis B vaccine than do non-stressed subjects.

Excess stress response has been implicated in heart disease, stroke, problems of the digestive tract and migraine. Studies in heart disease, where most research has been done, have shown the physical benefits of stress reduction teaching to those most at risk (Patel, 1987). Studies of patients in hospital also show that those who felt most in control and relaxed not only had fewer emotional problems but also had a shorter recovery time.

In relation to pregnancy, a Danish study showed the effects of distress on preterm delivery (Hedegaard *et al.*, 1993). In a population of 8719 women there was found to be a significant relationship between distress, established using a general health questionnaire, at 30 weeks' gestation and preterm delivery. No relationship was found between preterm delivery and distress at 16 weeks' gestation. This study obviously has implications for the management of stress in pregnant women, particularly in the later weeks. This research has not been confirmed by other studies, one of which found anxiety more common in women who did not go into labour until 42 weeks (Sharma *et al.*, 1993).

Recognising stress

What we most notice when we are stressed is change: in our feelings, behaviour and mood. Change is also one of the triggers of stress. Any alteration in our circumstances requires us to make some adaptation in response. In order to reduce stress we must begin by knowing how to recognise the symptoms and identify some of the causes. These symptoms may be physical, mental, emotional or produce behavioural changes. How the individual responds will depend on personality, experience and learned coping mechanisms. For some women physical symptoms may be ignored, and to somatise their symptoms will not produce any reduction in stress. They do not easily allow themselves to be sick. For others sickness may be the only refuge from overwhelming psychological pressure. Whilst none of the individual symptoms listed below are exclusive to stress, taken together they may show that someone is not coping well.

Examples of physical stress symptoms:
Tense muscles
Dry mouth
Nausea
Palpitations
Dizziness
Sweaty hands
Diarrhoea

Examples of emotional stress symptoms:
Anxiety
Irritability
Feeling depressed
Feeling insecure
Crying
Guilt feelings

Examples of mental stress symptoms:
Difficulty in making decisions
Difficulty in concentrating
Memory lapse
Feeling under pressure

Examples of behaviour changes:
Increased smoking or drinking
Appetite changes
Sleep pattern changes

It is clear that many of these changes may occur normally in pregnancy; there is a natural increase in the size and activity of the adrenal glands, nausea is frequently experienced and concentration may be affected by the change in focus from external to internal concerns. However it is the cluster of symptoms and the individual's own feeling of stress that are important.

The cause of the stress may come from outside ourselves or from within. External stresses such as poverty, poor housing or isolation, as well as particular life events, may seem obvious causes of stress. The threat to which we are responding is clearer even if change seems difficult or impossible. The Holmes and Rahe Schedule of Life Events (Holmes and Rahe, 1967) charts the possible seriousness of an event, for example, the death of a spouse is rated as 100, and divorce as 73. Whilst pregnancy scores 40 it may have a very different effect on the woman for whom it is a planned and wanted event and the woman for whom it may be unplanned, unwanted or both. Brown and Harris (1978), in their research into depression in women, found that it is probably the meaning of the event for the person that is important in establishing the level of tension and subsequent depression. Internal stress results from our perception of a situation. If something is perceived as threatening we activate our fight/flight response. It is often fear that frightens us. We may cope well with real situations but live in fear of what is imagined or dreaded. We most often feel frightened or stressed when we feel helpless. If we feel unable to respond to the perceived threat, we feel vulnerable and undefended. We may look outside ourselves for protection or guidance, and our expectation of others to look after us may be unrealistically high.

Personality too affects our ability to adapt to and reduce stress. Cardiologists Friedman and Rosenman (1974), in the course of their research into cardiovascular disease, found those whom they described as having Type A personalities to be at greater risk of heart disease. These people were very competitive,striving, easily angered and quick in movement. When they learned to relax more they became no more at risk than matched controls.

Since we cannot entirely avoid stress or change our personalities easily we need to be able to recognise when the stress is becoming damaging, learn to activate our coping skills, and how to reduce the effects.

Stress in pregnancy

Pregnancy may be the time of greatest change in a woman's life. A first pregnancy is a journey into the unknown, when every map seems to show a different route. The journey is also taken carrying all our history and experience and the feelings and expectations of others. It represents change not just in income and expenditure, home and social life, but change in self-image from woman to mother, man to father. It brings with it a loss of our old self and life with uncertain gains; a testing of our skills and maturity and the strength of our relationships. Such enormous changes may make us feel vulnerable and we need time and support to adapt to them. If there are other pressures in our lives this adaptation can be complicated, delayed or extremely difficult.

A woman in her second and subsequent pregnancies also faces changes; how to assimilate another child into the pattern of life, how to help her other children to adjust,as well as financial and social implications.

Pregnancy also causes physical stress.Because these are such common experiences, nausea, vomiting, fatigue and sleeplessness may be marginalised by both the woman and health professionals. She may feel that it is wrong to complain about these things, that they are the lot of the pregnant woman,but for her they may be distressing and disabling. They may be taken as a positive sign of pregnancy and almost welcomed, but they may be resented and feared, affecting her feelings about the infant who is felt to be causing the discomfort.

Signs of stress, depression and anxiety are commonly found in normal populations of women attending antenatal clinics. One study in south London showed 35% of women attending for the first time had high negative scores for depression on the General Health Questionnaire (Sharpe, 1988). Other studies have found high levels of worry, mood lability and insomnia (Raphael-Leff, 1991). Some of these are socio-economic in origin and not easily amenable to change, but many relate to the pregnancy itself. There are the doubts expressed about motherhood, the unanswerable question of 'what will it be like' as well as the very understandable fears of women who have experienced previous problem pregnancies or for whom this pregnancy is unwanted or untimely. There are also particular anxieties that arise at different times throughout the pregnancy.

Conception

Now that for many women conception and pregnancy is an option, there may be stress around making that choice and why we make it. The reasons for choosing to have a child at all or at that time may well affect her feelings about being pregnant, and there may be many pressures on a woman to become pregnant and to choose to continue the pregnancy. These might be her own anxieties about 'the biological clock', or pressure from others to fulfil some need of their own. She may find it difficult to tell anyone about whether she chose to be pregnant and assumptions may be made that she is pleased, when her feelings are ambiguous or confused. It can then be difficult to admit to feelings of ambiguity or uncertainty. This may be true of the first or subsequent pregnancies. The woman who is pregnant through aided conception may also have issues about whether or whom to tell. What motherhood means to that woman may be very relevant to how she feels about the changes in her body and her self-image.

Joanne was a 35 year old single woman in a senior management post in industry. She became pregnant by her married lover when not using contraception. The response of her partner was to assume that she would seek abortion immediately. When she said that she wanted time to consider her options, he withdrew and never made further contact. She was distressed to find that some friends also assumed that she would not continue the pregnancy. Her elderly widowed mother, whilst apparently offering support, rehearsed all the difficulties of single parenthood and reflected on her own difficulties postnatally. Joanne was left feeling that her choice to continue the pregnancy was selfish and unthinking. She began to feel depressed and unwell, concentration at work was difficult and she became uninterested in food although nausea was a minor problem. She felt she had to be positive about the pregnancy when talking to midwives and doctors as so many people had been so negative, and a junior doctor had expressed some surprise at her wanting to start a family 'in her circumstances'. She also feared that this negativity might in some way harm the baby. It was only when she could admit her own ambivalence about coping with single motherhood, and her anger at the response of her partner and some of her friends, that she could look at the reality of her situation and begin to feel more in control of making the changes that were needed. When the baby was delivered early although well, she again felt that she may have been in some way responsible because she had been uncertain about whether or not she wanted her. Her doubts about her ability to mother affected her feelings of capability in handling her daughter.

First trimester This is the phase of 'becoming pregnant'. The woman's mood may depend on how she feels about being pregnant. She may spend some days totally involved with the pregnancy and her hopes and fears, and others may be almost unaware of her state. Her response to the physical discomforts of early pregnancy may also be affected by her reaction to being pregnant. If she has experienced previous difficulties in pregnancy or the loss of a baby through miscarriage or stillbirth, these early weeks can be fraught with danger and she may be unwilling to even talk about the pregnancy until she is certain it will continue. Those women afraid of pregnancy or of its implications for their future may even deny the pregnancy to themselves and apparently live their lives as normal.

Early pregnancy may also see the resurfacing of painful past conflicts or experiences. The vulnerability and the enforced changed self-image of pregnancy may arouse many infantile responses that seemed well hidden. The woman's own relationship with her mother, her own childhood anger and frustration may surface in a way that feels overwhelming.

Ellen approached her GP asking for a termination of pregnancy at 12 weeks. She was feeling extremely unwell with constant sickness and abdominal pain. She had not been able to work as a secretary for more than occasional days since 2 weeks into the pregnancy. The illness and disability was the only reason she gave her doctor for seeking termination, and she refused to consider remedies the GP suggested. The GP was uncertain about this and referred Ellen to the counsellor. In the first session, the counsellor encouraged Ellen to discuss the whole situation of the pregnancy including her partner's reaction and the effect it might have on her whole life and the plans she had made. Ellen denied any anxieties about the future, insisting that it was only the sickness that had made her decide to seek termination. She did however agree to another counselling session later that week. The counsellor was aware of the need to explore the situation quickly given the time constraints. The fact that Ellen had readily agreed to another session suggested that she did want to talk about her situation. In the second session the counsellor addressed this apparent ambivalence, her determination to seek abortion and her willingness to continue counselling. Ellen said that she had recognised the need for counselling after it had been lacking in the past. When the counsellor pressed this Ellen began to talk about a previous termination when she was 17 years old. She had told no one about this and had tried to put it out of her mind. She felt she had been successful in doing this until she became pregnant again. She now believed that the sickness and pain that she was experiencing was retribution for ending the previous pregnancy and that she had no right to become a mother, as she had killed her other child. When she was able to look at the situation she had been in when she made the decision to terminate the first time, she agreed that she could not have coped with a pregnancy in a violent, abusive relationship with no family support. In trying to deny the first pregnancy, she had also denied the awful situation in which she, as a refugee and homeless, had been living.

Second trimester At this stage the woman becomes more aware of the baby as an individual, the demands from within become more obvious and her focus becomes more internal. This may be difficult for those around her, particularly a partner, when she seems to be absorbed by the baby, and they may feel excluded. Now the pregnancy also becomes public property and the woman is on the receiving end of comment, advice and warnings. There is often a very strong feeling of nurturing the baby at this stage, particularly as activity increases and so does appetite. If she has doubts about whether she is doing the right thing or if her physical health is poor, she may have great anxiety about protecting and nurturing her baby properly.

Third trimester A woman's coping resources may be very stretched by this stage of pregnancy. She may need help, for the first time since infancy, with simple tasks, may tire easily and feel very dependent. If she has had to stop work she may also feel isolated and withdrawn. It is a transition period from being the woman you know to the mother you are uncertain about becoming.

Depending on how she has felt about being pregnant or during the pregnancy, the woman may anticipate the end of it with relief or regret. She may enjoy the last weeks of not being a parent or be eagerly anticipating beginning. Some women who have doubts about their ability to be a good mother may become preoccupied with this during the last few weeks. Others may have great anxiety about the labour itself. If they have experienced difficulties and anxieties before or if they do not feel confident in the professionals they have met antenatally they may dread the whole experience. They may also be concerned about whether they will behave 'well' during labour or if they will 'let themselves down' by seeming out of control or by upsetting or angering those who attend them.

Postnatal period If all has gone well the immediate postnatal reaction may be one of relief and joy, exhaustion and elation. Later the woman will need to learn or relearn the skills of mothering. If this is accompanied by doubts about her ability to mother or by physical problems this early pleasure may be quickly lost in the need to just get by. Women are not always sure how they should feel postnatally and may suffer a lot of discomfort unnecessarily.

Between a half and two-thirds of women suffer from the 'blues' in the days after delivery. This may be related to the immense hormonal changes that the woman experiences but also to the upheaval of new motherhood. Other new mothers experience a more serious depression that will require professional help. It is estimated that one in ten women suffer from clinical depression after giving birth, but in fewer than a third is it actually recognised or treated.

The father's or partner's reaction to the birth and arrival of the baby may be very important in affecting the mother's state of mind. If they are positive and felt to be supportive, the woman may find the transition to motherhood much eased, but if they have their own issues about coping with parenthood and what they see to be this new role, they may be demanding that the mother help them to adjust. Some men take over the care of the child as a way of establishing their role and women sometimes see this as threatening to their own position and feel marginalised in their caring for the baby.

The resumption of sexual relations may also be stressful for some new mothers. They may feel sore and uncomfortable physically, be afraid of damaging the perineum, or simply not feel very sexual. Some women find great difficulty in combining the role of mother and lover and may need help to think through their own responses. For those women for whom this becomes a continuing problem it may be necessary to seek out professional counselling.

Reducing the stress

Methods available to the midwife Since stress is both a physical and emotional reaction to what has happened or is happening to us, and our interpretation of those events, we can explore various therapies that deal with all aspects of coping with the symptoms of stress. Some can be simply taught and learned and can be practised safely at home alone or with a partner; these include meditation, breathing techniques, relaxation exercises and visualisation. Other therapies need to be taught and supervised by a qualified therapist but are generally available, such as yoga, Alexander technique, t'ai chi and hypnotherapy.

Clear advice, information and giving the time and space to answer questions honestly and in a way the woman feels acceptable may be enough to reduce the anxiety of pregnancy significantly for some women. Simple remedies as can be seen in other chapters of this book may improve much of the physical stress. It may be possible for the midwife herself to offer massage or aromatherapy or reflexology with appropriate training.

Other women will benefit from more formalised counselling to deal with problems that are affecting their feelings about the pregnancy or about motherhood.

Counselling Counselling may be seen as a therapy complementary to conventional medicine in that so much of how we feel about ourselves affects how we feel in our bodies. Counselling as practised by a trained and qualified counsellor is a therapy that aims to help the client to clarify the problems, examine her resources for coping with them and her reasons for not feeling able to cope and to make choices for further action, in a non-judgemental and supportive atmosphere. As well as a relationship that is non-judgemental, warm and genuine, the counsellor offers time and a safe space in which to explore feelings. This may be difficult for health professionals to offer in the course of their normal work. They can, however, learn to offer a 'counselling approach'.

The counselling approach for health professionals There are certain principles of counselling that should be observed. It needs to be more focused and purposeful than just a chat with a friend, and the needs of the client must be uppermost. The counsellor needs to maintain a **therapeutic distance**, that is, a lack of emotional involvement. The therapist has not to be so distant as to fail to engage with the client, but should seek to avoid becoming personally affected. If the client presents problems very similar to those of the counsellor, this too may prevent the therapeutic distance being maintained. If the therapist shares her own feelings or solutions, this may either be seen as the counsellor requiring the client to support her, or her solution being the one that the client should also adopt or risk displeasing the therapist. Avoid **advice giving** in the counselling alliance. This affects the power balance and can make the client dependent and not seek out her own answers. When the advice proves to be wrong this also destroys trust in the therapy. The inexperienced counsellor should also avoid **interpretation**, that is explaining to the client the meaning of what she is thinking or feeling. This technique is used in some models of therapy but it has the risk of appearing judgemental and leaving the client feeling guilty or rejected. The basis of counselling is **listening and attending**, valuing what the client is telling you not just in words but in the unspoken communication. The relationship between client and counsellor is a microcosm of all the relationships the client experiences, and if the counsellor appears neglectful or lacking in concern this may confirm for some clients their lack of value.

The counsellor does not have to put everything right for the client. She may often become distressed in sessions from remembering or talking about painful issues, but this is what the counsellor is working with not trying to stop. It may be important just to acknowledge the importance of it for the client and help her to move towards a way of making it better for herself.

A model that may be helpful for the health professional counsellor is that developed by Egan (1982). His three stage model of the counselling relationship is:

1. Identifying and clarifying the problems.
The client sometimes just feels sad or disturbed or confused. She has not always identified the immediate cause of the feelings, they may have become overwhelming in themselves. To be able to work out the precipitating factors may help to clear some of the confusion. It may also give the client 'permission' to feel upset, to recognise the normalcy of thé response. It also helps to lead on to:

2. Goal-setting – developing and choosing goals.
In this the client chooses the end point of the counselling but also sets her own final goal. It may be just to get through the day without thinking about a loss or problem, or it may be that she would choose to think about something without feeling overwhelmed. It is important for the goal to be set by the client; it may be important for the counsellor to help make the goals realistic.

3. Action – moving towards the chosen goals.
The client may need some guidance in working out ways of achieving her goals. These should start with the most easily attained, so that the client may grow in confidence. Again the client should feel comfortable with the methods chosen, which may be based on a behavioural programme of

setting tasks to achieve or a cognitive approach of trying to think differently about a problem or situation.

These stages can be dealt with separately, although they overlap. It helps to assess the development of the relationship and the work being achieved. It also helps to keep it progressing. The fact that the client is setting the agenda is also important in helping her to recognise that she has the resources to cope and only requires the support and guidance of the counsellor.

Counselling skills can be learned and used by most health professionals, but it is important to recognise that it is a skill and not just something that anyone with the time can do. Clients can be greatly helped but also hurt by careless counselling.

The woman at risk

It is important to recognise that for some women, information, advice and basic supportive counselling may not be enough. It is possible to identify areas of increased risk of abnormal psychological reaction to pregnancy and childbirth: women for whom the pregnancy is unwanted either because of timing, her partner or her own issues; those who have experienced problem pregnancies or losses; and women who are experiencing difficult concurrent life events, are all more likely to be experiencing increased stress and distress. Those also at risk are women already showing some symptoms of stress such as alcohol or drug abuse, eating disorders, agitation or depression. We cannot assume, however that all these women will experience difficulties during pregnancy, or indeed that they will confide their anxieties to their professional carers. We must therefore be aware of the symptoms of extreme stress or psychological disorder, as well as giving women the opportunity both in time and space and in attitudes to express their feelings.

Some symptoms of disorder may be fairly obvious; paranoia, delusions; de-personalisation and de-realisation will usually be observed and referred to the psychiatric services. However there are more subtle changes that carers who are listening to the woman may notice and act on. She may become overly anxious about the pregnancy or concerned about potential or actual harm being done to the baby. Some women are also unusually concerned about the baby being abnormal. All these feelings are normal but become exaggerated in the woman who may be more at risk. Some women's state of mind may lead them to become obsessive, with compulsive cleaning or checking behaviour. Others may deny their pregnancy or their needs in pregnancy. All these women require time and skilled help to deal with their feelings, which may not be available in the antenatal clinic and should be referred for counselling, psychotherapy or psychiatry if they are willing to accept help.

The stress of the carer

A GP described the expectations of the professionals caring for a pregnant woman to be 'to produce a perfect, healthy baby and a mother who is delighted with the outcome'. This is clearly not possible in every case and sometimes outside the ability of the carer to influence. Realistic expectations not just for the woman but also for her carers is important in reducing the feeling of failure that can result from expectations that are not achieved. The carers have their own expectations of themselves and their role; these may not necessarily coincide with those of the woman or her partner and this can lead to tension and lack of communication. Throughout her pregnancy the woman who has become 'medicalised' may expect her carers to interpret for her the condition of her baby and its needs. The lack of her ability to make choices or to obtain information for herself may cause her to feel vulnerable. This vulnerability gives increased power to the carers in an area where 'knowing' gives power of itself. They may not always welcome this but it needs to be recognised if the power balance is to be addressed. We receive information and act on it best when we feel in an adult/adult relationship with our advisers; if we are caught in a parent/child relationship, whilst it may feel supportive at some level, we are handing over responsibility to the carer.

One great value of the carer, the midwife or the wise-woman, may be to provide a calm rational space when the mother feels agitated or uncontrolled. This may feel burdensome to the carer who is not feeling calm or controlled herself, and may produce stress itself.

The helplessness we have discussed, being experienced by the pregnant or labouring woman, may also be experienced by health professionals if they too feel they are unable to control or affect a situation. As carers we need to be aware of our own areas of stress and our coping mechanisms and to feel able to take action or seek help and support when appropriate.

Reducing stress: self-help therapies

Earlier in this chapter it has been shown that relaxation can reduce or eliminate the harmful effects of stress and tension.

Pregnancy is a stressful time for most women both physically and emotionally and most can benefit from techniques that aid physical relaxation. Here we will examine some techniques that are easily learned and can be safely practised by the woman alone or with a partner, with minimal support from a therapist. However midwives may appreciate a review of some of the techniques which could also be taught in parent education classes.

Breathing Breathing is automatic and usually involuntary, however it can be consciously controlled to help with mental and physical reduction of stress.

Our breathing reflects our state of mind and can be controlled to improve our feelings. We sigh when we are sad, we yawn when tired and hyperventilate when anxious or excited. Our tone of voice is also changed; high on an inhaled breath in anxiety, low and exhaled when low or depressed.

When we are calm and relaxed we generally breathe abdominally, that is using the diaphragm to contract and push down, making the abdominal muscles relax and lift. The lungs can then fill easily. This creates the optimum oxygen exchange. Diaphragmatic breathing has been shown to reduce high blood pressure and increase feelings of relaxation. Costal breathing, from the chest alone, is harder work and less efficient in taking in oxygen and expelling carbon dioxide. Costal breathing is part of our fight/flight mechanism. It may be effective in helping us to run a race but will not reduce tension.

Health professionals can help women and their partners to learn effective techniques to control breathing and thus increase a feeling of relaxation.

Abdominal breathing can be taught by the subject lying or sitting comfortably with one hand placed on the chest and the other on the abdomen. The midwife or helper should encourage the woman to inhale and exhale slowly, noticing where the movement comes from under the hands, and then push the abdominal muscles gently on inhalation and be aware of them pushing out again on exhalation, with little movement in the chest. The woman can be helped to be aware of breathing slowly and smoothly and try to reduce the number of breaths to around 12–15 per minute. It helps if someone else can count the number of breaths until it becomes almost automatic. If the mother is breathing too fast and finds it difficult to slow down, it may help to have the midwife or helper close by breathing slowly and evenly with her, until a better rhythm is achieved.

A simple and effective exercise is known as 'sigh out slowly' (SOS); here the breath is controlled after the inward breath and released slowly and gently on a sigh until the breath is all expelled; the inhaled breath is then left to take care of itself.

Relaxation During antenatal classes the midwife can advise women to try relaxing mental tension by involving themselves in an activity which they enjoy; listening to music, going for a walk, reading a book, may all encourage a sense of calm. Women sometimes need 'permission' to actually relax and devote time to themselves. Anything that is found to be relaxing may also be helpful as a distraction during early labour. However if women have become physically tense they may need to deal with this specifically with relaxation exercises. These can all be safely taught and practised. It may be helpful to use background music to aid relaxation and to cut out extraneous noise. There are some cassette tapes of relaxing music available. The advantage of these is that the music itself has no particular emotion attached to it as a famous or popular tune may have.

In pregnancy it is best to lie or sit comfortably in a well-supported position. There should be support under the neck and lumbar spine if semi-recumbent and if lying on the side a pillow under the upper knee will avoid strain on the lumbar-sacral spine. Good support prevents the woman becoming aware of discomfort and needing to keep changing position. She should choose a place that is warm and where interruption is least likely.

The midwife can help the woman to start by diaphragmatic breathing with the eyes closed, and once this is settled the woman can start to think of relaxing each area of the body in turn. It is helpful to have the midwife or a helper guide the subject around the body. She may begin with the right foot and concentrate on making it feel relaxed whilst still breathing steadily. Then move on to the rest of the leg and then the left foot and leg. Progress to the arms and then the spine. When the back muscles are relaxed try the head and neck, making sure that the teeth are not clenched and the eyes not screwed up. Stay as relaxed as possible and concentrate on breathing. To end the relaxation begin by moving the arms and legs slowly and then stretch and yawn. Sit up gently and stand for a few moments before moving around.

Edmund Jacobson (1938) developed the system of progressive tension and relaxation. With this method muscles are first tightened, held for a count of five and then relaxed. Again this is used progressively through the body. This helps the awareness of relaxation, but some people find it difficult to maintain regular breathing and start to hold their breath; they should be reminded of the SOS technique.

Meditation The technique of meditation is easily learned but does require considerable practice and repetition to become effective. It can however be both suggested and taught by the midwife, offering several possible techniques for the woman to find the one that suits her best.

Meditation in one form or another has existed in almost every culture and religion and is still valued as a method of developing self-awareness and potential, as well as offering a way of finding a calm centre in life. At a physical level it has the effect of reducing the respiratory rate, cardiac output and the activity of the sweat glands, all of which improve the experience of tension and anxiety (Hewitt, 1978). Those who are able to meditate regularly report a great feeling of relaxation and peace.

There are several ways of meditating and it may be necessary for the individual to try them all to discover the most effective for themselves. It is important, particularly at first, to be in a quiet, comfortable place, undisturbed. The three methods of meditation examined here are breathing, mantra and object focus, and may be used as a guide by the midwife.

Breathing Begin by becoming as relaxed as possible and take slow deep breaths. Start to become aware of the breathing itself, how the air feels in the nostrils and the sensation of the air filling the lungs. The feelings may change as the focus becomes more intense. If other thoughts begin to intrude, try to return to the sensation of the breathing.

Mantra This is the repetition of a word or phrase. It may be the name of a god or any sound that has no negative attachment chosen by the meditator or teacher. Buddhists use the word 'om', which means, all that is, past, present and future. The sound is repeated over and over closing out thoughts of anything else. It may be accompanied by holding an object, as with rosary beads, to aid concentration. At a simpler level the technique sometimes employed in labour, of singing or tapping out a simple song repetitively was based on this concept.

Object focus Here the image of a place or an object becomes the focus of concentration. The meditator chooses an image that feels positive and allows the mind to focus on this and explore all its possibilities. This can be helped by another person guiding the focus once the subject has become relaxed. A beach for example may be chosen and the meditator will start to explore mentally the feelings, smells and sounds associated with it. It is safest to ask the client to select their own scenario, to avoid associated fears or phobias, such as water or heights. About one-tenth of adults are unable to hold a mental picture and this method will be unsuitable. They may be able to use an actual object on which to focus, and maintain the relaxed concentration in this way.

To become practised and effective any meditation method needs to be repeated about twice a day for 10–15 minutes, until the subject can easily become relaxed and focus concentration. The benefits for stress reduction and peace of mind can be profound.

Visualisation This is exemplified by the phrase 'every day in every way, I'm getting better and better' (Emile Coué). It aims to encourage positive images about physical and mental activities and attitudes. The mind and body are so closely connected that our thoughts can effect our physical responses. Close your eyes and think of a lemon. Imagine you are holding it in your hand, smell it, squeeze it – now bite into it and suck – your mouth fills with saliva, no lemon is required. Visualisation harnesses this response to help deal with making actual events more positive.

Always begin by finding a comfortable undisturbed position and begin to breathe slowly and steadily, with the eyes closed. Try to picture a situation that the subject wants to explore. Some women are able to visualise their baby growing in the uterus, how it is looking and moving. For pregnant women, anxious about labour, visualising the birth of the baby with guidance from someone experienced, may help to encourage positive images. They can concentrate on feeling relaxed and imagining the baby sliding out through the birth canal gently and smoothly. Sheila Kitzinger advocated imagining the vulva in labour as a flower bud opening up.

It is sometimes helpful to begin with a simple sentence such as 'my body is good' and develop an image of the good body. This can then progress to 'my body is good and healthy'. It is important to keep the thinking in the present and keep it positive.In labour the thought 'I can do it, I will do it', may be most positive.

Breathing as a means of relaxation, meditation and visualisation can be learned and practised alone. Other techniques need specific training and supervision, such as yoga, autogenic training, Alexander technique and hypnotherapy.

Contra indications Although relaxation exercises are usually helpful and harmless, in certain circumstances they may be contraindicated or the midwife should be particularly aware of possible difficulties.

Those exercises requiring progressive tensing and relaxing of muscle groups may be unsuitable for anyone who should avoid raising their blood pressure, as the tensing phase can have this effect. It may be possible to do the exercises but with a short tensing phase. Depressed women may be better advised to choose action rather than physical relaxation. Palmer (1992) suggests they may be better using a mantra technique to distract from negative thoughts.

Midwives should also be aware that techniques involving deep breathing and breath holding can induce anxiety or panic attacks in women suffering from anxiety disorders.

Those women with extreme stress and anxiety or serious problems in their everyday life may find it very difficult to achieve any meditative state alone and may need guidance or a partner supporting and going through the exercise with them, or seek out one of the methods that involve a therapist being present. It is also important for women to recognise that although they may have done all they can to visualise a perfect birth, things can still go wrong and they must not feel that they have failed to visualise it properly and therefore have some responsibility for not helping their baby sufficiently.

Reducing stress: supervised therapies

It is not within the scope of this book to offer detailed information about the therapies that require formal training and supervision, but only to indicate their value to some clients, and where they may be usefully offered or practised by the midwife.

Autogenic training Developed by Schultz and popularised by Luthe (1963) and well described by Kermani (1992), this technique helps to bring about relaxation, encouraging the subject to think in a certain way. Particular phrases are learned that, with repetition, result in physical changes. For example, in a relaxed and comfortable position the subject begins to repeat 'my right arm is feeling heavy', 'my left arm is feeling heavy', 'both arms are feeling heavy'. This may need to be repeated for some time until there is a sensation of heaviness experienced. This in itself may be quite relaxing. The subject then moves on to use the same method for other parts of the body, for example the legs and the head. Sensations are added later such as feeling warm. Learning is progressive and should be supervised by a trained practitioner to bring about effective change, although it is practised alone.

Yoga Yoga, with its emphasis on both physical and mental benefits, is very suitable for pregnant women. The physical postures can be adapted and will encourage strength and suppleness (see Figs 1–4). The gentle stretching exercises maintain free movement and help posture. They can also relieve the backache suffered during pregnancy and after delivery, and other symptoms such as constipation (see Chapter 2). The breath control and meditation that accompanies the exercises, help to lessen the tension and increase a feeling of being in control.

Fig. 1. Yoga positions to facilitate breathing, encourage muscle relaxation and improve pelvic circulation.

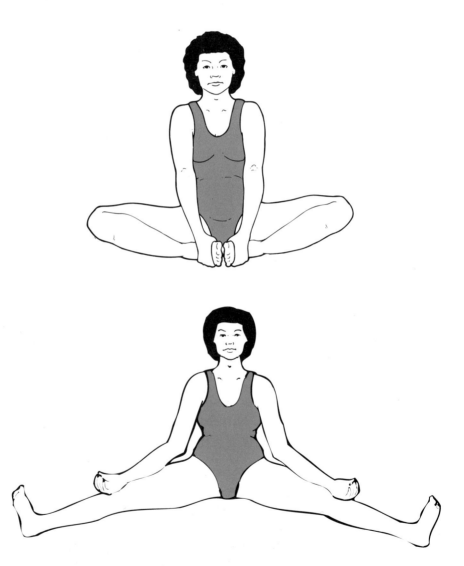

Fig. 2. Yoga position to relax chest and shoulders, improve breathing, tone pectoral muscles and may relieve heartburn.

Fig. 3. The knee–chest position, practised daily from 34 weeks' gestation, may encourage cephalo-version in a mother who has a breech presentation. The increased blood supply to the brain may also counteract tiredness.

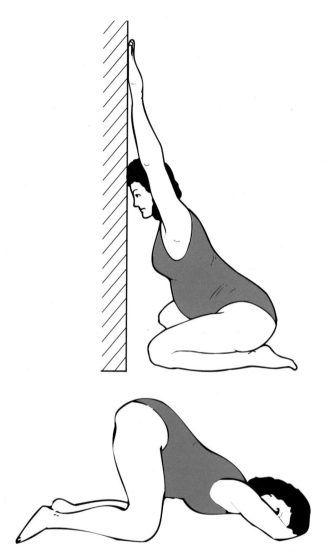

Yoga classes especially for pregnant women are available in some areas. Exercises should be taught and supervised by a qualified yoga teacher, and some in non-specific classes are willing to include pregnant women.

Alexander technique Developed by a nineteenth century actor, the Alexander technique is designed to correct bad postural habits, which may cause aches and pains, headache and tiredness. Some Alexander technique practitioners use it specifically to help in pregnancy when bad posture can cause discomfort, and also in childbirth to ease the pain and help recovery. It does require a trained therapist to help the woman learn better postural habits.

The full training as a therapist takes 3 years but it could be useful for a mid-wife to learn or at least to be able to refer women appropriately to a teacher.

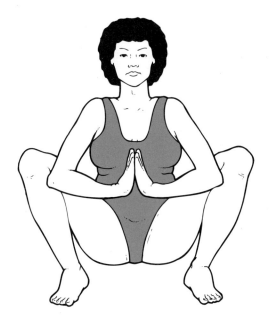

Fig. 4. The squatting position aids flexibility in preparation for labour. Also relieves pressure on abdominal wall, and may counteract leg cramps and ease the discomfort of varicose veins.

Hypnotherapy Hypnotherapy can be helpful in dealing with anxieties and emotional problems, as well as a way of tackling difficulties such as stopping smoking and tranquilliser abuse. It may also be used to deal with the pain and fear of labour (Guthrie *et al.*, 1984).

It is a way of entering an altered state of mind somewhere between sleeping and waking. This level of consciousness allows the unlocking of some control centre in the mind, that can then be affected by the guidance of the therapist. Stage hypnotism has given some people a fear that they may be made to do something that will make them seem foolish or out of control, however hypnotherapists are concerned to help the client achieve their goals, and believe that the client not the therapist makes the decisions about what those goals should be. For some women the fear of being out of control may be strong and they may feel that this therapy is not suitable for them, but they should discuss this with a hypnotherapist.

There are now a number of medically trained hypnotherapists who offer help to women with infertility problems as well as pregnant and labouring women. It is a therapy in which, when the client feels comfortable with the therapist, the benefits of increased relaxation and the control and management of pain can be very significant.

T'ai chi ch'uan T'ai chi ch'uan (or taijiquan) was originally developed in China as a martial art but has become popular in the West as a way of improving physical health, and improving the physiological processes of all the body's systems. It improves stamina, increases flexibility and promotes general good health.

Learning the art and science of t'ai chi is a lifelong process by which the practitioner practises consistently, reflects and learns from the practice. It involves completing a number of set moves in a routine. Each routine comprises a set of postures and movements which are developed with an understanding of the anatomy and physiology of the human body, combined with the principles of physics, such as centrifugal force, gravity, inertia, equilibrium of forces and circumferential action. These are combined into a set of harmonious movements which affect all parts of the body including the internal organs. The synchronisation of slow movements, concentration and breathing facilitates the flow of the 'chi' within the body and between the organs via the network of 12 meridians.

There are other therapies that may be helpful in reducing stress; biofeedback, a way of monitoring our physical processes, enables us to become aware of them and thus make changes by applying our mind; spiritual healing is when the healer affects the energy field of the client, to make it more positive; art therapy and movement therapy may also be useful ways of getting in touch with feelings and expressing them, to help in the release of tension and anxiety.

Environmental methods of stress reduction

Midwives working within maternity units may be able to influence the environment in order to help reduce the stress of mothers, their partners and staff.

Colour therapy is a relatively new idea in which colour is used to affect the mood of those in the environment. Blue and peach are regarded as particularly calming, and could be used as the dominant wall colouring or for coloured light bulbs. Emerald green is associated with intellect and bright yellow with logic, so that operating theatres or offices could be decorated with a predominance of these colours.

Aromas could be varied throughout the department, using refreshing but calming essential oils such as mandarin in a vaporiser through the day; sleep-enhancing camomile on postnatal wards in the evening and rosemary and basil to stimulate and aid concentration in theatres. Care should be taken to use electrical vaporisers, which although more expensive are much safer then those based on candles.

A homely atmosphere could be planned when decorating the delivery suite, with beds more like conventional ones, rocking chairs, and equipment stored behind cupboards until needed. This has long been advocated as a way of helping women to feel that a hospital birth can be as satisfying as a home birth, and it may help to reduce a mother's fear.

Staff attitudes are probably the most important means of inducing or reducing stress. A positive, friendly manner, offering women as much choice about their pregnancy and labour as possible, will result in better cooperation between staff and mothers and a feeling that they are part of a team. Many innovative units have introduced team midwifery, the named midwife concept and aspects of choice for mothers. It would appear however from the investigations that resulted in the 'Changing childbirth' document (1993) that there is still a long way to go in many areas.

Many of the therapies discussed here are available through health professionals or therapists may be contacted through national organisations.

Conclusion   The causes of stress, whilst having common elements, will be unique to the individual. Responses to stress are equally dependent on the circumstances, personality and experience of the individual. Methods of stress reduction must be appropriate, if they are to be effective. We need to acknowledge the stress, mobilise our coping mechanisms or learn to develop new ones. We can never eliminate fear, anger and anxiety from our life but we can hope to learn how to minimise the damage they do.

Training

Alexander technique
Professional Association for Alexander Teachers
14 Kingsland, Jesmond, Newcastle upon Tyne, Tyne and Wear NE2 3AL, UK

Autogenic training
Centre for Autogenic Training, 101, Harley St, London W1N 1DF, UK

Counselling
British Association for Counselling, 1 Regent Place, Rugby CV21 2PJ, UK

Healing
Guild of Spiritual Healers
36 Newmarket, Otley, Yorkshire LS21 3AE, UK

Hypnotherapy
The National Association of Hypnotists and Psychotherapists
145 Coleridge Rd, Cambridge CB1 3PN, UK

T'ai chi ch'uan
School of T'ai Chi Ch'uan – Centre for Healing
5 Tavistock Place, London WC1H 9SS, UK

Yoga
British School of Yoga
46 Hagley Rd, Stourbridge, West Midlands DY8 1QD, UK

British Wheel of Yoga
1 Hamilton Place, Boston Road, Sleaford, Lincolnshire NG34 7ES, UK

Further details of training in various branches of complementary therapies can be found in:

Maher G. *Start a Career in Complementary Medicine* Tackmart Publishing (1992)

References

Brown G.W. and Harris T. (1978) *Social Origins of Depression*. Tavistock.

Egan G. (1983) *The Skilled Helper*. Brooks/Cole, CA.

Friedman M. and Rosenman R. (1974) *Type A Behaviour and Your Heart*. Knopf.

Guthrie K. (1984) Maternal hypnosis induced by husbands during childbirth. *Journal of Obstetrics and Gynaecology*, **4(5)**, 93–95.

Hedegaard M., Henrikson T.B., Sabroe S. and Secher N.J. (1993) Psychological distress in pregnancy and preterm delivery. *British Medical Journal*, **307**, 234–239

Hewitt J. (1978) *Meditation*. Hodder & Stoughton.

Holmes T.A. and Rahe R.H. (1967) The Social Readjustment Rating Scale. *Journal of Psychosomatic Research*, **11**, 213–218.

Jabaaij L. (1993). Influence of perceived psychological stress and distress on antibody response to low dose rDNA hepatitis B vaccine. *Journal of Psychosomatic Research*, **37**, 361–369.

Jacobson E. (1938) *Progressive Relaxation*. University of Chicago Press, Chicago, IL.

Kermani E. (1992) *Autogenic Training*. Thorsons.

Lazarus R. (1966) *Psychological Stress and the Coping Process*. McGraw-Hill, New York.

Luthe W. (1993) Autogenic training; method, research and application in medicine. *American Journal of Psychotherapy*, **17**, 174–195.

Palmer S. (1992) Guidelines and contra-indications for teaching relaxation as a stress management technique. *Journal of the Institute of Health Education*, **30**, 25–30.

Patel C. (1987) *Fighting Heart Disease*. Dorling Kindersley.

Raphael-Leff J. (1991) *Psychological Processes of Childbearing*. Chapman & Hall.

Seyle H. (1956) *The Stress of Life*. McGraw-Hill, New York.

Sharma J.B., Smith R.J. and Wilkin D.J.W. (1993) Induction of labour at term. *British Medical Journal*, **306**, 1413.

Sharpe D. (1988) Validation of the Thirty Item General Health Questionnaire in early pregnancy. *Psychological Medicine*, **18**, 503.

Further reading

Bailey R. and Clarke M. (1989) *Stress and Coping in Nursing*. Chapman and Hall.

Berg V. (1981) *Yoga in Pregnancy*. Watkins.

Brennan R. (1991) *The Alexander Technique*. Element.

Dalton K. (1989) *Depression after Childbirth*, Oxford University Press, Oxford.

Department of Health (1993) *Report of the Expert Maternity Group*, HMSO.

Heardman H. (1982) *Relaxation and Exercise for Childbirth*. Churchill Livingstone.

Karle H. (1992) *Introductory Guide to Hypnotherapy*. Thorsons.

Liu D. (1986) *T'ai Chi Ch'uan and Meditation*. Penguin, London.

Machover I., Drake A. and Drake J. (1993) *The Alexander Technique Birth Book*. Robinson.

Madders J. *Stress and Relaxation*. Optima,

Mosse K. (1993) *Becoming a Mother*. Virago,

Oakley A. (1991) *Social Support and Motherhood*. Blackwell.

Sutcliffe J. (1991) *The Complete Book of Relaxation Techniques*. Headline.

Watts and Cooper (1992) *Relax – dealing with Stress*. BBC, London.

Weller S. (1991) *Easy Pregnancy with Yoga*. Thorsons.

Which Consumer Guides (1992) *Understanding Stress*. Hodder & Stoughton, Penguin.

Dianne Garland

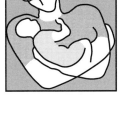

Chapter 6

The Uses of Hydrotherapy in Today's Midwifery Practice

Continuing advances in medical technology have totally altered both the nature and pattern of care offered to pregnant women today. The tide of social change in care provision will, in the next few years, move the power base from professionals to clients, particularly as a result of the most recent report on 'Changing childbirth' (Department of Health, 1993).

For many years pioneers of alternative maternity care have been striving to develop a gentler approach to labour and delivery. Frederick LeBoyer's 'Birth Without Violence' (1975) attempted to affect the way in which obstetrics was practised in Western countries. The technological age was advancing and LeBoyer's work was a starting point on the long road to change. Although the book was written nearly 20 years ago his words still have as much relevance today as they did then:

'We were wondering about how best to prepare the child . . . now we can see it's not the child that needs to be prepared. It is ourselves. It is our eyes that need to open, our blindness that has to stop. If we used just a little intelligence how simple things could be.'

Another French pioneer brought to the forefront the continuing medicalisation of childbirth and the need to relearn our cultural and social skills that are linked to childbirth. In 'Entering the World' (1984) Michel Odent supported the theory that in labour a known caregiver and an environment conducive to regaining and retaining a sense of dignity and identity would do much to enhance a woman's labour and delivery.

Midwives wishing to implement the use of water for labour and delivery are likely already to respect these values and attitudes for the care of women. For those who seek a deeper spiritual philosophy for the use of water the writings of Michel Odent (1990) and S. Ray (1986) can lead them into a fascinating exploration of birth.

Water does seem to possess powers of recuperation, for example visitors to Niagara or Victoria Falls cannot fail but to be inspired by the strength and beauty of the cascading water. For many people their holidays are spent by water, by the sea or mountain lakes, or even skiing, on frozen water. At the end of a long tiring day many people will seek seclusion and relaxation by taking a bath. Is it so surprising therefore that many women find water for labour so inviting?

Water births around the world

Reliable data regarding the number of centres undertaking water births around the world are difficult to obtain. It is however evident that approximately 30 countries have centres where water births may be conducted (Fig. 1). In many of these countries the service has been designed and often spearheaded by consumers.

In the United States the use of hydrotherapy is sporadic with the most renowned unit being Michael Rosenthal's in Upland, California. It seems that almost all centres around the world have two things in common: a trained birth attendant and a readily available supply of clean fresh water. In post-Communist countries and the Indian subcontinent water is an infinitely cheaper means of pain relief than pharmaceutical analgesia. Even in Britain costs are considerably less, with pethidine costing approximately 14 pence per ampoule, bupivicaine £1.27 per ampoule and water costing about 85 pence per tub. These would be approximate costs for an established water birth service and obviously do not take account of the expense of setting up the service.

Aquanatal swimming

It is not a prerequisite that women considering the use of water during labour should attend prenatal or 'aquanatal' classes. However these sessions at which exercises to music are practised in the pool may help women to determine whether or not they like the floatation sensation, as this environment may require a period of adjustment (Garland and Ford, 1989).

Exercising in water can be a pleasurable experience and a social event for pregnant and newly delivered women. It is a way of empowering them to regain control over their bodies and, as Oudshoorn (1990) writes, is designed to maintain general condition, muscle function and improve circulation. The mothers are encouraged to practise relaxation techniques, and controlled breathing and floating in water facilitates this. The combination of

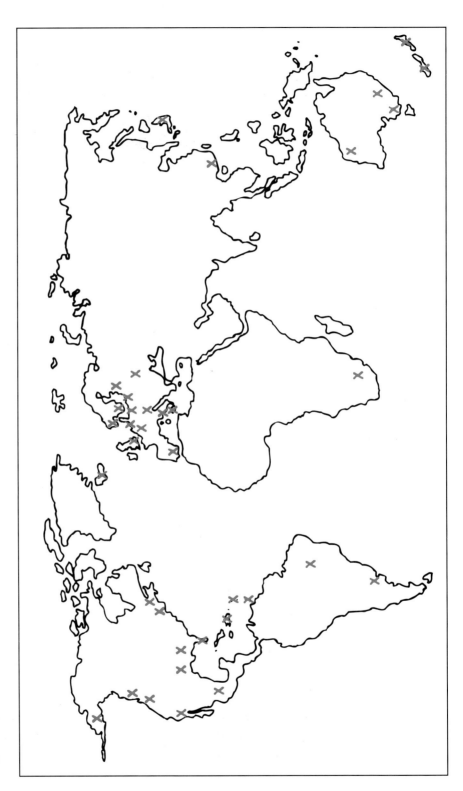

Fig. 1. Water births worldwide.

Fig. 6.2. Aquanatal exercises.

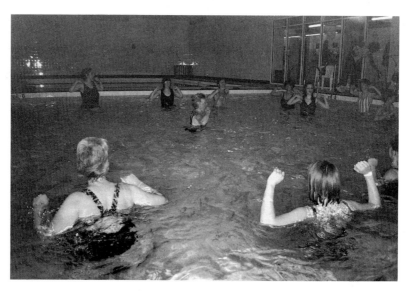

practising exercises and the water tension means it is especially effective in relieving aches and pains such as backache or the throbbing of varicosities.

In addition for some women, negative perceptions of self-image related to their enlarging shape may be overcome while in the water. Mothers-to-be gain a freedom of movement they may not have felt for some time, particularly towards term. In a non-threatening environment the 'hidden' body is free to move and relax without the full force of gravity.

Aquanatal classes may replace or augment conventional parent education classes, but in either case, being with other women with similar interests in the use of water for labour and delivery can facilitate a sharing of fears and aspirations about the situation. Where there are mothers present who have delivered previously in water this can also be helpful (Figure 6.2).

Postnatally it may be possible to continue the classes, or perhaps to run them concurrently for ante- and postnatal mothers. This may be a way of encouraging the women to continue postnatal exercises and so facilitate the shedding of extra weight and adipose tissue acquired during pregnancy (Baddeley, 1993).

Before commencing aquanatal classes midwives should consider the following issues:

- Pool suitability – graduated pools with a shallow and a deep end are preferable to enable non-swimmers to join in and to provide variation in water pressure for different exercises.
- The temperature of the water should be between 29°C and 30°C as this reduces tension and relaxes muscles. If the water is too hot the women may feel dizzy and faint or if it is too cool they may be susceptible to muscle cramps.

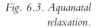

Fig. 6.3. Aquanatal relaxation.

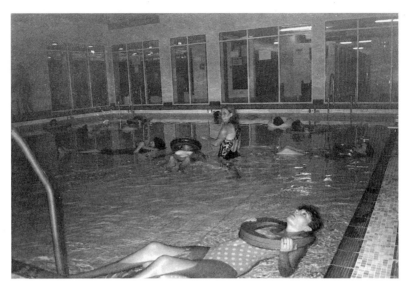

- Arranging for exclusive use of the pool during classes facilitates a more relaxed environment and ensures privacy. Clarification should be sought as to the cost of hiring the pool and whether this will include the entrance fee for the mothers or if they will need to pay for themselves.
- There should be at least two midwives present for the classes, one to demonstrate the various exercises at the side of the pool and one to be in the pool assisting the women. The midwives should hold either Amateur Swimming Association or specific 'Aquafit' certificates as well as a life saving certificate if there is no other life saver at the pool.
- Midwives must refer to the relevant professional documents such as the UKCC's 'Code of Practice' (1994) and the 'Scope of Practice' (1992).
- It may be necessary to review personal indemnity insurance cover as midwives may be conducting these classes outside their normal work parameters, perhaps because of their own interest, and would be considered to be working independently.
- Carrying out a local survey of mothers' wishes will determine the demand for aquanatal classes; various means of advertising the classes should be utilised.
- Careful screening of mothers wishing to commence the classes to ensure that anyone with a medical or obstetric problem obtains the approval of the obstetrician to do so.
- It may be necessary to arrange creche facilities.
- A portable, battery-operated cassette player should be available for music.
- There should also be a variety of floatation aids available such as rubber rings and inflatable neck supports.
- Comfortable swimwear for mothers and midwives.

**The use of water
for labour and
delivery**

The demand to set up a waterbirth service has often come from the consumers and midwives should of course act as the mothers' advocate, but it is easy to become so enthusiastic that the importance of adequate planning can be overlooked. The Midwife's 'Code of Practice' states that 'some developments in midwifery care can become an integral part of the role of the midwife' (UKCC, 1994). The Code emphasises that each midwife should acquire competence in new skills through adequate preparation. Midwives spend a great deal of time, following qualification, in developing advanced skills and knowledge, and this section addresses this in relation to water labour and birth.

In some maternity units delivering babies under water is seen as an extension of normal midwifery practice with practitioners regaining 'lost' skills such as physiological third stage management. Midwives are expected to seek out appropriate opportunities for gaining experience. Managers and supervisors in other centres have decided that this aspect of care should be viewed as part of the scope of practice (UKCC, 1992), and specify a requirement for midwives to attend lectures and conduct a certain number of water births under supervision. Each unit must develop the most appropriate way of training its staff, in conjunction with the midwives themselves, supervisors of midwives and medical colleagues. Many excellent study days and opportunities for networking are now available and midwives should scan the professional journals for relevant advertisements.

Midwives are also advised to communicate with those from other units where water births are an established part of the maternity service, in order to share achievements and examine potential or actual problems. Skill sharing is of paramount importance, locally, regionally and nationally, and because of the sporadic availability of water births so far, issues common to several units can be identified.

Similarly there needs to be good teamwork between the midwives and medical staff right from the start of the project. Some units have been able to devise protocols for water births jointly with midwives, obstetricians, paediatricians and microbiologists in the planning groups. Increasingly units offering water births are developing policies to cover as many issues as possible. Part of a study being undertaken at the National Perinatal Epidemiology Unit in Oxford, due for completion in 1995, involves collection of waterbirth protocol details from units around the country.

Reviewing currently available literature, both on maternal and neonatal physiology and on recent research trials, can enable revision of basic theory relevant to the practice of water birth and an exploration of statistical evidence on a variety of issues (Celfalo *et al.*, 1978; Brown, 1982; Burke, 1985; Gradert *et al.*, 1987; Dane, 1987; Milner, 1988; Spiby, 1993).

Simulation exercises are a useful means of discussing the management of practicalities such as assisting the mother in and out of the tub, or dealing with obstetric and paediatric problems in the bathroom, such as haemorrhage or shoulder dystocia. Positioning of necessary equipment in the bathroom, and health and safety issues such as care of the midwife's back can also be considered. If possible observation of a colleague conducting a delivery with the mother in water is a valuable exercise. Reflecting on the episode may raise additional issues.

Suitable facilities for conducting water labours and deliveries Some units who have attempted to set up facilities for water births have experienced major difficulties with finding suitable tubs and adequate space in which to put them. Several types of tubs are now available, both portable and those which can be installed into the plumbing system in the unit. The tubs may differ in shape and size but have similarities regarding depth, temperature maintenance and cleansing. Some units have specified the ease and speed of water drainage as being important in the event of maternal problems, but in reality it is more practical to ask the mother to leave the water rather than attempt to drain the tub.

When selecting a tub suitable for the labour ward, the following factors need to be considered:

- The weight of the pool when full of water, remembering that one gallon weighs ten pounds, and water birth tubs hold 100 gallons. It may be necessary to involve the engineers and building and works departments in hospitals. The weight of the tub has posed a particular problem for women who have hired pools for use at a home birth, only to find that the floor was not substantial enough to support the tub.
- The depth and width of the tub to allow the midwife easy access to the mother whilst providing space for the mother to move around in the water.
- Systems for filling and draining the pool and for filtering out debris such as meconium, blood and membranes. It may be necessary to check with the hospital engineers, especially for tubs which drain into the main hospital drainage system. A plastic, easily sterilised sieve or small fishing net could be used to remove some debris.
- Thermostatic control in order to maintain the water temperature (portable tubs usually have a thermo-cover included to maintain the heat until full). A thermometer such as those used in aquaria will help the midwife to check the temperature of the water once the mother is in the tub.
- A policy for cleaning the tub after use to avoid the risks of cross-infection. Disposable liners may be available for certain types of tub.
- Local availability of the tubs with an opportunity to observe the ease and speed of preparing them prior to hire or purchase.
- Cost – and the source of funding. In some units midwives have entered enthusiastically into innovative methods of fundraising.

If the midwife is caring for a mother anticipating a water birth in the home it is normally the responsibility of the family to sort out the practical

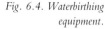

Fig. 6.4. Waterbirthing equipment.

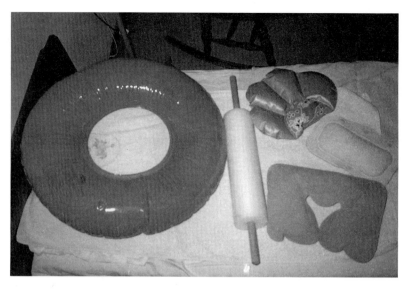

details and arrange for hire and arrival of the tub. This would include checking structural support of floors, covering, with child safety covers, of electrical sockets in the relevant room to avoid the effects of humidity, and insurance of the building and the contents in case of disasters.

An additional source of water may also be required in the home as most domestic water tanks hold between 40 and 70 gallons and tubs for delivery hold 100 gallons.

Other useful equipment Although continuous routine fetal monitoring should be unnecessary for women in the bath, a monitor suitable for use in water will be needed for auscultating the fetal heart. A battery-operated mucus extractor may also be required.

Floatation aids to ensure the mother's comfort should be available (Figure 6.4), and a battery-operated cassette player to enable the mother to listen to music will add to her comfort.

Fans to keep the mother and midwife cool can also be useful.

Preparation of mothers who wish to use water for labour and birth
As stated previously, aquanatal exercise is not a vital prerequisite for water labour and birth, but it is important to plan the care and discuss with the parents the relevant mutually agreed 'ground rules' for the event. For example the mother will need to understand that if the midwife requests her to leave the tub it is for a matter of safety. Parents should be offered sufficient information to enable them to make an informed choice about water birth, as with any other aspect of their care. Midwives should recognise that acknowledging their own limitations is not an admission of inadequacy but rather enables parents to understand the parameters of the situation and

engenders a feeling of trust and confidence. This is particularly so in the early days as units work to establish a waterbirth service. Some maternity units offer special waterbirth classes for interested parents to enable them to find out information and to discuss practicalities with midwives and with other parents. Other units see their waterbirth service as a normal part of the care available to all low risk women and incorporate the relevant information into conventional parent education classes.

Criteria for agreeing mothers suitable for water labour and delivery
In conjunction with the obstetric team it is important to identify selection criteria and to adhere to these when introducing the concept of water birth to parents.

Details of the medical and obstetric history should be examined to elicit any existing or potential problems. Towards term the progress of the current pregnancy should be reviewed and decisions made, according to locally agreed criteria, about mothers with complications such as hypertension, haemorrhage or anaemia.

Whilst women within a very wide spectrum of normality are recorded as labouring and delivering in water, there have also been anecdotal accounts of water deliveries of breech presentations, twins, and women who have had a previous Caesarean section. Individual units must identify those criteria for 'normality' which are most appropriate, and may reflect other policies within that unit, for example the care of a woman with a uterine scar.

Policies and guidelines Before introducing a service of water labours and births it is important to draw up protocols. Adverse publicity in 1993 regarding the temperature of the water has resulted in units working together to design universal guidelines.

Maternity units such as Maidstone in Kent have been offering water births for several years and have adapted their protocol in response to suggestions from midwives, mothers and medical staff and after reflection on early experiences. The following points for possible guidelines are based on those currently available at the Maidstone unit.

It is considered that the clinical judgement of the midwife is paramount; if a midwife feels it is necessary to ask a mother to leave a water tub for medical reasons the mother must understand the situation. This is explained at parent education classes and when parents are seen individually about their wishes for a water labour.

The unit's guidelines reflect the criteria of 'normality' as specified by the midwives, obstetricians and paediatricians. It is preferred that there should be no known or envisaged problems in labour and that the gestation of pregnancy should be at least 37 weeks. Mothers requiring induction of labour with either amniotomy or prostin pessaries may use the tubs if there are no other known problems. Labour needs to be established before immersion to

Fig. 6.5. Monitor.

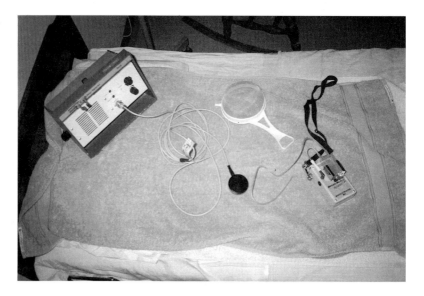

facilitate the enhancement of uterine activity, which does not seem to occur if the woman is in early labour (Lenstrup *et al.*, 1987).

Although women whose diastolic blood pressure is more than 90 mm-g at the onset of labour are generally discouraged from using the tubs, those who have had mild hypertension in pregnancy may use them, as evidence suggests that relaxing in water can reduce blood pressure. Mothers who have had a previous Caesarean section are not offered hydrotherapy as the effects of intrauterine pressure changes as a result of immersion in water have not been evaluated. Once the membranes have ruptures the mother may stay in the tub for up to 24 hours, as is the practice with other women without obstetric complications, although experience has shown that women do not normally need more than 5 hours in the water to complete their labours.

As the water is primarily used as a means of relieving pain in labour (Kroska and Carroll, 1982; Brown, 1982; Dane, 1987; Milner, 1988) the only other form of analgesia offered to mothers in the tubs is inhalational analgesia.

All maternal and fetal observations need to be carried out as agreed, with a monitor suitable for use in water being available (Figure 6.5); a baseline cardiotocograph may be useful in case of problems later in the labour (Gibb, 1992).

In order to keep the mother as comfortable as possible the flotation aids can be used to support her head and neck, and she should be encouraged to drink plenty to avoid dehydration in the warm room. Midwives too should be allowed to drink frequently as the room will naturally be even warmer than the normal labour rooms. These aspects must be discussed before water births are commenced, particularly in units where there is a policy of fluid restriction in labour.

Fig. 6.6. Water birth
equipment.

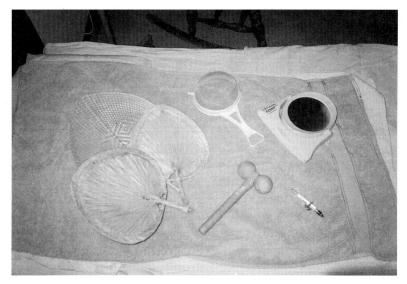

To prevent the risk of infection and to keep the water clear enough to observe any blood or meconium passed from the vagina, a sieve should be used to remove debris. As with other deliveries it is recommended that gloves are worn for any necessary examinations per vaginam. The temperature of the water is maintained between 33°C–40°C in the first stage and at a constant 37–37.5°C in the second stage, during which period it is recorded quarter hourly. It is likely that initiation of respiration in the baby may occur if the temperature is cooler than this in the second stage.

Due to the effects of water on skin elasticity it is probable that minimal control of the fetal presenting part will be required in the second stage and that perineal trauma will be slight. However when suturing is required it may be necesary to delay the procedure as the tissues of the perineum may initially be saturated with water.

As the baby is delivered he should be kept totally under the water to prevent respiration in response to the colder air, but he should be brought to the surface promptly as hypoxia may occur if the placenta begins to separate while the baby is submerged. There is no evidence to suggest a risk of water embolism, so if the mother wishes the cord can be clamped and cut after it has stopped pulsating. However, under no circumstances should the cord be under water when it is clamped and cut.

Most women should be able to expel the placenta spontaneously if the first and second stages have been normal, therefore it should not be necessary to administer an oxytocic drug. Third stage management may vary according to the condition and wishes of the mother, but it is often preferred that either the mother leaves the tub or that the water is drained out. If the mother remains in the water for the third stage blood clots will need to be collected using a sieve and estimated as either less than or more than 500 ml as it is not feasible to record the blood loss any more accurately than this.

In an emergency the mother should be asked to leave the water to provide appropriate treatment.

The Maidstone unit does not have a second midwife present at deliveries in water as it is not normal policy to do so for any normal delivery, unless the midwife requires assistance or is working with a colleague for educational purposes.

Midwives should take account of their own positions when leaning over the tubs. Balaskas and Gordon (1990) suggest that midwives should undertake back strengthening exercises in an attempt to prevent injury, and certainly the health and safety issues should be considered in advance.

The need for research and audit Reports that two babies had died as a result of their mothers delivering in water hit the headlines in late 1993 (*Sunday Times*, 17/10/93 and *Daily Telegraph*) and attention was drawn to the lack of reliable research and audit. Some units are actually auditing their own statistics, and some have been published (Burns and Greenish, 1993; Garland and Jones, 1994). It is noticeable that certain accepted medical practices have been adopted without initial research or later evaluation, yet this is a popular criticism levelled at any complementary therapy or alternative strategy in midwifery or nursing.

The need for reliable audit was highlighted by McGraw (1989):

> Throughout the struggles over [these] innovations in childbirth, proponents have all too often made broad sweeping and unsupported claims about the lasting benefits of these changes. Similarly opponents have frequently predicted dire calamities, also with limited supporting evidence, if such innovations are adopted . . . It is naive to assume that mere anecdotal evidence or assertions that [their] innovation is more natural will lead to its adoption by a medical profession that prides itself on its objectivity and scientific methods.

This statement, written some years ago, appears as relevant today as it did then. Whilst it is true that little pure research exists, much has been written by consumers and professionals. Only through research and audit in units where the service is already offered can water labour and birth be shown to be a safe option for low risk women. Such aspects as outcomes of labour, neonatal Apgar scores, and the rate of complications such as postpartum haemorrhage and maternal or neonatal infections need to identified and evaluated. Subjective data on client expectations and satisfaction would be especially valuable in the light of the 'Changing childbirth report' (Department of Health, 1993). In this report the Expert Committee highlighted the need for research into many aspects of midwifery, stating:

> There is a long history in maternity services of well intentioneed changes which are not backed up with proper research based evidence to support their introduction..This is also true for other techniques and practices such as water birth, homeopathy and aromatherapy . . . where women express

a wish for a particular form of care which has no proven benefits, this fact must be discussed with them openly and fairly.

Water birth has much to offer as a means of relaxation and analgesia in labour, and there may be other, as yet undiscovered, benefits to mothers and babies. It is certainly an additional choice for mothers, allowing them greater freedom and control in the labour and delivery.

Clients and midwives must continue to work together to establish a firm foundation on which to build for the future. Perhaps the research nearing completion at the National Perinatal Epidemiology Unit will enable midwives to evaluate waterbirth practices and plan for the future in the light of their findings. In the mean time midwives must be guided by their professional bodies in relation to accountability, by demand for water birth from the mothers for whom they care, and by the future development of the maternity services in Britain.

Useful addresses

Active Birth Centre
55 Dartmouth Park Rd, London NW5 1SL, UK

Mid-Kent Health Care Trust (study days)
Maidstone Hospital, Hermitage Lane, Maidstone, Kent, UK

National Perinatal Epidemiology Unit
Radcliffe Infirmary, Oxford, UK
(undertaking waterbirths' trial, due 1995)

References

Baddeley S. (1993) Aquanatal advantages. *Modern Midwife*, July/August.

Balaskas J. and Gordon Y. (1990) *Water Birth*. Unwin.

Brown C. (1982) Therapeutic effects of bathing during labour. *Journal of Nurse-Midwifery*, **27(1)**, 13–16.

Burns E. and Greenish K. (1993) Pooling information. *Nursing Times*, **89**, 8.

Daily Telegraph (15/10/93) Health chief alerted after babies die during water births.

Dane S. (1987) Help for mums in labour. *Evening Telegraph* (Peterborough) 9/2/87

Department of Health (1993) *Changing Childbirth*. HMSO, London.

Garland D. and Ford L. (1989) An aqua birth concept. *Midwives Chronicle*, July.

Garland D. and Jones K. (1994) Waterbirth, 'first stage' immersion or non immersion? *British Journal of Midwifery*, **2(3)**.

Gibb D. (1992) *Fetal Monitoring in Practice*. Butterworth Heinemann.

Gradert Y., Hertel C., Lenstrup C., Bach F.W., Christensen N.J. and Roseno H. (1987) Warm tub bath during labor: effects on plasma catecholamine on bendorphin-like immunoreactivity concentrations in the infants at birth. *Acta Obstetricia et Gynaecologica Scandinavica*, **66(8)**, 681–683.

Kroska R. and Carroll M. (1982) Use of water in labor. *Birth*, **9(1)**, 47.

LeBoyer F. (1975) *Birth Without Violence.* Mandarin,

Lenstrup C. *et al.* (1987) Warm tub bath during delivery. *Acta Obstetricia et Gynaecologica Scandinavica*, **66(8)**, 709–712.

McGraw R. (1989) Recent innovation in childbirth. *Journal of Nurse-Midwifery*, **34,** 4.

Milner I. (1988) Water baths for pain relief in labour. *Nursing Times*, **84(1)**, 38–40.

Odent M. (1984) *Entering the World*. Marion Boyers.

Odent M. (1990) *Water and Sexuality*. Arkana.

Oudshoorn C. (1990) Swimming classes for pregnant women. ICM paper.

Ray S. (1985) *Ideal Birth*. Celestial Arts.

Sunday Times (17/10/93) Fears grow over water births as more babies die.

UKCC (1994) *The Midwife's Code of Practice.*

UKCC (1992) *The Scope of Professional Practice.*

Further reading

Brown C. (1982) Therapeutic effects of bathing during labor. *Journal of Nurse-Midwifery*, **27**, 1.

Burke B. (1985) The shock of birth. *Nursing Times*, **161**, 11.

Cefalo R.C. and Hellegers A.E. (1978) Effects of maternal hyperthermia on maternal and fetal cardiovascular and respiratory function. *American Journal of Obstetrics and Gynecology*, **131**, 687–694.

Church L. (1989) Water birth: one centres observations. *Journal of Nurse-Midwifery*, **34**, 4.

Coghill R. (1992) To the water born. *Nursing Times*, **88**, 24.

Coyle A. and Hicks C. (1984) Elegance for pregnant mothers. *Nursing Mirror*, **159**, 5.

Garland D. (1992) An American tail, *Midwifery Matters*, **55**, Winter.

Garland D. (1993) The water babies. *Maternity and Mothercraft*, August/September.

Gorton Y. (1991) Waterbirth: a personal view. *Maternal and Child Health*, **16**, 8.

King S. (1992) Water wise. *New Generation*, March.

Lines M. (1992) Feet first. *New Generation.* December.

Lines M. (1993) Water birth; feedback from mothers and midwives. *British Medical Journal*, **1**, 6.

McCandlish R. *et al.* (1993) Immersion in water during labour and birth. *Birth*, **20**, 2.

Newton C. (1992) Bath rights. *Nursing Times*, **88**, 24.

Nightingale C. (1992) Waterbirths. *Midwifery Dialogue*, **6**, 1–2.

Reid Campion M. (1990) *Adult Hydrotherapy*. Heinemann.

Rosenthal M. (1991) Warm water immersion in labor and birth. *The Female Patient*, **16**, 35–47.

Sidenbladh E. (1982) *Water Babies*. Adam and Charles Black.

Skinner A.T. and Thomson A.M. (1983) *Duffields Exercise in Water*. Baillière Tindall, London.

Stoddart C. (1992) Home but not alone. *New Generation*, September.

Elise Johnson

Chapter 7 **Shiatsu**

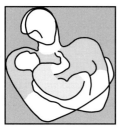

Shiatsu is a Japanese word meaning 'finger pressure'. It has evolved from an earlier form of Japanese massage called Anma (or Tuina in China). In order to comprehend the principles behind shiatsu we have to understand those of Chinese medicine, which was introduced to Japan as early as the sixth century by a Buddhist monk. The Japanese then developed their own method of manual healing, particularly concentrating on techniques of abdominal diagnosis and treatment. Shiatsu is actually a twentieth century art, since newer western medical knowledge of anatomy and physiology and physiotherapy techniques have been incorporated into it. It was recognised in Japan in 1964 as opposed to its former Anma massage, and has spread rapidly to the west since then. Now there are over 300 qualified therapists throughout the United Kingdom and this number is increasing all the time.

Details of the therapy
Unlike its predecessor Anma, which consisted of many techniques such as pushing and pulling strokes, tapping, rubbing, stroking and squeezing, done directly on the skin, shiatsu uses simple pressure and holding techniques in combination with gentle stretching, and is performed through loose fitting clothing. A qualified shiatsu practitioner will take a full case history and then a diagnosis before treatment. There are several forms of diagnoses (as there are styles of treatment). Many concentrate on 'hara' or palpation of the abdomen in order to assess the relative energy in each of the internal organs.

In other forms of shiatsu, pulses are taken. Whatever the style of diagnosis and treatment, they are all based on traditional Chinese medicine. The practitioner will then apply pressure, with either thumbs, fingers, elbows or knees along meridians (energy lines) and points in the body, according to the diagnosis made. This application of pressure tonifies, sedates, or 'moves' the 'Ki' (energy) in the body. Further refinements of treatment are carried out according to what the practitioner feels energetically in the body. Recipients feel a variety of sensations while receiving shiatsu, described commonly as a 'good hurt', dull aching, or pain disappearing under the therapist's fingers, as the energy is being rebalanced in the body.

How traditional chinese medicine works

Energy, known as 'Qi' in Chinese, 'Ki' in Japanese, is considered to be the motive force of all life. Without Ki there is no life. In ancient times it was noted that even though Ki flowed everywhere in the body, sometimes it seemed to flow near the surface. When there was illness, when the flow of Ki was disturbed, sometimes it manifested in the superficial areas of the body as pain, swelling, irritation and redness. It was then found that by rubbing or pressing these areas, one could eradicate the illness itself, even an internal one. These observations were systematised and the basis of meridians and points was founded. Therapies emerged such as acupuncture, moxibustion, cupping and massage. Whereas acupuncture utilizes needles to adjust the Ki energy, moxa uses heat and cupping uses cups shiatsu, on the other hand, uses touch to adjust the internal energies of the body. Since imbalance of Ki precedes obvious symptoms of a disease, shiatsu (like all oriental medicine) has a preventative role in the treatment of disease. However, the most common syndromes which shiatsu does help to treat are conditions such as musculo-skeletal problems (for example lumbago, fibrositis and sciatica), headaches and migraine, respiratory ailments, including coughs, catarrh and asthma, stress and tension, insomnia and digestive disorders. The gynaecological conditions that can be treated include infertility and menstrual problems. The common disorders of pregnancy which are amenable to treatment by shiatsu will be discussed later in this chapter.

The western explanation

In order to examine the physiological effects of finger pressure or shiatsu on the body, we have to examine the nature of connective tissue. Research done by two independent researchers in Japan, Yoshio Nagahama and Hiroshi Motoyama, has concluded that the meridians lie in the connective tissue, and more specifically in the superficial fascia.

An interesting insight into the nature of connective tissue is provided by James Oschman from Natural Science of Healing.

The connective tissue and fascia form a mechanical continuum, extending throughout the animal body, even into the innermost parts of each cell. All the great systems of the body – the circulation, the nervous system, the musculo-skeletal system, the digestive tract, the various organs – are sheathed in connective tissue. This matrix determines the overall shape of the organism as well as the detailed architecture of its parts. All movements, of the body as a whole, or of its smallest parts, are created by tensions carried through the connective tissue fabric. Each tension, each compression, each movement causes the crystalline lattices of the connective tissues to generate bioelectric signals that are precisely characteristic of those tensions, compressions, and movements. The fabric is a semiconducting communication network that can convey the bioelectric signals between every part of the body and every other part. This communication network within the fascia is none other than the meridian system of traditional Oriental medicine, with its countless extensions into every part of the body. As these signals flow through the tissues, their biomagnetic counterparts extend the stories they tell into the space around the body. The mechanical, bioelectric, and biomagnetic signals travelling through the connective tissue network, and through the space around the body, tell the various cells how to form and reform the tissue architecture in response to the tensions, compressions, and movements we make.

While this theory shows that connective tissue is capable of communication and energy conduction in the form of electron and proton transfer, it follows that the application of pressure anywhere in the body will generate small electric currents. This is explained more easily by the following scenario. Pressure applied to tissues can help to transform the tissue. Work done on organic gels, part of the cytoplasm of cells, shows that pressure will cause the gel to become a solution. Therefore, particle accumulations trapped in the gel state may be released at the same time as the gel becomes more hydrated. Hydration will make the tissue more energetically conductive. Shiatsu massage will not only induce small electric currents that will be conducted away from the point of pressure, but it will also help rearrange the tissues, making them more conductive (Matsumoto and Birch, 1988). The electric currents will have many physiological effects, just as they do in acupuncture, such as increase in microcirculation and vasomotion that will increase oxygenation of the tissues, and will help flush toxins, waste products, improving their overall function (see also Chapter 10). The end result of all this is that physiologically, shiatsu massage has the ability to regulate nerve function, strengthen the body's resistance to disease, flush out the tissue, improve circulation of blood, and make joints more flexible.

Fundamentals of giving shiatsu treatment

- Always be calm and centred. Deep breathing techniques are very effective in achieving this, as also are t'ai chi and Qi-Gong.
- Never use muscle power but rather use your body weight to lean into a point or meridian in applying pressure.
- Always use two hands while working. This is more relaxing and supportive for the recipient.
- Always use perpendicular pressure while leaning into a point.

Fig. 7.1. Gall Bladder 21

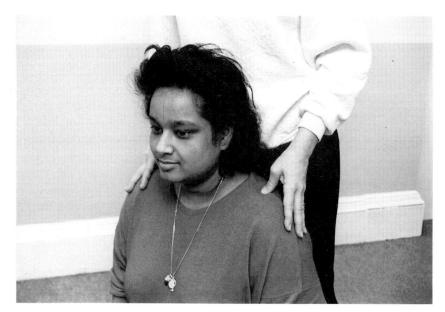

Fig. 2. Large Intestine 4

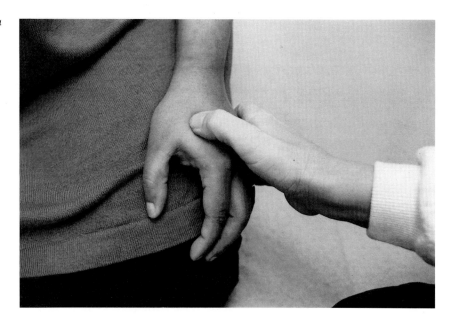

**Contra-
indications**

In general, most conditions are amenable to shiatsu treatment. Some conditions
that are contraindicated include active skin diseases, burns, fractures (above or
below the site is permitted), fever, herniated vertebral discs, infectious diseases,
open sores or scars, osteoporosis, tumours or cancers, although it is effective for
pain relief, thrombosis and varicosities (above or below the site is permitted).

During pregnancy there are not very many contraindications for shiatsu,

Fig. 3. Spleen 6

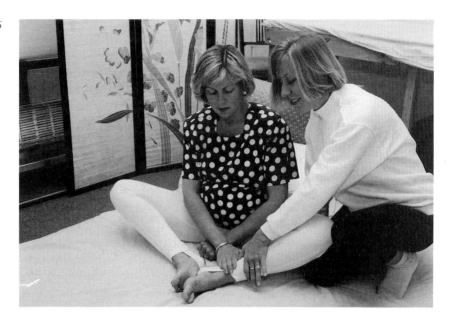

Fig. 4. Liver 3

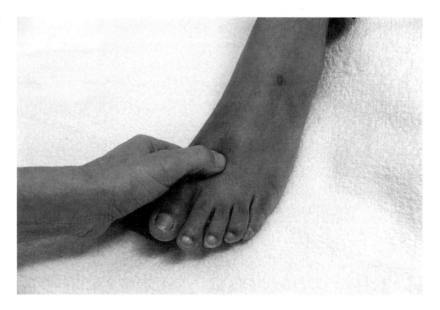

but rather specific areas of the body to avoid pressure on. Points to be avoided are Gall Bladder 21 (Fig. 1), Large Intestine 4 (Fig. 2), Spleen 6 (Fig. 3) and Liver 3 (Fig. 4). Only gentle work is advised on the lower back and sacrum, while the lower inner leg around Sp6 location should be avoided, especially during the first trimester. Shiatsu is not advised in the first trimester if there has been a history of miscarriage or if there are signs of imminent miscarriage.

Uses in pregnancy

Breathlessness	Increased frequency of micturition
Haemorrhoids	and vaginal discharge
Nausea and vomiting	Cramps
Carpal tunnel syndrome	Insomnia
Heartburn	Pain – lumbar and sacral pain
Oedema	Headaches
Chronic cough	Tiredness

Midwives would find a knowledge of shiatsu techniques a very useful adjunct to their normal practice. However while certain simple techniques can be learnt and used in conjunction with massage and other manual therapies, the midwife as always must recognise her limitations. Shiatsu can be enormously beneficial for pregnancy, labour and the puerperium, but unless the midwife is fully trained she should refrain from using some of the more involved techniques. Referral to a qualified, reputable practitioner would be preferable (see Chapter 1).

The remainder of this chapter deals with the application of shiatsu to pregnancy and childbirth in order to demonstrate the effectiveness of the therapy for the women in the care of midwives. If there is any doubt as to whether or not the midwife should be attempting the shiatsu movements, she should refer the woman to a practitioner.

Why is shiatsu of benefit in pregnancy?

Since shiatsu is a physical 'hands on' therapy, it can be extremely useful during pregnancy which is a very emotional time for women, due to hormonal changes. Physical touch can be very reassuring and calming. In terms of Oriental medicine, pregnancy together with the postnatal period is considered to be one of the 'gateways of change'. These occur at times of great hormonal fluctuations and are held to be stages where great care should be taken with one's health, because during them it is possible either to strengthen or weaken one's constitution to a great degree. One sees this when, for example, a mother develops a condition after one pregnancy which disappears after a subsequent one. By having shiatsu during a 'gateway of change', a woman's Ki can be bolstered thereby preventing any pathology from developing.

Gateways of change are birth, perinatal period (for the baby), puberty, onset of regular sexual activity – 'marriage' in the texts, pregnancy, labour and the postnatal period, and the menopause
(From course notes, JCM Seminars, London 1981)

Shiatsu allows the woman's Ki to flow freely during pregnancy, and facilitates relaxation. This is important for the mother and fetus, as she is advised to 'modify her mental outlook and lifestyle in order to ensure healthy development of her baby' (Zhejiang College of Traditional Chinese Medicine, 1987). In practical terms today, this means to be calm and free from emotional upsets. The Japanese call this fetal education or 'Tai Kyo'. In the Orient it is traditionally thought that one-third of a person's ultimate social, physical, and mental functioning is determined by their experiences in the uterus (Ohashi, 1983). It is also thought that fetal education is embodied in the effort to remain quiet. The fetus will grow in peace if there is a well-regulated circulation of Ki. Therefore it is most important for a mother to maintain a stable and smooth circulation of Ki so that the infant may gain a bright and cheerful disposition. This is surely one of Shiatsu's real strengths, to enable the mother's Ki to flow, with the resultant relaxation and relief of fatigue.

Shiatsu is also very useful in pregnancy because of its ability to tonify the body's Ki, for it is the Ki energy of the Kidney primarily and the Stomach and Spleen that most often becomes depleted during pregnancy. (It should be noted that in terms of Oriental medicine the organs and their functions are not identical to the Western definition of organ function, but have a much wider meaning. For example, this is why we use the capital letters 'K' in Kidney and 'S' in Stomach and Spleen to denote Chinese function and meaning. It is not within the scope of this chapter to go into the full oriental physiology of the organs, since that would entail a complete course of study in itself, but see the further reading list.) Most of the pathologies or conditions of pregnancy can be helped by addressing these deficiencies in the shiatsu treatment.

The Kidney energy of the mother provides the primary source of energy for the fetus growing within her, so it becomes utilised from the moment of conception. The mother's Kidney energy reserves will be drained further if she overworks and does not rest enough. Hence a variety of symptoms or disorders will occur such as lower backache, oedema, fatigue, breathlessness, chronic coughs, anxiety and insomnia, vaginitis and cystitis. It is interesting to note that in oriental medicine, as indeed in other complementary therapies, recognition is given to the relevance of all symptoms, even those which in Western terms seem coincidental, for example coughs.

The Spleen, with help from the Stomach, is the organ which is responsible for the production of Blood. Nourishment of the baby both during and after pregnancy depends on an adequate supply of the woman's Blood. In pregnancy Blood nourishes the fetus via the placenta, and afterwards the Blood helps make breastmilk. Therefore, the mother's Blood is constantly nourishing the baby and tonification of the mother's Spleen energy is necessary. Symptoms of imbalances in these organs are as follows: constipation, spasms in the legs, haemorrhoids, heartburn, nausea and vomiting and oedema.

Therefore it can be seen that shiatsu is a very effective way to tonify the particular energies that become depleted during the natural course of pregnancy. Acupuncture is sometimes used for specific pathologies (see Chapter 10) in pregnancy, although some of the ancient texts do not advise acupuncture during pregnancy (Zhejian College of Tradition Chinese Medicine, 1987) because often one tenses up at the time of insertion of needles and this could cause undue stress to the woman. Shiatsu does not seem to have this effect and is more relaxing.

Another special advantage of having shiatsu is more accessibility to the meridian to be worked. This is especially so if Shizuto Masanaga, the Zen style of shiatsu, is practised. Shizuto Masanaga extended the traditional meridian system throughout the body and in effect with shiatsu administered in this style there is more opportunity to work the appropriate meridian.

Shiatsu treatment during pregnancy

Generally it is considered safe to receive shiatsu from the beginning of pregnancy, with a caution not to use any of the contraindicated points. The areas of the lower inner leg, and strong pressure on the lower back and sacrum should be avoided.

Pregnant women will benefit from weekly shiatsu sessions with a qualified therapist with the relevant experience.

The following antenatal conditions during the 40 week gestation period are all suitable for shiatsu treatment, either during the antenatal examination given by the midwife if she is appropriately trained or during a complete shiatsu session given by a shiatsu therapist. (Aetiologies of each condition are explained below in terms of Oriental medicine.)

Breathlessness Not only does this occur by reason of the size of the pregnant abdomen which takes up so much room, but in terms of oriental medicine the Lungs are strongly related to proper functioning of Kidney Ki. Therefore during a session with a qualified practitioner, working the Kidney meridian throughout the body will support the function of the Lungs, which will also be assisted by opening up the chest with work on the Lung 1 point (Fig. 5). This is extremely effective to relieve breathlessness, especially during the last trimester. Midwives can also try pressure on Pericardium 6 (Fig. 6), which is a point that affects the chest.

Chronic coughs Many times while working with pregnant women one sees clients with chronic coughs. Treatment should be sought from a shiatsu therapist to tonify the woman's energy, since often this weakness in the lungs in oriental medicine is caused by weakened Kidney energy.

Carpal tunnel syndrome This is seen often in pregnancy, due to oedema causing compression on the median nerve. In order to avoid administration of diuretics by doctors, either several shiatsu sessions by a therapist or first aid shiatsu techniques by a midwife can be of help. Oedema during pregnancy is seen in oriental medicine as a disorder occurring as a result of a deficiency of

Fig. 5. Lung 1

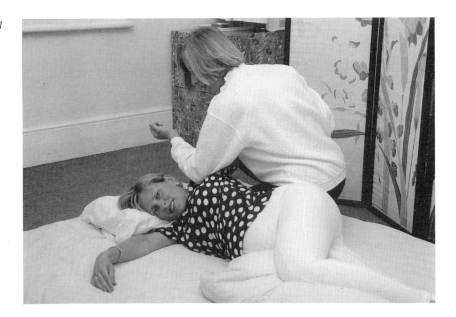

Fig. 6. Pericardium 6

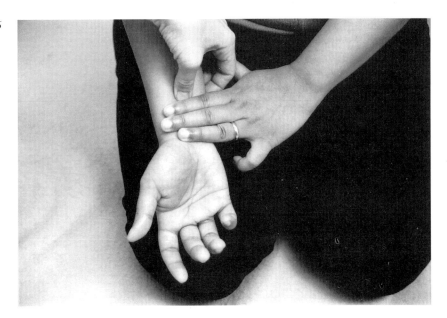

These points aid the relief of breathlessness

Spleen and Kidney energies causing retention of body fluid. Work on the Masanaga's meridians of Spleen and Kidney channels in the affected arm will help. Another effective technique is work on the Masanaga Kidney channel of the leg. Midwives mastering the fundamentals of shiatsu can perform this latter method and locally work Pericardium 6. Press firmly for 7–10 seconds, three times.

Constipation This can be very troublesome especially in the third trimester. Regular shiatsu treatments as well as attention to diet during pregnancy will prevent this, as one of the reasons in oriental medicine for constipation is the mother's depletion of Stomach and Spleen energy. The midwife could work gently but firmly down the Stomach meridian concentrating on pressing Stomach 36 (St 36) (Fig. 7), for 7–10 seconds, three times. Self shiatsu on Stomach meridian (Fig. 8) is also helpful.

Fig. 7. Stomach 36

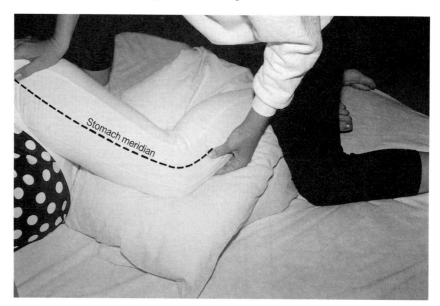

Fig. 8. Self shiatsu on stomach meridian

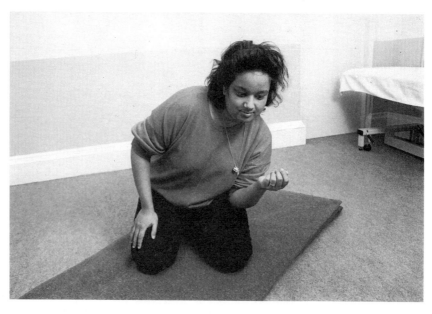

Can be pressed to relieve constipation

Cramps Leg cramps, or spasms of the gastrocnemius muscles, occur in the leg muscles through deficiency of Blood nourishing the tissues and deficiency of Kidney energy. Regular shiatsu can be a preventative or first aid treatment. Pressure to Stomach, Gallbladder and Bladder channels in the leg will help cure cramps. Midwives could demonstrate the Bladder 57 (Fig. 9) point while dorsiflexing the foot slowly, which the woman could press during a spasm.

Fig. 9. Bladder 57 – may help to ease cramps

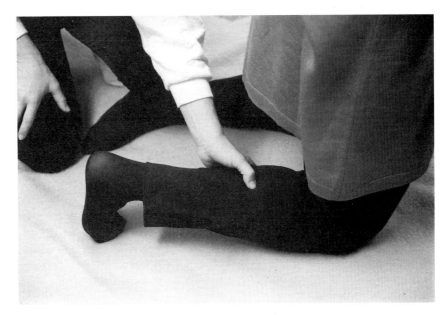

Haemorrhoids One reason for haemorrhoids to occur in pregnancy is due to the taxing of the Spleen energy. This is because in oriental medicine one of the functions of the Spleen is to hold Blood in the blood vessels, and to support the organs.

First aid techniques are as follows:

- Gentle but firm pressure on Governing Vessel 20 (Fig. 10), pressing firmly for 7–10 seconds, three times.
- Similar pressure on Bladder 57, Bladder 58 and Bladder 17. In the postnatal period Spleen energy can be improved by pressure on Bladder 57 and Governing Vessel 20 (GV 20).

Shiatsu is effective on points such as GV 20, and Bladder 57, which effectively tonify Spleen energy, and help lift 'prolapsed anus'.

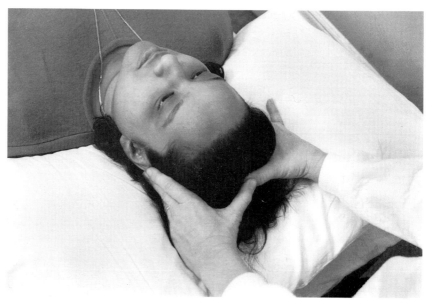

Fig. 10. Governing Vessel 20 – first aid for haemorrhoids

Heartburn This can be very problematic in late pregnancy and a frequent source of discomfort which is very responsive to shiatsu treatment. Besides Western medical advice on avoidance of fried and fatty foods and eating small frequent meals (this is practical advice to mothers with weak Stomach Ki also), shiatsu treatment is very effective. Heartburn occurs in oriental medicine because of the weakening of Stomach Ki, which thereby is caused to rebel and travel upwards causing heartburn.

Symptomatic treatment is as follows. Work Stomach meridian firmly. Midwives with some shiatsu training can do this effectively. The trained midwife could also teach the mother to work Conception Vessel 22 and work down the Bladder Channel (Fig. 11). Press Stomach 36, and Pericardium 6.

Suzie was a 34 year old with two other children aged 3 and 1 year old, who came for shiatsu treatment at 33 weeks' gestation. She had been suffering from severe heartburn with acid regurgitation most often in the day, and especially on eating. The diagnosis in the session was weak Stomach and Spleen energy. The meridian was felt to be very depleted in the leg and was very sensitive to touch, especially Stomach 36. Slow, gentle but tonifying firm pressure was administered to the Stomach, Kidney and the Spleen meridian (avoiding strong pressure on the inner lower leg) with great sensitivity displayed by Suzie. Symptoms improved immediately after treatment and relief lasted for about 4–5 days. Self shiatsu at home on the Stomach meridian and Conception Vessel 22 also improved symptoms. Several more sessions before the end of the pregnancy kept the symptoms down to a minimum.

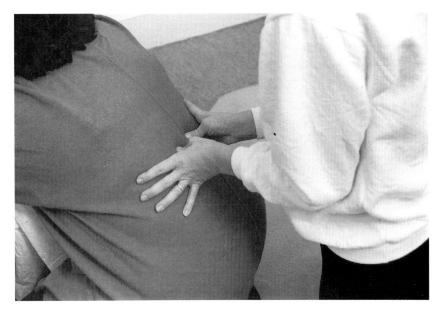

Fig. 11. Working down
the Bladder Channel
concentrating on the
associated points of the
stomach and spleen

Increased frequency of micturition and increased vaginal discharge
Both of these conditions can often be found in the first few weeks of pregnancy and also the last trimester. These occur because in terms of oriental
medicine there is a switch of the mother's Kidney energy as it is redirected
towards the fetus. Typical symptoms include frequent, copious micturition,
heavy legs, bloating in the first few weeks of pregnancy, and increased vaginal discharge. Sometimes a first aid measure which can be performed by the
midwife involves working on the Kidney channel in the leg, both Masanaga
and the traditional location.

Insomnia This is commonly experienced at the end of pregnancy because of
increased movements of the fetus and frequency of micturition.
'Overthinking' and anxiety about the expected baby often cause insomnia
and if this is the case, regular shiatsu sessions with a therapist can help by enabling the mother to relax. Sessions are recommended to be performed in the
evening and it is best to include a lot of work on head, neck and shoulders.

Nausea and vomiting In terms of oriental medicine there are several
reasons for this condition. It occurs due to depletion of Stomach Ki during
the time that the pregnant woman is nourishing the baby. The natural direction of the Stomach energy in the body is in a downwards flow, but when
the Stomach energy is weak there is a tendency for it to 'rebel' upwards,
hence nausea occurs. Alternatively it may be due to the fact that the Liver
energy stagnates (usually because of weakening of the mother's Kidney

Fig. 12. Treating the bladder channel will tonify the stomach and spleen energies

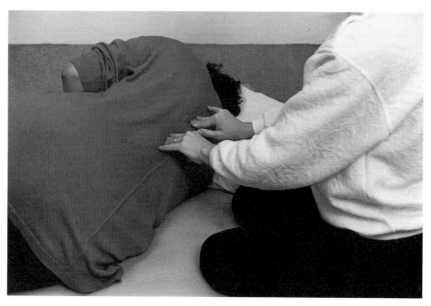

energy in supporting the growing fetus) and leads to rebellious Stomach Ki. This stagnation of Liver Ki happens as result of the sudden cessation of menstruation when one becomes pregnant. There is a swift change in metabolism which causes the Liver Ki to stagnate which in turn 'invades the Stomach and Spleen', hence once again nausea occurs.

In practice, whatever the aetiology, the midwife can assist in tonifying the mother's Stomach meridian down the leg with gentle but strong focus on Stomach 36 and by pressing firmly for 7–10 seconds, three times.

Research by Dundee *et al.* (1988) showed research study efficacy of the use of the Pericardium 6 point in the reduction of troublesome sickness. This work has been repeated by other researchers in relation to pregnancy (Hyde, 1989) and the sickness resulting from chemotherapy for carcinoma (Stannard, 1989).

It is now possible for mothers to purchase wristbands from health stores and chemists which are designed to work on the P6 acupressure point, in order to relieve sickness. Midwives may prefer to advise mothers to use these or perform shiatsu themselves on Pericardium 6. A shiatsu therapist will work down the Bladder channel with the woman either sitting or lying on her side (Fig. 12). Treating the Bladder channel will not only tonify the Stomach and Spleen energies via their associated points, but will also tonify the Kidneys because of the strong relationship between the Bladder and Kidneys in oriental medicine.

Mothers can be advised to eat biscuits frequently because this stimulates peristalsis which descends the Stomach Ki that is rebelling.

Amanda was 10 weeks pregnant when she came for shiatsu treatment and was feeling quite nauseous, although not actually vomiting. Her symptoms were better for eating, worse with fatigue. She was always running around after her 2 year old and 4 year old children. She was anaemic and quite tired and had been prescribed iron tablets. Occasionally if she was very tired she would feel nauseous in the evening, at about 5 p.m. After the first treatment which consisted of Stomach meridian work, pressure on Stomach 36, Bladder meridian work and Pericardium 6 pressure, she felt immediate relief which lasted for about 4 days. She was advised to drink ginger root tea, which has the effect of warming the Stomach and Spleen, thereby strengthening it.

She was also advised to rest more, eat frequent small meals, and to avoid rich, greasy food which further aggravates stagnation of Liver Energy. After the next week of similar treatment, relief went on for 6 days. She was advised to make rice congee, which is a rice soup made from six parts water to one part rice and is cooked slowly for several hours. Camomile tea was advised for settling the stomach instead of tea or coffee. This advice was heeded and Amanda managed to cope with the reduced nausea until her body had adjusted to the hormonal changes of early pregnancy.

Oedema Oedema is a disorder, in terms of oriental medicine, occurring in pregnant women with depletion of Spleen and Kidney energy, causing retention of body fluid which further depletes the Spleen and Kidney energy. The Spleen and Kidney energies become drained or exhausted towards the end of pregnancy, and thus the function of transportation and transformation of body fluids becomes impaired and fluid accumulates in the tissues, primarily in the extremities and lower half of the body. This condition is ideally suited for treatment by the shiatsu practitioner on all Kidney meridian locations in the body, especially Masanaga locations in the leg. Midwives could try working the Bladder meridian (Fig. 13) with the woman sitting or lying on her side. Alternatively first aid treatment involving pressing points Kidney 7, Stomach 36, Bladder 23 and Kidney 3 can be effective.

Most of the severe cases that this author has treated have been found in women aged 35 and over. This is not surprising since Kidney energy naturally declines with age. Also, many cases of oedema were found in women who did not rest enough. Kidney energy becomes depleted through overwork and not resting.

Loretta, a journalist aged 38, was in her third trimester and suffering from severe oedema of pretibial areas and ankles, forcing her to buy larger sized shoes. Her blood pressure was within normal limits, she had no headaches but had slight proteinuria. She was under considerable pressure of deadlines for her newsletter, drank one or two

Fig. 7.13. Bladder meridian

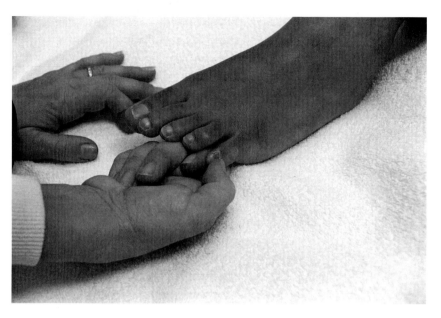

cups of coffee daily, and attended various after work conferences.

One shiatsu session focused on the traditional Kidney meridian location in the leg, and Masanaga location, and also in the arms and chest, after which, there was significant reduction of oedema. Advice for more rest was slightly adhered to as was the advice to stop drinking coffee. Weekly sessions controlled the oedema from progressing further and indeed markedly improved it.

Lumbosacral pain and sciatica This is found frequently because of the increase in weight on the mother's spine and due to Kidney Ki deficiency, which governs the lower back. Consequently, deficiency of Kidney energy causes lower back pain. Mothers will often instinctively rub the pain to make it better and it is this very reason that shiatsu is so recommended for this pain. Work by an experienced shiatsu therapist is recommended. This will involve working on the Bladder channel of the back in side or 'sitting position' with focus on Bladder 23, and also firm but gentle pressure on the Masanaga Kidney meridian in the sacral area, upper thigh and lower leg. This is of particular value in labour, and work on the Bladder channel could be performed by the midwife or taught to the birth companion.

Headache Headaches should be treated by a shiatsu practitioner who can assess the cause and treat the mother accordingly. However the midwife should be vigilant in observing the mother for pre-eclampsia and would normally seek advice, in the first place, from the obstetrician.

Tiredness This is very responsive to complete shiatsu treatment by a qualified practitioner. Weekly sessions are extremely beneficial, especially during the last six weeks of pregnancy. Work will be focused on the Kidney, Stomach, and Spleen channels.

Uses in labour

> Shiatsu is a technique used in labour either for
> induction for prolonged pregnancy
> augmentation of contractions,
> as an analgesic,
> or for the expulsion of the placenta.

The midwife should be familiar with the ways in which a qualified shiatsu practitioner can help the mother, as some women may wish to be accompanied by their practitioner in labour. Teamwork is vitally important and communication early in pregnancy will help to develop the partnership.

Midwives are able to use a limited number of simple Shiatsu techniques if they can justify their use, but may wish to refer to an expert for specific conditions and appropriate treatment.

Induction for prolonged pregnancy and acceleration of labour

Shiatsu techniques are a favourable method of inducing labour for postmaturity. Firstly, if anxiety is a factor, complete shiatsu sessions in the week during which the mother is overdue will help to foster relaxation and tonify her energy. The shiatsu practitioner will then use all the points previously contraindicated. Strong downwards pressure on Gall Bladder 21 then pressure on Spleen 6, Bladder 67 and Large Intestine 4. These points can be pressed safely from the estimated due date onwards, and this treatment is most effective if performed daily. Midwives should remember that induction of labour falls outside their normal practice and therefore only those who have shiatsu training should perform these techniques after consultation with medical staff.

Augmentation of contractions If the first stage of labour has started and the contractions have begun to slow down, then pressure on Spleen 6, Large Intestine 4, together with Bladder 3l, Liver 3 and Gall Bladder 21 can help to stimulate uterine activity. Strong thumb pressure on all the points is required as well as strong downward palm pressure on sacral points (Fig. 14).

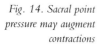

Fig. 14. Sacral point pressure may augment contractions

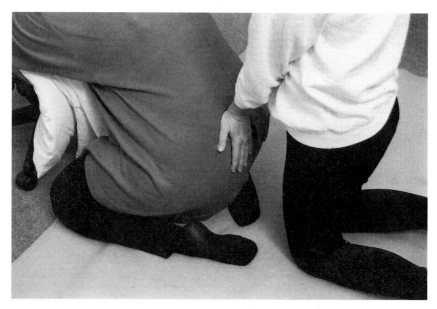

Joanne was a 45 year old primigravida who was admitted with spontaneous rupture of membranes at 36 weeks' gestation. She was hoping to have an active birth, moving around freely, adopting different positions without continuous monitoring unless it was necessary, preferring a small tear to an episiotomy but hoping to deliver with an intact perineum and giving birth without drugs if possible. The midwife explained that she would work with her to achieve this but it was probable that the obstetrician would suggest that an oxytocic infusion be commenced to stimulate contractions as labour had not begun. It was at this point that Joanne suggested shiatsu, as her husband had benefited from recent treatment for back and joint problems. It was arranged that the shiatsu practitioner should join them in the delivery suite.

The obstetrician had no objection to the shiatsu treatment but agreed with Joanne that she should receive oral prostaglandin to stimulate contractions. There was no regular uterine activity, just occasional tightenings when the shiatsu practitioner commenced treatment, with Joanne in a semi-recumbent position. External cardiotograph monitoring was recommended to ensure fetal well-being during shiatsu. The initial aim of the treatment was to establish contractions, then to stabilise and strengthen them. The midwife and Joanne observed the therapist begin to work points beginning on the legs with Spleen 6 and moving to Large Intestine 4 on the hands and Gall Bladder 21 on the shoulders. Tiny magnets were also taped to the skin over the Spleen 6 points on the lower legs. Magnets are widely used in Japan as a means of stimulating the acupuncture points, since they are shown to have electrical properties. About 30 minutes after the therapy commenced weak, irregular contractions were palpable and observations satisfactory.

Four hours later a reassessment of the cervix was performed which was found to be rigid and closed. The midwife explained that to avoid an oxytocin infusion being sited, there needed to be considerable change by the next vaginal examination. Over the next hour further shiatsu treatment was given on the Gall Bladder 21 (GB 21) and Large Intestine 4 (LI 4) points. The points on Joanne's left shoulder and hand were treated as these had previously been noted as having optimum effect. A further point at the end of the toe Bladder 67 (BL 67) was used in between contractions to assist cervical dilatation. The length, strength and frequency of contractions increased considerably under the influence of the shiatsu treatment and by the time of the next cervical assessment Joanne was in established labour, which progressed to a normal delivery 7 hours later.

Exhaustion during labour If the woman becomes exhausted during labour, work on the Stomach meridian and Bladder meridian on the back and legs between contractions can be helpful. The reason for this is two-fold; it will not only revitalise tired legs but will also increase the vital energy of the woman to enable sufficiently strong contractions to occur for dilatation of the cervix.

Analgesia in the first stage of labour If labour is prolonged, shiatsu pain relieving techniques should be supplemented between contractions. Pressure to Gall Bladder 30, Gall Bladder 3l, Stomach 36, and Bladder 60 points will help to restore circulation and relax leg muscles (Fig. 15). For effective pain relief during a contraction, strong pressure on Bladder 60 is very useful and effective. Additional points of Spleen 6, Large Intestine 4, Liver 3 and Conception Vessel 4 are also beneficial.

Analgesia in occipito-posterior position Shiatsu is an excellent analgesic for the occipito-posterior position, which is regularly associated with very tedious and painful labour. The midwife could perform this technique and should use strong downward palm pressure or thumb pressure into the sacral foramen at the beginning of the contraction, maintaining it to the height of the contraction till it subsides. This can be done with the woman in either a standing position, sitting leaning over a beanbag, or lying on her side (Fig. 16).

*Fig. 15. Bladder 60 –
pressure can be effective for
pain relief in labour*

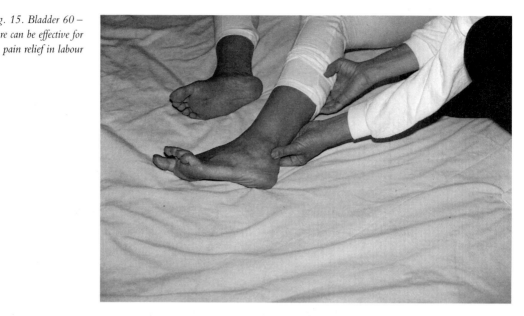

*Fig. 16. Easing the sacral
pain of an occipito-posterior
position*

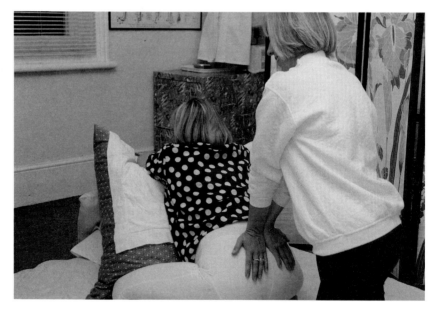

*Ester, a 33 year old shiatsu therapist, was in her second pregnancy.
Following spontaneous rupture of membranes at term, she arrived at
hospital in established labour. She remained ambulant until
contractions were occurring every 2 minutes. On vaginal
examination the cervix was found to be 2 cm dilated. The midwife
suggested that Ester enter the birthing pool for pain relief and*

relaxation. Ester asked her husband to use strong palm pressure on her sacrum as she hung on to the side of the pool. Once she left the pool, her husband continued applying thumb pressure around the sacral grooves while she was on all fours, and leaning over the beanbag chair.

Ester found this technique combined initially with water then on 'all fours' to be very effective in easing the pain and she delivered a 3.5 kg baby in the 'all fours' position with no trauma to the perineum.

Analgesia in the second stage of labour During the second stage one midwife can support the mother's occiput with pressure around the occipital ridge with one hand and another person can use very strong pressure on the Bladder 67 point, squeezing between thumb and index finger or using the nail to press the point. If it is impossible for one person to do this, two people can do it between them. Bladder 67 runs down both legs from the sacrum along the same lines as the autonomic nerves. Intense pressure applied here tends to block sensation in the sacral and pelvic area, thus relieving pain.

Retention of the placenta Midwives could, with limited training, and in an emergency,press on Gall Bladder 21, Bladder 60, Large Intestine 4, and Spleen 6 points to facilitate separation of the placenta. However, without adequate training this could be a case of a little knowledge being dangerous. If a shiatsu practitioner is present in the labour room she or he could apply treatment which would be effective in separating and expelling the placenta. It should be recognised too that the mother who is accompanied by a shiatsu practitioner is likely to want to avoid active management of the third stage. It is therefore possible that except in cases of a morbidly adherent placenta, patience and time will work naturally and shiatsu may not be required.

Shiatsu in the puerperium

Can be used for:
Postnatal depression
Insufficient breast milk

Postnatal depression The woman who is susceptible to the 'blues' or extreme tiredness would be advised to consult a qualified therapist as soon as she feels able. The practitioner may treat the woman even while she is breastfeeding, lying on her side. The importance of adequate rest during the puerperium cannot be emphasized enough. The postnatal period, described earlier as one of the 'gateways of change', is a crucial time in a woman's life, when she must take care of herself and replenish all the energy given out during the birth process. The Chinese place so much importance on this period they also call it 'doing 40 days', where the mother is advised only to care for the baby and to rest; all members of the family and community members take on responsibility for the household chores, so that the mother will fully recover her energy. This is not always possible to achieve today, but the midwife should encourage the woman to rest more. The euphoric energy immediately felt after birth soon wears off and the true state of energy of the mother emerges. Rest, plus several shiatsu sessions can help to boost the mother's Ki so that postnatal depression is less likely to develop. If rest is not possible during the night because of an unhappy, crying infant, shiatsu for the neonate may be helpful.

Insufficient breast milk One of the reasons for this condition is depletion of the mother's Blood after birth and exhaustion of energy. Shiatsu sessions from a qualified therapist will aid relaxation in order to build the mother's Ki. Concentration on work on the Stomach and Spleen meridians will help build up quality reserves of milk, as will work on the Kidney meridian which helps build vital energy.

Shiatsu massage for the neonate

Shiatsu baby massage is actually a combination of Swedish massage and shiatsu techniques, mainly done directly on the baby's skin using oil. In many cases the relaxation of the baby achieved through the massage will help the mother to rest and relax as well. Learning how to massage the infant can be extremely useful to both mother and baby. If the neonate is happy and relaxed, it will sleep thereby enabling the mother to rest.

In terms of Chinese medicine a woman's Ki and blood go into making breast milk. Tired exhausted mothers do not make adequate breast milk. The baby may suck and suck and still not be adequately satisfied; the consequent intake of air in such excessive breast feeding will create colic, leading to pain and crying. The mother naturally tends to try and feed the baby more in order to satisfy her, leading to more severe colic. A vicious cycle is produced and the mother will find herself drained through having to get up constantly during the night to try and placate the baby. Conversely if the baby is happy and relaxed with the help of massage, the mother can rest and produce adequate quantities of breast milk to satisfy the baby.

In Dr Montague's book *Touching* (Montague, 1971) he writes:

> . . . the more we learn about the effects of cutaneous (skin) stimulation, the more pervasively significant for healthy development do we find it to be. Stimulation of the skin, cuddling, rocking, massage – increases cardiac output, promotes respiration and develops the efficiency of the gastrointestinal functions of the infant.

Fig. 17. Abdominal massage for the relief of neonatal colic

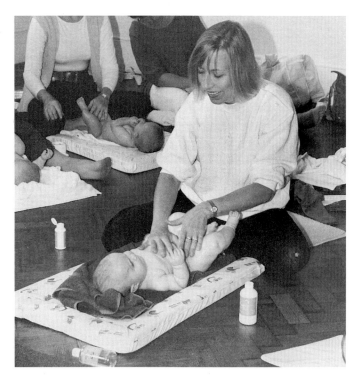

Conditions helped by shiatsu baby massage	Colic Sleeplessness Vomiting, possetting

Colic In the early days there are many occasions when the baby will cry and not settle. For the breastfeeding mother requiring analgesia this may be explained in terms of Chinese medicine as 'cold producing' (Scott, 1991). This 'cold' is then transferred to the mother's milk and passes through to the baby via breast feeding. Cold contracts and it is this that produces the pain in the infant's digestive system. Other foods that are cold in nature are bananas, dairy products, grapes and their derivatives, e.g. champagne! When such foods are eaten by the breast feeding mother, the cold quality of them is also transferred to the baby via the breast milk, thereby causing digestive pain to the infant.

When abdominal massage is performed on the baby in combination with the techniques below it will help to 'move and warm' the Ki of the abdomen and strengthen the digestion thereby relieving colic (Fig. 17).

The shiatsu practitioner, appropriately trained midwife or the mother should use relaxed fingertips and hands to massage the abdomen in a clockwise direction, hand over hand, following the natural flow of peristalsis of the digestive tract. With the pad of the index finger gently press Conception Vessel 12 three times, then massage with the fingertips the left side of the baby's abdomen over the descending colon. This process is repeated three times followed by clockwise abdominal massage. Massage up the infant's Spleen meridian in the inner leg and down the Stomach meridian on the lateral thigh. Press point Stomach 36 gently three times.

Sleeplessness A complete daily body shiatsu massage can help relax the baby and increase circulation, fostering sleep. This is most effective to induce sleep an hour after the last feed before bedtime.

Vomiting and possetting Where there is no organic malfunction of the digestive tract such as pyloric stenosis or hiatus hernia, then shiatsu massage can help the baby who vomits. In addition to daily massage the techniques described for the treatment of colic with the addition of the point Stomach 34 can be helpful. The mother should be advised to keep the infant in as much of an upright position as possible directly after a feed.

The following conditions are also amenable to shiatsu baby massage during the first and second years of a baby's life.

Constipation, diarrhoea, teething, earache, restlessness, bedwetting, poor appetite, insomnia, excess catarrh, coughs

---

Information about mother and baby shiatsu massage classes (Fig. 18) is available through the Shiatsu Society.

Conclusion

Although a full shiatsu training is 3 years long it would be useful for one or two midwives within a maternity unit to undertake that training. They would be able to offer at least a limited service to mothers. Other midwives could attend specific short courses for midwives to enable them to learn the techniques sufficiently to use them safely to complement their normal midwifery practice.

Midwives may also wish to forge links with local reputable shiatsu practitioners with experience and a special interest in dealing with mothers and their babies. Practitioners could be encouraged to communicate with the maternity unit and could be invited to conduct ante or postnatal classes with the midwives. Shiatsu has a great deal to offer for pregnancy, labour and the postnatal and neonatal period. It is a non-invasive and pleasurably relaxing treatment. Midwives can work to increase their understanding of its value for mothers and babies so that clients can obtain the best care possible.

Fig. 18. Mother and baby shiatsu massage class

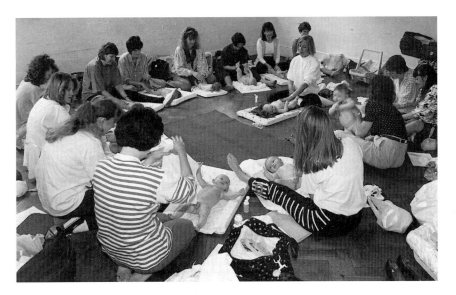

Training   As yet there is no licensing of shiatsu practitioners, therefore legally anyone can practise shiatsu. The Shiatsu Society has been set up to ensure standards of practice. This is an umbrella organisation for all the styles of shiatsu and includes the National Professional Practitioners' Register (set up in 1986) and Assessment Panel. Being a member of the Shiatsu Society (MRSS) guarantees a certain level of competence in practice. The Society's guidelines for training stipulate a minimum study period of 500 hours over a period of at least 3 years. This includes study in Western medicine including anatomy, physiology, and pathology. In order to qualify for inclusion on the Professional Register and to gain MRSS designation, candidates must pass theoretical and practical examinations.

Shiatsu training includes exercises to develop and maintain one's own Ki such as Qi-Gong, lower abdominal breathing and meditation; learning the basis of oriental diagnosis and principles of oriental medical theory; Zen shiatsu theory; shiatsu techniques, use of hara, location of classical and Masanaga meridians, and tsubo function and location; Western medical study of anatomy, physiology and pathology.

Midwives interested in gaining a professional qualification should contact The Shiatsu Society for further information.

Introductory courses offered by most schools can assist in the fundamental use of one's body weight in giving shiatsu.

Referring to a shiatsu practitioner

To find a local qualified shiatsu therapist, consult:

The Shiatsu Society
5 Foxcote, Wokingham, Berkshire RG 11 3PG, UK
Tel: 0734 730836

The Society holds a list of registered practitioners who are subject to a code of ethics and practice.

The Shiatsu Society provides a list of training schools. For training in London, Norwich, and Newcastle contact:

The Shiatsu College
UK Central Administration Norwich, 20a Lower Goat Lane, Norwich NR2 1EL, UK
Tel: 0603 632555

References

Dundee J.W. *et al.* (1988) P6 acupressure reduces morning sickness. *Journal of the Royal Society of Medicine*, **81**, 456–57.

Hyde E. (1989) Acupressure therapy for morning sickness – a controlled clinical trial. *Journal of Nurse-Midwifery*, **43(4)**, 171–178

Matsumoto K. and Birch S. (1988) *Hara Diagnosis: Reflections on the Sea*. Paradigm Publications, MA.

Montague A. (1971) *Touching*. Harper and Row, New York.

Ohashi W. (1983) *Natural Childbirth the Eastern Way*. Ballantine Books, New York.

Oschman J. (1987) *The Connective Tissue and Myofascial Systems*. Aspen Research Institute, Berkely.

Scott J. (1991) *Acupuncture in the Treatment of Children*. Eastland Press Inc.

Stannard D. (1989) Pressure prevents nausea. *Nursing Times*, **4(85)**, 33–34.

Zhejiang College of Traditional Chinese Medicine (Ed B. Flaws) (1987) *Handbook of Traditional Chinese Gynaecology*. Blue Poppy Press, Boulder, CO.

Further reading

Flaws R. (1983) *The Path of Pregnancy*, Paradigm.

Lundberg. (1992) *The Book of Shiatsu*. Gaia Book Ltd.

Maciocia G. (1989) *Foundations of Chinese Medicine*. Churchill Livingstone.

Masunaga, Shizuto with Wataru Ohashi (1977) *Zen Shiatsu*. Japan Publications.

Ross J.P. (1984) *Zang Fu, The Organ Systems of Traditional Chinese Medicine*. Churchill Livingstone.

Helen Stapleton

Chapter 8

Women as Midwives and Herbalists

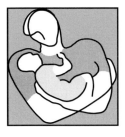

The use of herbs in midwifery picks up the threads of an old tradition when midwifery practice utilised the art and skills of prescribing the appropriate herbal remedies within the context of the ordinary, everyday occasions of life; of which childbirth was but one aspect. The 'herstory' of women healers as part of our heritage in Western society is at variance with the increased dissonance between 'women's talents and women's fate as it reflects the evolution of institutions that lack a feminine voice' (Achterberg, 1990). It might also be that the feminine voice has been silenced to facilitate the emergence of a large and exploited body of women who increasingly service these institutions from the humble position of de-skilled handmaidens. The majority of workers in healthcare systems in the industrialised world today are currently women; without them the day care centres, hospitals, laboratories, hostels, homes, GP surgeries and many other social agencies would collapse. Despite this highly visible presence, women generally now have very limited professional autonomy and with few exceptions, as is evident in midwifery, are legally or politically restricted from practising even the full range of skills acquired during training. This present lack of balance between the art and science of our healing tradition may be reflected in the current enthusiasm for rediscovering what has always been; as in the case of herbal medicine and its historic fusion with midwives' work.

Healing with the use of herbs is undoubtedly the earliest form of medicine, practised primarily amongst women everywhere since human existence has been recorded. For the most part, these ordinary, unremarkable women continued a timeless tradition of 'women's work' in attending labouring women, the sick and the dying. These were the 'wyse wimmin'; the unlicensed doctors, pharmacists, abortionists and midwives who travelled from place to place, collecting and cultivating herbs, learning from each other and passing on their wisdom, experience and knowledge as nameless keepers of an oral tradition.

One such historical figure whose life and practice during the Middle Ages has been well researched was Trotula, a distinguished teacher and physician at the famous Medical School of Salerno, Italy. Amongst remaining writings attributed to her is a treatise on gynaecology and obstetrics: 'Passionibus Mulierum Curandorum' (The Diseases of Women), also known as Trotula Major (Brookes, 1993). Trotula (the same Dame Trot of Chaucer and children's tales) was a skilled diagnostician in a time when actual knowledge of the inner workings of the body was largely left to the imagination as dissection was rarely, if ever, performed. Her reliance on the skills of urine and pulse diagnosis, in conjunction with careful consideration of the patient's features and choice of words, remain integral to the practice of many non-European systems of medicine in current use today. She wrote on a variety of topics directly related to women, which she subsequently made available to them at a time when such activities would have been considered highly subversive by the Establishment. The diversity of her subject matter reflected her understanding of the complexity of women's situations and difficulties, as is expressed when she makes suggestions in a herbal recipe for counterfeiting virginity. Trotula personified the balance so critical but yet so rarely visible in contemporary health workers; a knowledge and appreciation of the importance of science, attention to the 'magical' aspects of healing embedded in the mind, an empathy with the suffering and distress of illness and a willingness to engage compassionately with those who sought her advice.

This flowering of women practitioners, in a time before the avenues of healing work were abruptly closed to them, was possible because they lived at a point in history when religious and cultural beliefs did not focus on gender as a determining factor of ability. The increasing misogyny of the later Middle Ages blocked the more prestigious and politically important routes for women to obtain the formal academic qualifications necessary for them to continue as bona fide practitioners in their own right. This trend, albeit in a diluted form, continues to restrict the practice of both herbalists and midwives today.

Despite the constraints fettering the freedom of these practitioners, herbal medicine continued to be practised throughout the countryside and even up to the 1800s most people, when sick, still consulted herbalists. As women healers were further decimated or usurped, the developing fields of chemistry and physiology were subtly supplanting herbal traditions by subsuming them into a 'science'. Only with the rise of the pharmaceutical industries in the late nineteenth century did the intimate alliance between botany and medicine begin to falter. We still owe a considerable debt of gratitude to these persecuted witches for their accumulated empirical knowledge, as many of the herbal remedies tried and tested by them continue to hold their place in modern pharmacology. Significantly, witches were also known as 'herberia', meaning 'one who gathers herbs' (Walker, 1983).

Birthing the spirit . . .

In treating an ailment, the herbalist/midwife would not only administer a medicinal plant but would most likely also perform a ritual of some kind. Sharing symbolic content is not dismissed as an irrelevance to healing in those cultures where categories of sickness are not reduced to the mere physical imbalances so revered in Western medicine. The Mexican curanderas are women who continue to embody this powerful tradition, the majority of whom are herbalists, bone setters and midwives, but who also speak of themselves as servants of the divine. When engaging in healing rituals, it is not the ego-centred 'I', but rather this divinity who speaks and heals through the charged and dramatic chanting:

> I am the woman who swims in the sacred,
> I am the woman who sees the inside of things,
> I am the woman who came out of the earth . . .
> The woman of the essential healing fruits
> The woman of the sacred healing plants
> The woman who seeks so it says . . .
> The woman who explores by touch so it says . . .
>
> (Estrada, 1981)

As Jacqueline Vincent Priya cogently explains, this understanding of the 'other' aspects of healing work is inherent in health systems derived from a more holistic perspective, where physical illness is not necessarily distinguished from other kinds of misfortune (Vincent Priya, 1992). Within this context, physical symptoms of any kind may equally be the result of physical, social, emotional, spiritual or ancestral influences and may require a combination of different techniques to restore health. Such measures might include herbal medicines alongside individual or community ceremonies, into which the relevant religious or magical rituals are interwoven. This view of the world, as perceived by the inhabitants of many so-called 'primitive' or 'developing' countries, positively encourages the subjective feelings of sickness, unlike the tenets to which biomedicine adheres in holding that an individual is not ill in the absence of demonstrable, organic pathology.

Not forgetting nature . . .

The earth continues to provide a bountiful supply of healing prescriptions. Across cultures, in most areas of the world, herbs are used as antiseptics, coagulants, analgesics, diuretics and emetics; they aid digestion, lower fevers and staunch bleeding, whilst their ceremonial use eases the transitory moments of dying and of being born. The dawn of humankind regarded woman as a prodigious source of this mysterious healing wisdom and power. Through her creative juices and rites it was she who facilitated, sustained and curtailed life, thereby assuming the role of gatekeeper to dreams, visions and the world beyond the senses. Hers was a more equal and harmonious relationship with the earth as women 'not only collected and consumed what grew in nature', but reciprocated by planting and making things grow (Mies, 1976). It was this organic process of growth, formed from the mutually sustaining ecological partnership between women and nature, which informed this herstorically unique tradition.

Midwives were the great priestesses of the ancient worlds, encouraging women during their first major challenge: the birth ceremony. Through massage, herbs, prayer and sweat baths they prepared women to embrace the goddesses accompanying the sun from its celestial height to its setting low over the earth. This symbolic journey initiated them as warriors on their own 'battlefield' of childbirth where death was a not infrequent companion. The women who continue to carry out these functions in non-Western societies are also seen to be serving the needs of the whole community, becoming powerful mediators for its continued well being. Jules Cashford suggests that cultures such as our own, which either do not have or do not seem to acknowledge a mythic image of this feminine principle, may be seen to have desacralised Nature with subsequent loss of feeling, instinct, spontaneity and intuition as valid expressions of the sanctity and unity of life (Cashford and Baring, 1991). With this as a backdrop, small wonder that the birthing rituals of Western women are the medicalised, sanitised and deeply unsatisfying experiences so often described.

Towards a new way of being

The worlds of midwifery and herbal medicine are currently reflecting the evidence of these changing values. Within midwifery, the publication of two major policy documents, the Winterton report (1992) and the report of the Expert Maternity Group (1993), demand that midwives are encouraged to meet the challenges required in working as autonomous practitioners to transform midwifery services. The implementation of these recommendations is likely to have profound implications both for our profession and within a wider social context as the women and families with whom we work begin to 'consider autonomy as an essentially negotiable entity . . . ' (Manders, 1993).

Whilst the approval is of a more guarded nature, herbalists have also recently received a more positive, if cautious, affirmation with the publication of *Complementary Practices; New Approaches to Good Practice* (British Medical Association, 1993). In this report, the BMA Board of Science and Education studied the different forms of non-conventional therapies as it might any public health issue where measures are examined which would protect consumers of such therapies from possible harm. Herbal medicine is included as one of the five main therapies recognised as 'discrete clinical disciplines' most amenable to statutory regulation and thereby greater accessibility for the interested public. Seriously undermining this increased freedom of choice is EC legislation which has already removed a number of herbal medicines from the UK market and which also threatens the availability of vitamins, minerals and dietary products. At the heart of this conundrum is whether herbs and many other commodities presently classified as foods should be reclassified as medicines, with the associated requirement to show acceptable, 'scientific' proof of efficacy and safety.

Included on the list of herbs banned as medicines in one or other European Community country are those which have been used for centuries throughout Europe to great benefit and with no recorded ill-effects. In many cases, there is no demonstrable evidence that they pose serious health risks, but merely that they contain minute amounts of a toxic substance. This is also true, however, of many of the plants which constitute our daily diet including potatoes, bananas, almonds, lettuce, beans, peas and parsnips, not to mention beer, tobacco, coffee and tea. With a recent statement to the effect that by identifying particular herbs (such as those listed below) the European Community seem to be showing an increasing awareness of the inconsistencies of the position they have adopted and the need for further discussion.

Herbalists are seriously challenging the list prepared by the Committee for Proprietary Medicinal Products (CPMP; the European Community equivalent to the Department of Health). When paracetamol, a drug well known to be liver toxic, is freely available to the public, why should herbal medicines such as coltsfoot, angelica, comfrey, borage, parsley seed and pulsatilla be banned for use by the qualified medical herbalist? There are parallels between midwives and herbalists in this situation in what may be seen as an erosion into the sphere of clinical practice being dictated by an outside agency. Midwifery is only just beginning to show signs of recovery from this, as once limitations have been enforced, practitioners seem to incorporate rather than continue to challenge these changes.

Why herbal medicine?

Given the rich ethnic diversity of this country's inhabitants, herbal medicine can no longer be considered to exist within a cultural vacuum. Until recently, Western ethnocentrism has proved an insurmountable barrier in evaluating indigenous medical systems. In 1976 the World Health Organization calculated that traditional medicine was the main health source for approximately 75% of the world's population. Through frequently updated directives, this organisation continues to recommend the use of local health measures rather than encourage a dependence on expensive and often inappropriate biomedicine. With many of our clients using herbs as an integral part of their health care, it behoves us as professionals to respect intelligently this different knowledge. As with orthodox medicines, many herbs which have potent but beneficial effects also hold the capacity to exert unwanted or toxic effects if consumed at inappropriate dosages, if prepared incorrectly or if taken at vulnerable times, e.g. pregnancy (see Appendix 1, p. 176).

The use of herbal medicine throughout a woman's years of growing and birthing babies not only extends her nutritional and botanical 'vocabulary', but also introduces her and her midwife to safe, effective remedies for many common ailments. Encouraging women to self treat in this way simultaneously inspires the process of personal empowerment so necessary in effectively challenging the powerful prohibitions which still surround childbirth today.

Herbal medicine is participatory medicine. It is distinguished from the 'pill culture' of orthodox medicine by its messiness, stickiness and the awakening of a whole new range of sensations in the palate varyingly described as cleansing, bitter, refreshing, soothing, disgusting, pungent or vile. The initial reactions clients have to taking herbal medicines are often revealing of the extent to which the palate has shifted away from these strong, earthy, natural flavours to accommodate the artificially sweet, mushy, bland and uniform textures which typify a Western diet. The multi-faceted nature of herbal medicine requires a knowledge of basic pharmacy, which is really no more than the skills acquired by any good cook; it encourages the development of the skills of an amateur botanist and naturalist, whilst also inspiring a greater understanding of a wide range of ecological issues.

Herbs as everyday foods or medicinal meals

The availability and restorative properties of everyday basic foods such as porridge (oats), barley, horseradish, mustard, garlic, onions, alfalfa sprouts, celery, seaweeds, asparagus, chicory, endive, potatoes, carrots, artichokes, walnuts, almonds, pumpkin and sesame seeds (tahini), watercress, honey, fresh leaves of dandelions, parsley, coriander, dill, chickweed or young nettle tops all offer even the most reluctant an opportunity to begin to think herbally. It may be a useful and normalising process to begin the exploration of using herbs by regarding them essentially as food items at one end of the same continuum which also holds the potential for their transformation into medicines. This approach embraces a period in history which preceded the Cartesian dualism so fundamental to Western biomedicine. It was a time when many classifications were more holistic; where food was medicine and this common knowledge was a legacy enjoyed by people untroubled by the specialisms so divisive in orthodox medicine today. Herbs can be seen as the 'original food' containing all the essential vitamins, minerals and trace elements required by the body. This has great relevance as an ever increasing range of our food is increasingly denatured through the widespread use of fertilisers, pesticides and irradiation. Although herbs suffer in a similar way from environmental degradation, there are sources available for the purchase of organically grown herbs and the amounts required for regular consumption are relatively small. As many herbs are amenable to grow in tubs or windowsill containers, it requires comparatively little effort for even city dwellers to enjoy a year round supply of many culinary staples such as sage, thyme, chives or mint, all of which also incorporate useful medicinal properties.

How do herbs work?

Herbal medicine is health rather than disease orientated, with the aim of enhancing constitutional strengths rather than concentrating on the disruptive effects of illness. As individual needs are distinctive and reflective of a unique physiology, the highly personal experience of suffering is paramount in formulating a prescription which focuses on this person rather than on their complaint. Plants used for both nutritional and medicinal purposes are more in harmony with the natural, physiological rhythms of the body than the orientation of pills, vaccines or other synthetic substances promising instant relief of symptoms. In this way, consideration is given to the overall process rather than the discrete, mechanical functioning of isolated (bodily) parts.

This philosophical concept of holism is further mirrored in the way herbalists use the whole plant for its total medicinal value, rather than the fragmented approach of biomedicine which concentrates on isolating only the active constituent for administration. The lower concentration and more dilute solutions of the complex mixtures of chemicals present in the whole plant also greatly reduces the risk of side effects. Using all parts of the plant in this way tends to ameliorate the effects of the more potent constituents thus facilitating better tolerance. Another feature of herbal medicine which helps to keep effective doses low and hence reduces the likelihood of side effects is illustrated by the concept of synergism. This can be seen where the different ingredients of a single herb or prescription might otherwise interact, thereby increasing the effective response beyond what would be expected from the sum total of the individual constituents. For example, tiny amounts of cayenne (*Capsicum minimum*) will enhance the effectiveness of any other herb included in the prescription by increasing their rate of distribution through the blood vessels. Similarly, the flavanoids found in hawthorn (*Crataegus* spp.) can be isolated, extracted and will still have beneficial effects on the heart, but use of the whole plant in its natural form allows smaller doses, which are even more effective, to be given (National Institute of Medical Herbalists, 1991).

A knowledge of pharmacology, or the effect of drugs on the body, is integral to the study of herbal medicine. Within biomedicine, this fascinating exploration has been narrowed down to an absurd and artificial examination of the effects of isolated chemical constituents on isolated cells, structures or functions of the body. An attempt is then made to reassemble these fragmented observations and extrapolate from this the likely effects upon 'real' people with demonstrable illnesses. This approach favoured the development of synthetic drugs from the templates provided by plants and resulted in the extraction of ergotamine from ergot of rye, morphine and codeine from opium poppies, atropine from deadly nightshade, pilocarpine from jaborandi, reserpine from rauwolfia, digoxin from foxgloves, aspirin from willow bark, quinine from cinchona bark, anti-ulcer drugs from liquorice, anti-cancer drugs from periwinkle and yew and so on.

Offering a sharp contrast to the explicitly material and physical application of orthodox pharmacology, a traditional pharmacology 'must start with the human experience of an agent, a well charted catalogue of effects on mind and body as well as spirit.' (Mills, 1993). This view never loses sight of the 'whole' nor of the axiom that not only is this whole greater than the sum of its parts, but actually plays a decisive role in determining them. Carol MacCormack refers to this 'one' as all things; as incomplete without the least of them and yet with all the parts retaining their full identity. She goes on to urge that 'once this concept, so congruent with Bohm's theory of wholeness and the implicate order is grasped, it frees us from Cartesian dualism' (MacCormack, 1991; see also Bohm, 1980)

The medicinal property ascribed to a particular herb then, is not that of a single, active constituent, but rather an entire orchestra of ingredients working synergistically and thereby reinforcing the overall positive effect of the herb. The incredible complexity of this vast array of chemical components, all possibly interacting with one another in a (mostly) unknown and infinitely variable manner, has posed something of a dilemma for the needs of orthodox medicine regarding standardization, predictability of action and the need for replication. Yet, as clinical pharmacology knows full well, this state of affairs is illusory as is demonstrated by the administration of digoxin or insulin with its variable results on different patients, with the acknowledgement that tailoring the dose to the individual's real life situation will inevitably be necessary. The herbalist, in common with most alternative practitioners, begins from accepting the premise that although life is infinitely variable, it does follow a distinct pattern. It is also acknowledged that although fluctuations exist, they are within workable limits.

A few considerations for pregnancy . . .

The general health of the woman and her partner (or other sperm donor if this is practical) could usefully be assessed in terms of nutrition, exercise, attitudes, the quality of existing relationships, domestic and working environments etc. before pregnancy is contemplated. Life being what it is, the confirmation of pregnancy frequently serves as the trigger for stimulating thought in this direction. As gestation is a time of growth and nourishment, only herbs supporting this process should be used. Included in this list would be all of the herbs-as-food mentioned earlier, plus those more traditionally considered as such: chamomile, lime blossom, red clover, lemon balm, rosehips, cleavers, raspberry leaves, vervain, St John's wort, nasturtium, calendula and borage flowers, thyme, basil, peppermint, ginger, orange blossom and scullcap.

It is important to emphasise that we are healthy and perfect most of the time; that healing begins by doing 'nothing' other than honouring this innate ability to heal ourselves. It should also be remembered that pregnancy is a natural state which a woman's body is perfectly able to accommodate without the need for any intervention, be it herbal or otherwise. Women need every encouragement to believe that it is their own powerful bodies which have carried and birthed their babies; that it is they and not alternative medicine that has accomplished this extraordinary miracle.

The routine use of herbal medicine in pregnancy is generally not advocated unless treatment for an existing complaint has been instigated prior to conception, in which case the advice of the practitioner should be sought. Although most health problems are self limiting, the appropriate use of herbal remedies during pregnancy ensures that acute episodes of illness do not become established as chronic and debilitating patterns of ill health. Whilst it is an established and commendable principle that pregnant women (and those still in the planning and breast-feeding stages) abstain from taking medicine of any variety, there are notable exceptions to this. In women whose constitutions may be weakened by previous childbirth, poor nutrition, unhappy relationships, unemployment, homelessness, chronic ill health or other stresses associated with the overcrowding and poverty of modern living, pregnancy may be perceived by the body as an intolerable stress. In such cases herbal support from a qualified practitioner may be warranted throughout pregnancy.

Jill was a 29 year old mother of two, who came at 16 weeks' gestation for herbal treatment of recurrent urinary tract infections. In her first pregnancy this had led to hospitalisation for pyelonephritis. Her second pregnancy followed a similar pattern although hospitalisation was avoided by the continuous use of antibiotics from 24 weeks through until her mid-stream urine returned clear at 8 days postpartum.

Her second son, a healthy term baby, was born at home as planned. After discussion with the midwives she and her partner decided against the administration of vitamin K. Unfortunately at 5 weeks, this baby became seriously ill and required a blood transfusion because of vitamin K deficiency. It was eventually postulated that this had been caused by the prolonged use of antibiotics affecting the intestinal mucosa and interfering with the production of intrinsic factor. She had not been warned that her baby was at any greater risk from not receiving vitamin K.

Jill's past medical history included bladder problems as a child manifesting in bed wetting and incontinence until 12 years of age. All investigations at the time were negative and symptoms ceased spontaneously until her first pregnancy. Family history also revealed that her father underwent a unilateral nephrectomy for kidney stones and recent ultrasound indicated the presence of stones in his remaining kidney.

A recent mid-stream urine showed positive growth for which antibiotics had been advised but which Jill had refused to take. The usual measures outlined later in the chapter for the management of cystitis were instigated, as was ingestion of a clove of garlic daily, which the whole family enjoyed rather than suffer the secondhand effects. Herbal treatment included using herbs such as golden rod, lemon balm, roses, plantain and thyme in the form of a tea with additional support from a tincture including horsetail, agrimony, uva ursi and marshmallow. The aim was to strengthen the mucous membrane of the urinary tract and gently stimulate the immune system whilst reducing the irritation in the genitourinary system with soothing demulcents. A base oil containing essential oils of hyssop, pine and lavender was prepared and massaged over the kidney area four or five times weekly from 30 weeks onwards.

Two acute episodes of cystitis were treated using tincture of purple cone flower with parsley piert. One further episode at 32 weeks, precipitated by Jill omitting her medicine for a whole week as she had felt so well, required a course of antibiotics. These were taken in conjunction with vitamin C and acidophilus with bifidus capsules.

Jill went on to deliver her third baby boy at home after a quick labour in her 43rd week of pregnancy and was subsequently transferred to the care of the health visitor for non-herbal care, with the advice to continue the tea for a further 6–8 weeks.

Herbal preparation for pregnancy

When considering health issues at this time, there is a myopic tendency to focus exclusively on the interval between confirmation of pregnancy and the birth of the baby. A herbal approach would extend this time to around 13 months in order that time be allowed for 'preparing the ground' for the demands of pregnancy and birthing, whilst also making space to 'tend the fruit(s)' afterwards. Due attention is thus paid to the heavy demands of parenting and the reshaping of relationships.

The time before a pregnancy is conceived may be well spent in 'spring cleaning' the internal environment of the body in order that the 'ground' referred to earlier is well prepared. As with any growing organism, it seems reasonable to expect that the more attention given at this stage will see results in the development of a healthy baby and in anticipating an uncomplicated birth. The depletion states so commonly seen in new mothers and which adversely affect such processes as healing of the perineum and the establishment of lactation, may also be minimised.

Certain principles are essential to this concept and would be incorporated into a herbal approach. They would include an evaluation of existing bodily functions such as absorption, elimination, relaxation, regeneration, growth, repair, nourishment and reserve capacity as well as an appreciation of the role of the circulation in maintaining homeostasis. Attention is directed towards the liver, kidneys and adrenal glands as these organs are particularly vulnerable to the stresses of pregnancy. These same precepts may be usefully applied where there has been difficulty in conceiving or in maintaining a pregnancy in the absence of any demonstrable pathology.

Mandy, a 35 year old woman, asked for help in conceiving following a 2 year period of infertility.

Her menarche occurred at 13 years of age with a 'regularly irregular' cycle established by her mid teens and which had remained unchanged. One pregnancy had been terminated 8 years previously and was currently a source of great emotional pain and grief. A referral by her GP to her local hospital for blood tests and an ultrasound scan had been inconclusive. She was now awaiting laparoscopy. Assessment of her partner's sperm for motility and volume showed that it was normal.

There had been many episodes of pelvic inflammatory disease during her early twenties following use of an IUD. Current complaints included both occupational stress and that directly related to the consequences of her infertility, skin rashes and osteoarthritis in both feet from years of classical ballet since her teens. There was no other relevant medical or family history. She was not taking any medication apart from vitamin B complex which had been found helpful for dysmenorrhoea. Anticipating pregnancy, I suggested she commence Folic Acid – 400 mcg daily – and to continue until 12 weeks pregnancy (Expert Advisory Group, D.O.H., 1992).

Dietary advice focused on her patterns of binge eating, particularly fatty and sugary foods and her high caffeine intake of four cups of tea and six cups of coffee daily. Treatment over the following 3 months focused on balancing her cycle with the use of tinctures of chasteberry and other herbs such as capsicum, cleavers, liquorice, valerian, St John's wort and helionas root to improve circulation, nourish and soothe the organs of the reproductive system and activate the lymphatic system whilst gently repairing a rather frayed nervous system. A tea made from equal parts of lime blossom, catnip, borage and lemon balm was consumed concurrently.

She conceived at the beginning of the fourth month and was advised to stop the main mixture but to carry on with the tea and chasteberry tincture. Two episodes of spotting with fresh blood at 8 and 10 weeks were remedied with an increased dose of chasteberry which was discontinued in week 15. A pregnancy tea comprising equal parts of lemon balm, nettles and raspberry leaves was enjoyed from about 30 weeks of pregnancy until 2 months postpartum.

A beautiful baby boy was born at home as planned; an ecstatic event in water following a 5 hour labour. The puerperium was uneventful with breast feeding continuing for 7 months. She is now pregnant again and has achieved this spontaneously, 12 months after weaning.

If a conception is planned for late spring/early summer, fortuitous use may be made of the greedy spring herbs, all of which draw up huge quantities of nutrients from the soil to fuel their dramatic growth rate. Examples might include chickweed, comfrey leaves, ground ivy, purslane, samphire, sorrel, nettles, cleavers, lambs' lettuce, wild asparagus, watercress and dandelion leaves. All of these plants, storehouses of essential vitamins and minerals, are powerful cleansing agents in the body, and the leaves when picked young can be used raw in salads or soups. Sorrel and samphire are traditional ingredients in the French 'soupe aux herbes' and the attention this culture gives to the liver in particular and to eating in general, is well recognised! Spring tonics are not just nutritious foods; they are tonics in the true sense of the word in that they stimulate the liver, invigorate the digestion and thereby increase the body's vitality by promoting more effective assimilation and elimination. Like most tonics, they need to be used regularly for maximum benefit, i.e. three to five times weekly. A reminder might be in order here that this is not the time to 'diet' but rather to use to full advantage the impulse of change conferred by pregnancy to review (unhealthy) eating patterns.

During pregnancy . . . problems and herbal solutions

Examples of conditions that occur during pregnancy and labour and the puerperium are discussed in this section. The list is not intended to be comprehensive but rather to give a flavour of a herbal approach which is safe and accessible.

List of problem conditions discussed below

Morning sickness	Exhaustion in labour
Threatened miscarriage	Perineal care
Varicose veins, haemorrhoids and constipation	Pain
	Engorgement and mastitis
Anaemia	Sore nipples
Heartburn	Heavy bleeding
Infections	Lactation
Mood changes or fatigue	

In parallel with much of medicine, the use of particular herbs is equally affected by the vagaries of fashion as by the results of any research. The herbs suggested are commonly available and mainly indigenous plants. The idea is to encourage a greater familiarity with our native flora and also to listen to the wisdom of the body over the words of any book; if the herb works for you, make a note of the circumstances and try it again.

Complicated or life-threatening conditions such as eclampsia or full-blown postpartum haemorrhage have been deliberately omitted as the knowledge and experience required to treat complicated or chronic conditions is beyond the scope of this chapter. What follows is intended to familiarise the midwife and interested lay person with commonly used herbs and their common applications during women's childbearing/rearing years. Looking herbally at health issues which arise around this time is essentially not so different from what might be expected at any major life change. What is so exciting and challenging is recognising that the judicious use of herbs may help to make the journey through pregnancy and birth less troublesome, whilst also facilitating an easier transition to mothering.

Accurate data about herbs known to adversely affect pregnancy is scarce, often contradictory and vague. What is available has mostly been gleaned from anthropological studies and older herbals by popularisers of folk medicine rather than by practising herbalists. Consult modern herbals with this proviso as the contents may reflect an exercise in information gathering rather than any real knowledge based on working experience. For a list of herbs to generally avoid from the planning stages of pregnancy to the cessation of breast feeding, see Appendix 1, p. 176.

Morning sickness There is a connection between nausea in early pregnancy and low blood sugar. Maintain blood sugar levels by frequent snacking, two to three hourly, on high protein/unprocessed carbohydrate foods such as oatcakes with tahini, miso soup with wholemeal bread, peanut butter on rice cakes etc. Regular exercise will encourage the body to eliminate toxins which may contribute to headaches and nausea. Increase the intake of dietary iron and vitamin B complex (see Appendix 4 (ii), p. 179). Avoid foods which are spicy or greasy; even the smell may be nauseating. Tea and coffee should be avoided as the tannins in the former inhibit the absorption of iron and the stimulating effect of caffeine contained in both may provoke nausea and headaches.

Herbal remedies Drink a cup of anise, fennel, meadowsweet, spearmint or peppermint tea with a dry cracker on waking. Keep a thermos of hot water or the electric kettle and a choice of teas by the bed to avoid having to get out of bed on an empty stomach.

Before sleeping, enjoy an infusion of chamomile, hops or lemon balm with a small carbohydrate snack. Sip infusions made from grated fresh ginger root or Iceland moss when nausea is particulary bothersome or if compounded by travel sickness. If available, powdered ginger root may be taken in capsule form. A cup or so of raspberry leaf tea daily, besides being a pregnancy tonic recommended from the second trimester onwards, is also effective. All of these infusions may be frozen and sucked as ice cubes if preferred. Some also 'marry' well in combinations for example ginger and chamomile. Chew or suck slippery elm tablets available from most health food shops.

It is not uncommon to find the beneficial effects of remedies quite short lived for this particular problem. What often works is drinking the herbs in rotation over a cycle of a few days in order to avoid incurring the tolerance which temporarily renders the herb ineffective. In persistent cases, a visit to a qualified herbalist may be necessary for more specific herbs such as wild yam or gentian roots. Many of these more powerful herbs are restricted from over-the-counter use and are administered in the form of tinctures. Very small doses in the form of drops is often all that is required.

Threatened miscarriage The outcome for women with a history of repeated miscarriage will be greatly improved if treatment has been given for varying lengths of time before pregnancy is attempted. This will enable nutritional deficiencies to be corrected, lifestyle habits to be addressed and any specific problems to be diagnosed. Both partners may require treatment.

Once bright red blood loss occurs, especially if accompanied by cramping, it is generally acknowledged that the pregnancy cannot be conserved. It is recommended that a scan be performed on any woman reporting fresh blood loss at any stage of the pregnancy, particulary in the second and third trimester.

Folklore has it that if the miscarriage results from a fetal abnormality or misplacement of the placenta, herbal remedies will not impede this natural process.

Herbal remedies Crampbark, as the name suggests, is specific for the relief of muscular tension and is a useful remedy where there is no suggestion of an underlying hormonal dysfunction. As a preventative, it may be taken in the form of a cup of the decoction daily throughout pregnancy or as drops: 10–20 drops at 30–60 minute intervals until symptoms subside.

Black haw bark, closely related to crampbark, is specific as a sedative and relaxant to the uterine muscle and may be taken in the same way.

Helionas root is a powerful tonic particularly where women report a history of repeated miscarriage and the suggestion emerges of irritability of the uterus or poor tone in the cervix. A decoction of the root is prepared and a half teacup consumed twice daily or five drops of the tincture twice to three times daily is recommended.

Chasteberry has a balancing action on the activity on the female sex hormones making it a herb of choice where miscarriage threatens around the time when placental functioning begins. It is generally administered in the form of a tincture, 10–20 drops at 15–60 minute intervals until symptoms have subsided.

Raspberry leaf tea may be consumed throughout pregnancy in the form of one to two teacups daily when miscarriage has threatened or where a previous pattern exists. As a 'partus praeparator', the astringing, tightening properties of this herb suggest its application be reserved for the last trimester in primiparous women or from the middle of the second trimester in multiparous women. As the toning action lends itself to the process of involution, infusions can be enjoyed for 1–2 months after childbirth.

Wherever possible, encourage women to rest in bed and spend a little time doing pelvic floor and appropriate visualisation or relaxation exercises. Support this process with soothing infusions of lime blossom, scullcap, orange blossom or lemon balm. In cases of severe anxiety, a herbalist might recommend the addition of valerian root.

If it seems apparent that a miscarriage has occurred and women would prefer to allow the process to complete itself naturally without recourse to an evacuation of the retained products of conception, in the absence of infection or haemorrhage the following herbal support may be advised:

- To control bleeding drink infusions of raspberry leaf, Lady's mantle, plantain or freshly picked shepherd's purse. Tincture of golden seal may also be administered at a dose of 10 drops four to six times daily.
- Recommend that the diet contain plenty of iron rich foods (see Appendix 4 (i), p. 179) and a clove of raw garlic daily as a protective measure against infection. Crushing and mixing the latter with yoghurt, tahini or peanut butter before spreading on bread or a cracker will reduce any tendency toward digestive upset. The superlative antiseptic effects of garlic are nullified by heat; cooked garlic has negligible medicinal effects.

Varicose veins, haemorrhoids and constipation Varicosities may occur in the legs, vulva or at the anus as haemorrhoids. A tendency towards them is often inherited but much can be achieved through implementing lifestyle and dietary changes. Leg cramps or spasms may be an accompanying feature which may indicate a deficiency of calcium in the diet.

Yoga positions which hold gentle, inverted postures such as lying in the dorsal position with the feet and legs raised above the hips are recommended. Relax in this position for 10 or 15 minutes and repeat twice daily. Fully inverted poses such as the plough, shoulder and head stands should not be attempted without expert guidance.

Regular swimming or a daily brisk walk stimulates the circulation, aids digestion and encourages regular bowel function.

Constipation, if a feature, may be lessened or eliminated by ensuring that the diet comprises a wide variety of fresh fruits, vegetables, unrefined carbohydrates, grains, nuts and pulses with a minimum of 2 litres of water daily. Ordinary tea and coffee should be avoided as should bran. The latter absorbs fluid from the colon, hardens the stool, and aggravates constipation. Linseed, acting as a gentle aperient, may be used as an alternative to bran and sprinkled over food or mixed with water.

The inclusion of raw garlic and onions are strongly recommended as powerful circulation tonics with the former having marked antihypertensive properties (Foushee *et al.*, 1982). The addition of both fresh parsley and nettles in the diet, whether directly in salads or soups or enjoyed as herbal infusions, will gradually improve the elasticity of the veins.

Herbal remedies Lotions, compresses or creams made from comfrey, marshmallow, marigold, plantain, yarrow or hawthorn berries can be used.

If staining of the skin is not worrisome, use a decoction of oak and witchazel barks combined with any of the above herbs as a local wash or sitz bath for particularly painful veins or haemorrhoids. Grated raw potato may be applied directly to haemorrhoids to ease swelling and pain. For longer term treatment and particularly following defecation, use pilewort cream combined with an equal quantity of comfrey cream. Add 10 drops of essential oil of Cypress to 30 grams of cream where rectal bleeding is an accompanying feature.

Decoctions of dandelion root have a gently laxative effect thereby counteracting any tendency toward constipation. Regular infusions of lime blossom or fresh ginger root soothe and strengthen the tone of the venous system with overall improvement in the entire circulatory system.

Anaemia In the majority of cases where an uncomplicated iron deficiency anaemia presents, concerted dietary efforts may be all that is required:

- Ensure the diet is wholefood based with an abundance of fresh, green leafy vegetables including seaweeds, watercress, dandelion leaves, nettle tops, lamb's lettuce, parsley, chicory, sprouted grains and seeds, spring onions and chives.
- Include plenty of dried, dark fruits such as hunza (or other unsulphured) apricots, figs, raisins, currants and of course, prunes. Soak overnight in plenty of water and eat as a breakfast compôte. Add blackcurrants, blackberries, loganberries etc. as seasonally available.
- Incorporate wholegrains present in bread, chapattis and oatcakes; also nuts (almonds), fish (shellfish, pilchards, kippers, salmon), legumes (pea and bean families) and include vecon concentrate in soup stock.
- Use cane molasses as a sweetening agent in place of honey or sugar.
- Offal, particularly liver, although rich in stored iron may also contain residues of waste toxins. Locate an organic source if possible.

Iron absorption is seriously compromised by the ingestion of bran which forms insoluble phytates in the digestive system thereby inhibiting the uptake of available dietary iron. The drinking of tea and coffee worsens the situation especially if these are consumed with meals.

Vitamin C facilitates iron absorption and is found in most fresh fruits and vegetables but particularly in the following: kiwifruits, potatoes, fresh oranges, rosehips freshly gathered in the autumn, parsley leaves, broccoli, Brussel sprouts and cauliflower.

Floradix, a concentrated iron preparation from vegetable sources, is a useful alternative to ferrous sulphate. Unfortunately, its tendency to fermentation makes it unsuitable for women with a history of thrush (*Candida albicans*), for whom a better recommendation would be chelated iron, generally available from wholefood shops.

Herbal remedies   Decoctions of yellow dock root combined with infusions of leaves from nettles, parsley, comfrey and peppermint.

Heartburn   Employ the usual measures such as eating small, regular, frequent meals which are well chewed and enjoyed in a calm, unhurried atmosphere. Avoid drinking whilst eating but do ensure an adequate fluid intake between meals. Eliminate any foods which aggravate (e.g. spicey, greasy or unfamiliar) and be mindful that common culprits include coffee, alcohol and cigarettes.

Herbal remedies   Add carminative seeds of anise, caraway, dill or fennel to cooked food. These can also be chewed or enjoyed as decoctions after a meal. Infusions of Iceland moss, lemon balm, chamomile or meadowsweet may be consumed throughout the day. In severe cases, a teaspoon of powdered slippery elm bark mixed with water and honey, or flavoured with a little cinnamon or ginger soothes the oesophageal and gastric mucosa whilst also neutralising gastric acid. Slippery elm is commonly available from wholefoods shops in the form of tablets or lozenges which should be slowly sucked or chewed before swallowing. Follow with a small glass of fluid.

Infections   Where a history of any urogenital infection exists, employ the usual measures such as wearing loose, cotton underwear which is changed daily; avoid all refined sugars (and in the case of *Candida*, all yeast-containing products), tea, coffee and alcohol; drink at least 2 litres of water daily; gently wash the genital area after urinating, defecating or sexual intercourse.

As with any infections, these are more likely to occur when the body defences are not functioning to full capacity. Lowered resistance may be due to a number of things such as chronic tiredness, emotional shock, poor diet or chronic constipation, all of which need to be remedied if recurrence of infection is to be prevented.

Partners of sexually active women require concurrent treatment even in the absence of symptoms. The use of condoms is advisable for male partners until laboratory investigations return negative cultures.

If antibiotics are required, concurrently take a course of yeast-free acidophilus with bifidus capsules and vitamin C (1 gram daily for a week) in conjunction with liberal helpings of live yoghurt to rebalance the intestinal/vaginal flora and reduce the likelihood of initiating the common cycle of cystitis–antibiotic treatment – *Candida* infection.

Herbal sitz baths or washes can be used instead of soaps or body shampoo. Use clean hands for washing yourself rather than damp flannels which simply encourage the spread of infection. Vaginal deodorants have no place in women's hygiene but especially where the genital area is troubled.

As acute infections of the urinary and genital tracts may be implicated with the onset of premature labour, the expertise of a qualified herbalist should be sought if symptoms persist.

Herbal remedies The ubiquitous garlic holds pride of place in treatment: ingest at least a clove daily in the manner previously described. Any partners of sexually active women should indulge in a similar fashion.

Cystitis Cook pearl barley with double the usual quantity of water; strain off and drink the remaining fluid as barley water to which may be added a little lemon juice. Where this has been a recurring problem, alternate infusions of nettle and marigold and drink one or two teacups daily throughout pregnancy. Consume a minimum of 1 pint of tea (infusion) brewed from equal quantities of thyme and marshmallow with either cornsilk, couchgrass or horsetail. A decoction of liquorice root may be added to the mixture for its soothing and aromatic qualities. Where fever or haematuria are present, use equal parts of yarrow, agrimony, plantain and uva ursi, two to three cups daily for no longer than 7 days. Where kidney pain is present or there is a past history of pyelonephritis, refer early to a qualified herbalist.

Herpes The use of nerve tonics such as oats, St John's wort, vervain, damiana and lavender are indicated and taken as an infusion; two or three teacups daily. Decoctions prepared from roots of dandelion and burdock will support this action by acting as internal cleansers and restoratives. Sitz baths of herbs such as lavender, thyme, marshmallow, marigold and witchazel will all provide local relief. Ointments from marigold or St John's wort, combined with either comfrey (where the skin is friable) or chickweed (when itching is present), may be liberally applied. Infused oils of any of these herbs may be used instead of ointments. Essential oils of Ti tree, melissa or geranium may be added directly to the sitz bath or 5–15 drops per 30 gram base cream or per 30 ml base oil. Diluted tincture of myrrh, if applied to the blisters, will sting but will encourage them to dry up quickly.

Candida Most commonly isolated from the vagina, mouth or nipples, but may be systemic or may first appear as a red, angry 'nappy rash' in a new born infant. Many of the recommendations for cystitis and herpes above are applicable and may be tried. In a breastfeeding mother, anticipate an infective 'loop' between her and baby. Both will need treatment.

Immune system restorative herbs such as purple cone flower, marigold, thyme or wild indigo are indicated in persistent cases. Use these in combination with mucous membrane restorative herbs such as golden rod, ground ivy or plantain. A clove of peeled, raw garlic wrapped in muslin, well oiled and placed in the vagina will act as an effective local antiseptic. Change once or twice daily, being careful not to nick the flesh of the clove when peeling as the juices will sting the inflamed mucous membrane.

Mood changes or fatigue Pregnancy is a time when the sensitivities of both mother and baby are very powerful. Herb baths using the flowers of roses, lavender, borage, daises or chamomile all nurture this aspect.

Women and midwives often need encouragement to take their 'soul' needs seriously; to make space for music, art and contact with nature, all of which are too often considered an irrelevant indulgence in the mainstream of antenatal 'care'.

Given the influence that food has on emotions and moods, concentrate on high protein snacks and eliminate all refined carbohydrates, especially anything containing white sugar.

Herbal remedies Infusions of raspberry leaf in combination with equal quantities of either peppermint or spearmint will calm and lift the spirits. The addition of the bitter tonics such as burdock, blessed thistle or orange peel help to maintain emotional balance. Where sleep is of poor quality, an infusion of hops or scullcap before bedtime will facilitate a more restful night. In addition, a qualified herbalist might prescribe a little tincture of rosemary or motherwort for overwhelming symptoms.

Exhaustion in labour This is relatively uncommon when women have been encouraged to follow their natural rhythms in eating, drinking and taking short naps.

Herbal remedies Infusions of fresh ginger root either alone or added to raspberry leaf tea with a little honey will enhance stamina and mental focus. As ginger stimulates local local circulation, do not use when birth is imminent or within an hour afterwards. An infusion of rosemary, either added to the bath water or sipped as a tea, acts as a stimulating tonic where fatigue and a sense of hopelessness threaten. It may be combined with vervain. Ginseng, either as a decoction, the root chewed whole or in tincture form, increases vitality and physical performance during long, arduous labours. A substantial body of research supports many of the traditional claims for this herb, including its effective use in supporting the body to better withstand stress (Fulder, 1987). Ginseng should not be taken in conjunction with caffeine or other stimulants or where there is a history of hypertension or headaches.

Perineal care Massaging the perineum from 37 weeks of pregnancy onwards invites women and their partners to give some attention to an often neglected, but very important part of the body. As with so many aspects of pregnancy care, there is a dearth of research on this subject, although it seems plausible that regular applications of nourishing oils such as wheatgerm or avocado combined with sweet almond oil encourages suppleness, elasticity and a sense of familiarity and deepening trust.

Encouraging a hopeful, optimistic attitude is particularly important where a woman's previous experience of childbirth has left her feeling miserable and anxious after months or years of pain or infection and the inevitable build up of scar tissue in the perineal area.

A perineal tear where the edges approximate well does not need suturing if the mother can rest in bed for a few days, eat well and use the perineal soaks suggested below. Low haemoglobin and zinc status compromise tissue healing. To raise haemoglobin levels, employ the dietary and other recommendations for anaemia. Dietary sources of zinc include ginger root, parsley, potatoes, garlic, turnips, carrots, beans, muscle meats (lamb chops and steak) split peas, corn, nuts, egg yolk, wholewheat, rye, oats, buckwheat and fresh oysters.

Herbal remedies Following birth, where the perineum is swollen, torn or bruised, use a warm decoction of oak and comfrey barks, to which is added an infusion of marigold and lavender flowers. Where damage to the deeper muscle layers is evident, or where there is a risk of infection developing, add a tablespoon of slippery elm and golden seal powders mixed in equal quantities. Strain off the liquid, add sufficient water to a large washing-up bowl or bidet, and soak the perineum for 20 or 30 minutes twice daily. Where sutures have been inserted, limit the soaks to once daily. Encourage pelvic floor exercises during the soaking time to draw a little of the healing fluid into the vagina.

Pain When women are supported and encouraged to labour in a familiar environment where they feel safe and secure, pain is generally within the expectations of a normal labour. Within this context, it serves as an early warning signal that all is not well.

Herbal remedies Motherwort is a useful herb for allaying anxiety and tension, particularly in early labour or for 'false' labour pains. As it is very bitter, it is best taken in tincture form: five to ten drops in a small glass of water and repeat once or twice hourly.

The sedative effect of scullcap makes it a useful herb throughout labour, acting by generally easing and dispersing the tension accompanying and accumulating with pain. It may be drunk as an infusion or sipped from a glass of water to which has been added one teaspoon of the tincture.

St John's wort is a useful remedy for relieving the crampy, spasmodic pains which are a specific feature of some labours. Use in the form of an infusion or add 20 to 30 drops to a glass of water. It combines well with scullcap.

Infusions of catnip leaves are an effective remedy for afterpains helping to relieve cramping uterine spasm and facilitating the flow of lochia.

Engorgement and mastitis Anticipate mastitis at the engorgement stage and act accordingly, as herbal treatment is sure but slow acting.

Herbal remedies In cases of uncomplicated engorgement, use the leaves of a green or white cabbage as a lining inside the bra. This will draw heat from the breast, cooking the cabbage as it does so. Change when limp. Cold poultices from grated raw potato or carrot have a similar effect.

Hot compresses of parsley or comfrey, prepared by tying a handful of the leaves into an old piece of cotton material and immersing in simmering water for 10 minutes, are also effective. Allow to cool until just tolerable before applying to the breast(s).

Immersing the breast(s) in an infusion of marshmallow root and fennel seeds prepared and left to stand overnight before reheating and leaving to cool makes a delightfully soothing, slippery soak for tender, inflamed breasts.

In stubborn cases, give 20–40 drops of purple cone flower tincture at hourly intervals until symptoms subside.

The ingestion of garlic in breastfeeding mothers significantly improves suckling time, with the obvious effect of improved drainage and reduction in engorgement. Research into the sensory qualities of human milk, found that babies sucked more efficiently and for longer periods when the milk was flavoured with garlic (Mennella and Beauchamp, 1991). Garlic also has the antiseptic effect described earlier, an important consideration in avoiding the unnecessary use of antibiotics.

Sore nipples If thrush is suspected, employ the measures suggested earlier.

Herbal remedies As it is difficult to remove all traces of creams and ointments from the nipple/areola, treat conservatively where possible by washing the nipples well with infusions of marigold or comfrey and expose to the air or sunlight. The application of crushed ice made from either of the above herbs and applied just before feeding is an effective local painkiller and also draws out soft, small or partially inverted nipples. Ointments from comfrey or yarrow are particularly effective in healing cracked nipples and relieving pain. The clear gel of a fresh aloe vera leaf will soothe and heal sore nipples but care must be taken to wash it off properly before nursing as the bitter taste will prevent the baby latching on correctly. The underside of geranium leaves soothes and heals cracks if placed in direct contact with the nipple inside the bra.

Heavy bleeding Once the initial emergency has been effectively dealt with, employ the measures suggested above for 'Threatened miscarriage' (see p. 166).

Herbal remedies Two to three teacups daily of infusions of Lady's mantle or freshly gathered shepherd's purse, combined with raspberry leaf and nettles is recommended for 3–4 days following birth where heavy blood loss has been sustained. Continue infusions of raspberry leaf and nettles for a further 4–6 weeks.

Lactation Establishing lactation in a first time mother requires enormous amounts of patience and time for midwives and mothers.

Herbal remedies Supporting herbs for this process include infusions of comfrey, milk thistle, red clover, alfalfa, nettles, fenugreek and hops. Borage, blessed thistle, wood betony and oats (as porridge) all act as antidepressant herbs, lifting the spirits as well as ensuring an abundant milk supply. Fennel seeds make a delicious tea to be sipped throughout the day before chewing and swallowing the seeds. Besides improving milk flow, fennel has the added bonus of relieving infant colic.

Training

Training for membership of the National Institute of Medical Herbalists may currently be undertaken either as a full-time course attending 3 days per week over 4 years or as a part-time correspondence course to accommodate those with occupational or family commitments. Discretionary grants may be available from local authorities upon enquiry. Besides the usual academic pre-entry requirements, students are required to pass examinations in key subjects throughout the course. Five hundred hours of clinical attendance must be certified before the final exams may be taken. The letters MINIH or FNIMH indicate an accredited member of the institute.

For further information contact:
The School of Herbal Medicine,
Bucksteep Manor, Bodle Street Green, Nr Hailsham,
East Sussex BN27 4RJ, UK
Tel: 0323 833812

Details of a qualified local herbalist may be obtained from:
Hon. General Secretary, NIMH
9 Palace Gate, Exeter, Devon EX1 1JA, UK
Tel: 0392 426022

A B.Sc. in Herbal Medicine will commence at Middlesex University (North London) in the academic year 1994–95. This will comprise the usual 4 year undergraduate syllabus with the requirement of a further year for those wishing to qualify for application for membership to the National Institute of Medical Herbalists. For further details, contact the university directly.

References

Achterberg J. (1990) *Woman as Healer*, p. 1. Shambala Publications.

Bohm D. (1980) *Wholeness and the Implicate Order*. Ark.

British Medical Association (1993) *Complementary Medicine, New Approaches to Good Practice*. Oxford University Press.

Brookes E. (1993) *Women Healers Through History*, pp. 36–39. The Woman's Press.

Carper J. (1992) *The Food Pharmacy*. Positive Paperbacks.

Cashford J. and Baring A. (1991) *The Myth of the Goddess; Evolution of an Image*, p. xi. Viking Arkana.

Davies S. and Stewart A. (1987) *Nutritional Medicine*. Pan Books,

Ehrenreich B. and English D. (1973) *Witches, Midwives and Nurses, A History of Women Healers*, p. 13. The Feminist Press.

Ernest E. (1987) Cardiovascular effects of garlic: a review. *Pharmatherapeutica*, **5**, 83–89.

Estrada A. (Ed.) *Marina Sabina: her Life and Chants*. Ross Erikson Inc.

Expert Advisory Group (1992) *Folic Acid and The Prevention of Neural Tube Defects*. Department of Health.

Expert Maternity Group (1993) *Changing Childbirth*. Department of Health.

Foushee D.B. *et al.* (1982) Garlic as a natural agent for the treatment of hypertension. *Cytobios*, **34**, 145–152

Fulder S. (1987) *The Root of Being*. Hutchinson.

Lau B.H. *et al.* (1983) Allium sativum and atherosclerosis: a review. *Nutritional Research*, **3**, 119–128.

MacCormack C.P. (1991) *Holistic Health and a Changing Western World View. Anthropologies of Medicine* (Eds B. Pfleiderer and G. Bibeau, Vol. 7.

Manders R. (1993) Autonomy in midwifery and maternity care. *Midwives Chronicle*, October, p. 373.

Mennella J.A. and Beauchamp G.K. (1991) Maternal diet alters the sensory qualities of human milk and the nursling's behaviour. *Pediatrics*, **88**(4), 737–743.

Mies M. (1976) *Patriarchy and Accumulation on a World Scale*, pp. 16, 17. Zed Books, London.

Mills S. (1993) *The Essential Book Of Herbal Medicine*, p. 261. Arkana, Penguin Group.

National Institute of Medical Herbalists (1991) What is medical herbalism? Draft paper.

Vincent Priya J. (1992) *Birth Traditions and Modern Pregnancy Care*. Element Books.

Walker B. *The Encyclopedia of Myths and Secrets*, p. 1076. Harper and Row.

Winterton (1992), Report from The House of Commons, Health Committee. Second Report. *Maternity Services*, Vol. 1, HMSO, 1992.

Further reading

Bairacli Levy J. de (1982) The natural rearing of children. In: *The Illustrated Herbal Handbook*. Faber and Faber.

Brooke E. (1992) *A Woman's Book of Herbs*. The Woman's Press.

Grieve, M. (1980) *A Modern Herbal*. Penguin.

Griggs B. (1981) *Green Pharmacy, A History of Herbal Medicine*. Jill Norman and Hobhouse Ltd.

Hoffman D. (1991) *The New Holistic Herbal*. Findhorn Press.

Mills S. (1993) *The Essential Book Of Herbal Medicine*. Arkana, Penguin.

McIntyre A. (1992) *The Herbal for Mother and Child*. Element Books.

Ody P. (1993) *The Herb Society's Complete Medicinal Herbal*. Dorling Kindersley.

Parvati J. (1977) *Hygeia, A Woman's Herbal*. Freestone.

Weed S. (1986) *Wise Woman. Herbal for the Childbearing Year*. Ash Tree Publishing.

Appendix 1
Herbs to avoid in the first trimester, but where possible during the entire time from planning to the cessation of breast feeding a baby

Although there is no definitive list, the following herbs, some of which are known emmenagogues, should be avoided. The term emmenagogue refers to herbs likely to induce a period; thus these may also be referred to as abortifacients. Some herbs such as squaw vine, blue and black cohosh, are commonly referred to as 'partus preparators' and may be indicated in the last few weeks of pregnancy, in a stalled labour or in anticipation of postmaturity. Senna, cascara and other purging laxatives should also be avoided. Included are some herbs which may be prescribed by a qualified herbalist for specific problems and for a limited time.

Common name	Latin name
arbor vitae	*Thuja occidentalis*
barberry	*Berberis vulgaris*
beth root	*Trillium erectum*
black cohosh	*Cimicifuga racemosa*
blue cohosh	*Caulophyllum thalictroides*
cinchona	*Cinchona* spp.
cotton root bark	*Gossypium hebaceum*
golden seal	*Hydrastis canadensis*
greater celandine	*Chelidonium majus*
juniper	*Juniperus communis*
marjoram	*Origanum vulgare*
meadow saffron	*Crocus sativus*
motherwort	*Leonorus cardiaca*
mugwort	*Artemesia vulgaris*
pennyroyal	*Mentha pulegium*
poke root	*Phytolacca decandra*
rue	*Ruta graveolens*
sage	*Salvia officinalis*
squaw vine	*Mitchella repens*
tansy	*Tanacetum vulgare*
wormwood	*Artemisia absinthum*

Appendix 2
Herbal pharmacy – including the buying, storing and the making of infusions

Herbs should look fresh and smell lively, so wherever possible, gather them fresh or buy them dried from a reputable supplier with a good turnover of stock. Label and store in a dark glass jar or brown paper bag out of direct sunlight. Use the aerial parts (leaves, stems and flowers) within 6–12 months and the hard, woody parts, (seeds, berries, barks and roots) within 2–5 years. Freshly picked herbs such as lemon balm and basil will freeze well.

Herbs are amenable to administration in a wide variety of ways such as poultices, baths, douches, inhalants, gargles, ear/eye drops, capsules, pills vinegars, syrups or even wines. Nowadays, the most common techniques include infusions (teas), decoctions, tinctures and infused oils.

Infusion (tea) The standard measure uses 1 oz (30 grams) of dried plant material to 1 pint (500 ml) of water. For freshly picked herbs, use 2 oz to the same quantity of water. This method is appropriate for the softer parts of the herb – flowers, soft stems, leaves and small seeds whose active constituents are readily soluble in water. Pour the boiling water over the herb, cover and leave to steep for 10 or 15 minutes. Strain, press out the herb to obtain maximum fluid and drink with enjoyment, preferably without sweetening.

Some herbs (notably the 'mint' family) have different actions when consumed hot or cold; sage tea prevents sweats if consumed cold but if drunk hot, it acts as a diaphoretic (encouraging sweating).

Decoction This method is used for hard, woody parts of plants where the active constituents are only released at the higher temperatures achieved by boiling.

Use the same measurements as for an infusion but bring cold water to the boil and simmer for 15–20 minutes before straining and drinking.

All water-based preparations of herbs should be drunk within 24 hours. If making more than is required for immediate use, keep warm in a thermos flask or refrigerate and reheat.

Tincture This is the most common form in which herbal practitioners currently administer herbs. They are prepared from either dried or fresh plant material carefully weighed out and left to macerate in varying strengths of alcohol or glycerine for 2 or 3 weeks before pressing out.

Infused oil Not to be confused with essential oils, suitable plants such as marigold, St John's wort, comfrey or chickweed are covered with a cold pressed oil such as sunflower, almond, or olive and either left in strong sunlight for 3–4 weeks or heated over a bain marie for a couple of hours. They can then be directly applied to the skin or used as a base for creams, ointments, pessaries or suppositories.

Appendix 3
Botanical names of herbs referred to by common names

Common name	Latin name
aloe vera	*Aloe vera*
anise	*Pimpinella anisum*
agrimony	*Agrimonia euphatoria*
black haw bark	*Viburnum prunifolium*
blessed thistle	*Cnicus benedictus*
borage	*Borago officinalis*
burdock	*Arctium lappa*
capsicum	*Capsicum minimum*
caraway	*Carum carvi*
catnip	*Nepeta cataria*

chamomile, German	*Matricara recutita*
chasteberry	*Vitex agnus-castus*
chickweed	*Stellaria media*
cinnamon	*Cinnamomum zeylanicum*
cleavers	*Galium aparine*
comfrey	*Symphytium officianalis*
cornsilk	*Zea mays*
couchgrass	*Agropyron repens*
crampbark	*Viburnum opulus*
damiana	*Turnera diffusa*
dandelion	*Taraxacum officinale*
dill	*Anethum graveolens*
fennel	*Foeniculum vulgare*
fenugreek	*Trigonella foenum-graecum*
garlic	*Allium sativum*
gentian	*Gentiana lutea*
ginger	*Zingziber officinale*
ginseng	*Panax ginseng*
golden rod	*Solidago virgaurea*
golden seal	*Hydrastis canadensis*
ground ivy	*Glechoma hederacea*
hawthorn	*Crateagus* spp.
helionas	*Chamaelirium luteum*
hops	*Humulus lupulus*
horsetail	*Equisetum arvense*
hyssop	*Hyssopus officinale*
Iceland moss	*Cetraria islandica*
Lady's mantle	*Alchemilla vulgaris*
lavender	*Lavandula officinalis*
lemon balm	*Melissa officinalis*
lime blossom	*Tilia europea*
linseed	*Linum usitatissimum*
liquorice	*Glycyrrhiza glabra*
marigold	*Calendula officinalis*
marshmellow	*Althea officinalis*
meadowsweet	*Filipendula ulmaria*
milk thistle	*Carduus marianus*
motherwort	*Leonorus cardiaca*
myrrh	*Commiphora molmol*
nettles	*Urticia dioica*

oak bark	*Quercus robur*
oats	*Avena sativa*
orange blossom	*Citrus aurantium*
parsley	*Petroselinum crispum*
parsley piert	*Aphanes arvensis*
peppermint	*Mentha piperata*
plantain	*Plantago lanceolata* or *major*
purple coneflower	*Echinacea angustifolia*
raspberry leaf	*Rubus idaeus*
red clover	*Trifolium pratense*
rosehips	*Rosa canina*
roses	*Rosa* spp.
rosemary	*Rosmarinus officinalis*
scullcap	*Scutellaria laterifolia*
shepherd's purse	*Capsella bursa-pastoris*
slippery elm	*Ulmus fulva*
St John's wort	*Hypericum perforatum*
spearmint	*Mentha* spp.
thyme	*Thymus officinalis*
uva ursi	*Arctostaphylos uva-ursi*
valerian	*Valeriana officinalis*
vervain	*Verbena officinalis*
wild indigo	*Baptisia tinctoria*
wild yam	*Dioscorea villosa*
witch hazel	*Hamamelis virginiana*
wood betony	*Stachys betonica*
yarrow	*Achillea millefolium*
yellow dock	*Rumex crispus*

Appendix 4
Dietary sources
of iron and
vitamin B

(i) see list (on next page) for iron-containing foods by comparison

(ii) The B group of vitamins are found in similar food sources such as brewers' yeast, animal meats, wholegrain cereals and vegetable proteins. Whilst chemically distinct, they work in relationship to one another in the body. Although deficiencies are relatively rare, except for B_{12} in people on vegan diets, pregnant and breastfeeding women require increased amounts of all B vitamins.

Folic acid is now recommended as a pre-conception supplement because of its central role in the development of the central nervous system. The best food sources include green, leafy vegetables, eggs, wholegrain cereals, (organic) liver and kidneys. See also the recommendations of the Expert Advisory Group as listed in the references.

List of iron-containing foods

FOOD	mg./100 gm	FOOD	mg./100 gm
Curry powder	75	Sardines in tomato	
'Vecon' concentrate	70	sauce	4.6
Cockles	26–40	Muesli	4.6
Ground Ginger	17	Sprats	4.5
Egg Yolk	13	Oat cakes	4.5
Liver	11	Figs, dried	4.2
Molasses	11	Shredded wheat	4.2
Soya beans	8	Apricots, dried	4.2
Parsley	8	Almonds	4
Chives	8	Ginger biscuits	4
Weetabix	7.6	Spinach	4
Lentils	7.6	Gingerbread	3.8
Peaches, dried	6.8	Malt bread	3.6
Red kidney beans	6.7	Pilchards	2.7
Chick peas	6.4	Wholemeal bread	2.5
Whitebait	5.1	Chapatis	2.3

Plate 1
Calendula officinalis.

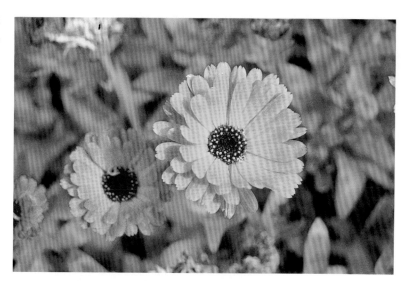

Plate 2
Alchemilla vulgaris.

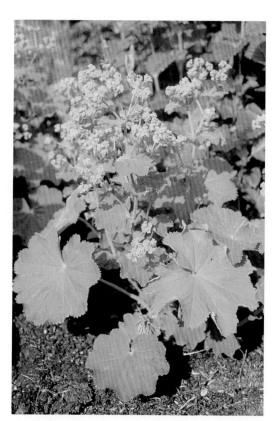

Plate 3
Hypericum perforatum.

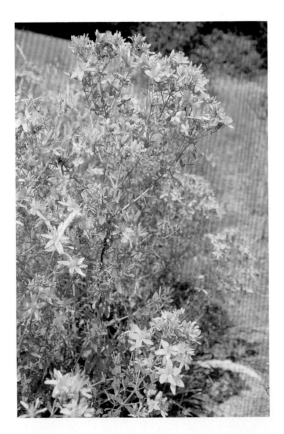

Plate 4
Matricaria recutila.

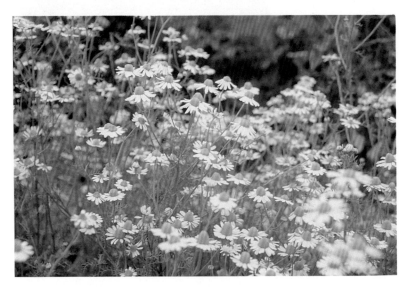

Plate 5
Rubus idaeus.

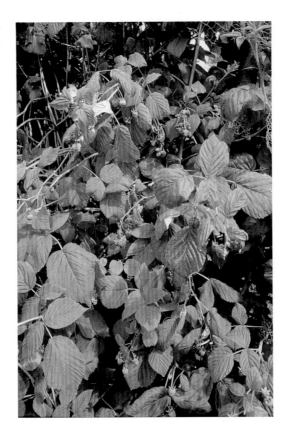

Plate 6
Vitex agnus castus.

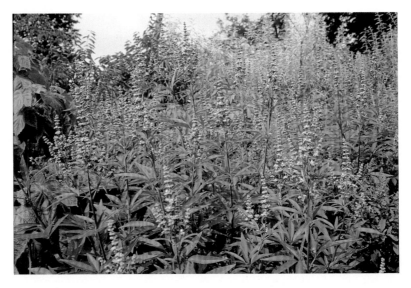

Plate 7
Lavendula augustifolia

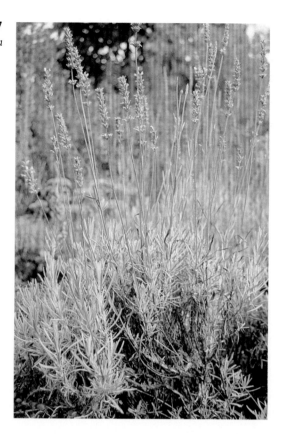

Bridget Cummings

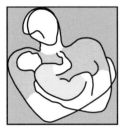

Chapter 9

Homeopathy for Pregnancy and Childbirth

Introduction

This chapter aims to give credence to the women who have chosen the homeopathic system of medicine. It also hopes to encourage midwives to appreciate the art and science of homeopathy; perhaps to find out more about homeopathy and, hopefully, to support fully its use as part of the woman's choice for pregnancy and birth.

Homeopathy is a pharmacological system of medicine using set principles and laws for administering specially prepared medicinal substances to correct individuals' disease. Homeopathy offers a safe, gentle and effective method of preventative, as well as curative, medicine. It promotes normal physiological processes and can stimulate the body's defences, in order for it to heal or correct itself. Health is seen as the well-being of mind, body and spirit. Ill-health is seen as disharmony within the whole person shown by the symptoms expressed. Its holistic and individualised approach can obviate weak areas of health and help remove these tendencies, optimising the health potential of the unborn baby whilst treating the mother.

Choudhury (1988) considered susceptibility to be the primary cause of disease and certainly the state of the mother and baby plays an enormous part in the progress of the pregnancy, birth and puerperium. Mental and emotional health as well as the mother's approach to birth is also included in her 'susceptibility'. To treat susceptibility ideally both parents would benefit from homeopathic consultation preconceptionally.

During pregnancy labour and the postpartum period homeopathy can be used safely and effectively to treat common ailments. Provided there are no irreversible mechanical problems, homeopathy can promote a normal labour with minimal pain and discomfort. The specially prepared minute dose of the remedy ensures elimination of its toxicity whilst enhancing its curative effects. It is so dilute that no molecules of the original substance remain. Women are most commonly attracted to homeopathy during childbearing for this aspect alone.

Homeopaths do not prescribe when the progress of the pregnancy and birth is normal and healthy. Like midwives, homeopaths believe in nature and letting it work when things are going well. It is only when nature shows itself to be in need of assistance, in the form of symptoms expressed in the mother and observed by the carers, that a remedy is prescribed.

This shows the importance of knowing what 'normal' is. Birth is a normal physiological process and midwives view birth as normal until proven otherwise.

The midwife is the expert in normal birth and has an important role to play in the enhancement of primal health. When a carefully selected remedy is prescribed, homeopathy can help avoid obstetric intervention or drugs and hence 'side effects', iatrogenic disease or adverse reactions from orthodox medicine are prevented. The remedy addresses an imbalance, whether emotional or physical . It works on an energy level and can stimulate vitality and the ability of the mother to cope. A knowledge and understanding of the principles and laws of homeopathy increases the sensitivity and perception of the midwife to the needs of the mother choosing this model of health and disease.

Midwives are trained under traditional 'medicine' and may find it difficult to accept homeopathy. Dr Donald Foubister (1989) found the ignorance about homeopathy in the medical profession hard to believe. This was especially noticeable in the education of medical students, where direct chemical or physical effects of drugs alone are taught.

Treating birth as a physical science, examining the biochemistry and biophysics, ignores the fact that birth is inseparable from its mental, emotional and social aspects. Obstetrics can intervene on a physical level, using fluids, drugs and instruments, but if the root cause is mental or emotional then this approach can be very traumatic (Tew, 1990).

The midwife is in a position to allow free expression of anxieties and other emotions and to allay fears. If her skills, support and nurturing are not enough to change the situation then homeopathy is an ideal, noninterventionist therapeutic tool. Rather than ignoring the mental and emotional symptoms, homeopathy uses them as the most important indicators as to the selection of a necessary remedy. Homeopathy can be incorporated successfully alongside sensitive midwifery care, by appropriately trained carers.

Peter, a first baby, was born naturally at home. He screamed and fretted at the breast and did not latch on. All 'calming' and encouraging methods were used to little or no effect.

This continued for a week at which point expertise from La Leche League was also sought. The mother was expressing her milk and feeding Peter using a spoon. Sometimes Peter would 'drip feed' at the breast. After discussion Anne, the mother, realised that the initial breastfeed after the birth had been extremely tense, so much so that Anne had screamed out 'in pain'. This had happened at the next attempt also. It was concluded that Peter was frightened at the breast and it was this emotion which needed to be cured. Anne agreed to try Aconite 30c. One tablet was crushed and given to the baby and the mother also had a dose. The result was immediate in that Peter calmed down, slept for a long stretch and awoke to latch on perfectly. The baby breastfed beautifully from then on.

The foundations of homeopathy

Dr Samuel Hahnemann (1755–1845) of Germany was the founder of homeopathy. He chose the name from the Greek words *homois-* 'similar' and *pathos-* 'suffering'. Whilst translating a medical text (Cullen, 1789) he was sceptical about the given reason why the Peruvian Bark (from which quinine is made) brought on the symptoms of malaria. These symptoms disappeared as soon as he stopped taking the Peruvian Bark. He realised that the drug that was known to cure malaria also produced symptoms like malaria! He gathered together many other examples of cures and in each case found that the drug used could also produce symptoms similar to those that it had cured (Handley, 1990). Hahnemann had discovered the principle that 'like cures like' or the 'Law of Similars'. In the fifth century BC Hippocrates had found that there were two ways of healing – by 'opposites' and by 'similars'. Hahnemann made the law of similars practical.

Orthodox medicine uses 'opposites'. For example, in constipation a medicine will be given which produces diarrhoea. Homeopathy uses 'similars'. For example, a remedy known to produce constipation in its crude form would cure the constipation if given in a small dose.

The symptoms caused by too much of a substance are the symptoms that can also be cured with a small dose of that substance, for example too much radium causes cancer whilst a small dose cures cancer.

Another instance from everyday life is seen when cutting a strong onion. An acrid runny nose, a particular soreness in the throat and stinging, running eyes may be experienced. A homeopath will prescribe *allium cepa* (the remedy made from onion) for the person who has a cold and bad throat with those particular symptoms. Similarly, strong coffee can give headaches and unusual activity of the mind and body. It is often drunk to 'keep us going!' A homeopath may prescribe *coffea* where there is insomnia of that nature. In relation to childbirth, a crude dose of *Ipecacuanha* (Ipecac root) will produce constant nausea and vomiting with much saliva but a clean tongue. A minute dose of *Ipecacuanha* will relieve vomiting during pregnancy if the symptoms match.

Hahnemann went on to discover that minute doses of homeopathic remedies were safer and in fact more effective. Many years were spent experimenting and verifying the Law of Similars. In order to discover the curative potential of medicines, Hahnemann concluded that they should be tested on healthy people – these 'provings' (see Glossary) or drugs tests are still being done today amongst homeopathic students and practitioners but to a far lesser degree, as the information recorded by the early homeopaths is still applicable today. Homeopathy stands strong on its original foundations. Women continue to look for a more natural method of healing. The interest shown during pregnancy and birth suggests a reflection of the desire to keep in control and be active in the childbearing process (Spiby, 1993).

Homeopathy has been, since 1948, the only complementary therapy to be part of Britain's National Health Service, although osteopathy is now included since the Osteopathy Act 1993. In 1952, the Faculty of Homeopathy in London was established by an Act of Parliament and recognised homeopathy as a safe alternative form of medical treatment.

The Medicines Control Agency license the manufacturers of homeopathic medicines. Following the thalidomide disaster, the Medicines Act 1968 was brought in to legislate for the safety, control and regulation of medicines. Homeopathic remedies are included under this Act.

The general public can of course buy homeopathic medicines over the counter at pharmacies, health food shops and natural medicine centres. These can be useful in acute situations. However, it must be noted that although these are termed 'homeopathic' they cannot be so called until the remedies have been prescribed according to the law of similars. Then and only then is the medicine truly 'homeopathic'. Hence, although safe for women, results will be non-existent if the remedy is inappropriately prescribed. Here, it is the prescriber who is at fault, not homeopathy. This shows the importance of accuracy of prescription and appropriate advice for women. How much easier it would be for women to consult their midwife for an accurate and precise prescription, or at least a referral to a centre for homeopathic advice or consultation. The fear of the homeopath failing to recognise abnormal states in parturient women can be allayed by the fact that women normally attend routine antenatal care (Dhunny, 1993). For chronic prescribing, an in-depth study of homeopathy and its applications is necessary, therefore this is the area where an experienced homeopath should be consulted for the best treatment.

Joanne, a 32 year old gravida 4, suffered from haemorrhoids from 30 weeks' gestation. She was emotionally very sensitive and often irritable. The 'piles' were very painful and she was also constipated. The urge to open her bowels was ineffectual and the 'piles' were large and protruding. She enjoyed coffee to drink mostly and spicy foods. In all of her pregnancies she had had haemorrhoids and described the pain with them postnatally as 'the worst part'.

The midwife gave an acute prescription of nux vomica 30c *(poison nut) to be taken in the morning and evening for a few days. She was advised to stop taking the* nux vom. *when there was an improvement. Both the midwife and the mother were expecting temporary relief, recognising that treatment would have been useful before this pregnancy. The report from the mother was that the 'piles' reduced and 'went'. They were expected to return after giving birth but this did not happen! Constipation was also relieved.*

Professional issues

The midwife needs to be informed, educated, flexible, safe and accountable. The care given must be evaluated in order that the best care and the provision of choice is offered to childbearing women (Spiby, 1993).

It has been suggested that a midwife practising homeopathy within the NHS would provide the mother with the 'best of both worlds'. The in-depth knowledge of midwifery and homeopathy with the safeguard of professional accountability and insurance cover is ideal in protecting the public (Royal College of Midwives, 1993). Homeopathic training is of a high standard amongst colleges, requiring students to train for up to 4 years (Goodliffe, 1990). However, under English Common Law, anyone can practise as a homeopath so long as they do not claim to cure or masquerade as a doctor!

Most women consult a homeopath because their own general practitioner was unable to suggest any safe treatment for the particular problem (Furnham and Smith, 1988). There is a need that is not being met under 'orthodoxy'. There are, for instance, no national guidelines or regulation for the use of homeopathy within the NHS, so each hospital devises its own rules (Rankin-Box, 1991).

The Midwife's Code of Practice (UKCC, 1994) offers guidance to midwives wishing to undertake further training in alternative therapies. But there are no requirements within these guidelines for the practitioner actually to undergo specific training.

Dana Ullman (1989) cautions professionals that homeopathy is not learnt by weekend workshops or even several weekends. Study over a couple of years with a good teacher can offer the practitioner the beginnings of mastering the art. Like midwifery, study is life-long. But for acute situations, where the condition is self-limiting, the midwife can quickly learn to use remedies. A good way to ensure that quality homeopathy is being offered to women and babies, is for the midwife to become educated in it. Some parents will have the opportunity to learn about homeopathy for the home from adult education evening classes or tutorials with their local homeopath. Others will turn to their midwife for advice. Short courses for midwives covering all aspects of homeopathy and its application to pregnancy and childbirth would be welcome and are being considered by some educational institutions. Ideally, this should include a research project into the effectiveness of homeopathic remedies in this specialised area.

Remedy sources

The medicines are derived from the following sources:

Animal Kingdom – e.g.:	*Apis* (bee)	
	Cantharis (Spanish fly)	*Canth.*
	Sepia (cuttle fish)	
	Lachesis (snake)	*Lach.*
Plant Kingdom – e.g.:	*Arnica montana*	*Arn.*
	Belladonna	*Bell.*
	Chamomilla	*Cham.*
	Pulsatilla nigrens	*Puls.*
Mineral Kingdom – e.g.:	Calcarea carbonate	*Calc. carb.*
	Silica	*Sil.*
	Natrum muriaticum (salt)	*Nat. Mur.*
	Phosphorus	*Phos.*
Disease products (nosodes) – e.g.:	Tuberculinum koch exotoxin	*Tub.*
	Diptherium	*Dipth.*
	Pyrogen (pus)	*Pyog.*
Healthy tissues and secretions (sarcodes) – e.g.:	Thyroid	
	Pituitrin	
	Ooverinum	

There are also metals, such as gold (aurum, *aur*) and, imponderables, such as X-rays and magnetism.

Homeopathy is wide ranging and continues to develop. Like Hahnemann who continued his research and improvements on his work until his dying day, his successors continue to make valuable discoveries, so diversifying the *Materia Medica*, whilst its laws and principles remain the same. This makes medicinal help more likely for most people. More than two thousand remedies are now recognised by the homeopathic pharmacopoeia, recent provings include chocolate, granite, hydrogen and scorpion.

Releasing the medicinal properties from the inert substance

Hahnemann originally gave measured doses of the drugs without further processing but he found that the reaction was too marked or excessive, or it was inadequate due to poor preparation. He aimed to process drugs to give better results by reducing toxicity whilst enhancing their curative ability. He also considered the individual and varied sensitivity and reaction to drugs.

He developed a step-by-step dilution and succussion (vigorous shaking) processing method which he called potentisation or dynamisation. In 1838, Hahnemann wrote that homeopathic dynamisations genuinely bring to life the medicinal properties which lie hidden in natural solids when these are in a crude state (Hahnemann, 1821).

Potentisation

After initial preparation of the raw material, the remedies are made by serial dilution and succussion in a solution of alcohol and water. This is done a few (three to four) times or up to many thousand times. The liquid dilution is then used itself as a remedy or soaked into tablets or granules for convenience. The diluted remedies are described as being 'potentised', in recognition of the dynamic healing power they can stimulate. Hahnemann described the self-healing energy of the person and that which his dynamic remedies stimulate as the vital force (see Glossary). Frequently, the remedy dilution is so great that no chemical trace of the original substance remains.

The process of dilution and succussion apparently imprints the characteristic energy pattern, or blueprint, of the original substance onto the water in which it is diluted. This may be likened to the transmission of television signals, where the original scene is converted into an electromagnetic energy pattern (a signal) which can then be broadcast to your receiver (Society of Homeopaths, undated).

Evidence in support of microdoses One of the more controversial aspects of homeopathy is the fact that infinitesimal doses (microdoses) of a substance – so diluted that no molecules of the original substance remain – can have any impact on a person receiving such a homeopathic dose.

Sceptical people will always point to the placebo effect as an explanation for the homeopathic success stories they have encountered. Whilst homeopaths and their clients know that this medical science is certainly no placebo, it is well worth recording scientific evidence of microdoses working on biochemical, plants, bacteria, animals and minerals, none of which are known for falling prey to the placebo.

The use of minute quantities is recognised outside of homeopathy in the field of hormonal treatments, for example, the concentration of free thyroid hormone in the blood is one part per 10 000 million parts of blood plasma. Coulter (1981) cited evidence for the infinitesimal dose as below.

Biochemical Investigations William Boyd's experiments, published in 1954, were to show if a microdilution of mercury chloride added to flasks containing starch, distilled water and diastase would affect the rate of hydrolysis of the starch. The amount of mercury chloride was 61x or 10^{-61} (see 'Potency scales', p. 189). In theory, this should appear to be just distilled water. The outcome, after several rigorous repetitions and attention to detail to avoid error and bias, was that the mercury chloride 61x accelerated the rate of hydrolysis.

The *Pharmaceutical Journal* (September 1954) quoted the President of the London Faculty of Homeopathy that this 'would prove to be one of the greatest medical advances recorded'. Reports also appeared in the British newspapers.

Botanical investigations In 1968 Wannamaker conducted experiments to test the effect of sulphur microdilutions on the growth of onion plants. The microdilutions were found to have a significant effect on the weight and dimensions of the onion bulbs and seedlings and also their calcium, magnesium, potassium and sodium content.

Bacteriological investigations Junker investigated the effect of microdilutions of various substances (including caffeine, lemon juice, hydrochloric acid, and copper sulphate) on paramecia cultures and found they affected the degree of daily growth of the cultures.

Zoological investigations J. and M. Tetau experimented with thuja intoxication of rats. The rats were first taught a conditioned reflex and then injected with thuja until so intoxicated that there was a loss of reflex. A test group of these rats was then injected with thuja in microdilution (9c) and returned to their normal state more rapidly than the remaining control group.

Investigations using physics Gay and Boiron found that the dielectric index (a measurement of electrical charge of the water) of distilled water was altered by adding to it a small amount of sodium chloride 27c. By dielectric testing they were able to select the bottle with the microdilution of sodium chloride out of 99 other bottles containing only distilled water.

Drug quality is determined by quantity

Maupertius, a mathematician, discovered the 'Law of Least Quantity' which has been accepted in science as a fundamental principle of the universe. He describes it thus: 'The quantity of action necessary to effect change in nature is the least possible.' The prescriber in homeopathy applying the Law of Similars must use the 'minimum dose' to achieve good results without aggravating the patient's symptoms and so avoid unwanted effects (Close, 1981).

Homeopathic remedies cannot cause side effects or addiction. This area of the infinitessimal dose is the most controversial aspect of homeopathy, along with the principle that the medicinal power of a substance increases with the dilution and succussion.

Fincke (1821–1906), a homeopath, said:

> The quality of action of a homeopathic remedy (i.e. one which has been selected according to the rules of homeopathic prescribing) is determined by its quantity'. 'Thus the Law of Least Action must be acknowledged as the posological principle of homeopathy. (Close, reprinted 1981.)

With reference to birth, in particular during labour where erratic contractions lead to obstetric augmentation using oxytocic drugs, the minimum dose of such drugs seems appropriate. Available data so far do not show that augmentation using oxytocics is beneficial to mother and baby but that simple measures such as mobility, eating and drinking are just as effective (Enkin *et al.*, 1990). Where this does not work, researchers of effective care in pregnancy and childbirth have recommended a mode of care not dissimilar to homeopathy. 'Logic would dictate that, in such circumstances, the smallest effective drug dose should be given, in the most effective manner' (Enkin *et al.*, 1990).

Individual sensitivity to oxytocin varies from woman to woman and it is unclear how large the initial dose or the increments should be and at what interval they should be implemented. Solid research evidence is lacking. Homeopathy avoids these risks by using the minimum dose of an individualised prescription based on the law of similars and the fixed principles of homeopathic medicine. The specially prepared potency and number of doses is determined by the physician according to the needs of the individual.

Potency scales Remedies may be prescribed in a number of different strengths, or potencies. The lower potencies have been subjected to less dilution and succussion than the higher ones and are not, broadly speaking, as powerful and long lasting in their effects. It is the lower potencies, such as the sixth (e.g. arnica 6), which are found and bought 'over the counter'. These lower potencies are most useful for self-care situations. They can be repeated as often as necessary in an acute situation. High potency remedies are usually prescribed by experienced, qualified homeopaths. The higher potencies are used more in chronic cases and are not suitable for self-prescribing.

The two most commonly used scales likely to be met by the midwife are as follows.

The decimal scale is shown by the letter 'x' after the amount of dilutant, e.g. 6x. This scale 'x' means that the dilution is of one part of the original substance with nine parts of alcohol and water to make ten parts, i.e. 1+9 = 10 dilution. So 6x (scale 'x') means that the medicine was diluted one part to nine parts (1:9), then shaken (succussed), diluted again 1:9 and shaken and this procedure was repeated six times.

The centessimal scale is shown by the letter 'c' after the number of dilutions, e.g. 30c. This means that the medicine was diluted one part to 99 parts to make 100 parts, i.e. 1 + 99 = 100, then succussed; then diluted again 1:99 and shaken; and this was repeated 30 times.

Experienced homeopaths may use further scales. The M scale refers to a dilution of 1:1000 and when a medicine is labelled LM, it was diluted 1:50 000.

The midwife will most commonly come across the 6x, 12x, 6c, 30c and 200c potencies.

Sarah was a primigravida, admitted to hospital for induction of labour for postmaturity, and accompanied by her homeopath. An amniotomy was performed which led to regular painful uterine contractions. Sarah took arnica *at this time in preparation for labour and delivery.*

The fetal position was found to be occipto-posterior and Sarah experienced long, painful contractions and backache, which started in the sacral area. Kali carb *200c was given as it is renowned for relieving backache.*

Progress was slow and the obstetrician suggested an oxytocic infusion, which Sarah declined, but she did accept intramuscular pethidine for pain relief. Sarah suffered leg cramps and was given mag phos *6x, and* kali phos *30c to combat tiredness. The* kali carb *was repeated as the backache increased.*

Eventually, as Sarah went into the transition stage, she became frenzied, biting the pillow, thrashing about and swearing, and chamomilla *200c was given with good effect. The* arnica *was repeated for overexertion, and shortly afterwards Sarah delivered a baby girl, without trauma to either herself or her daughter.*

Principles of prescribing

Successful prescribing is achieved through following the principles of homeopathy laid down by Hahnemann in the sixth edition of *The Organon of Medicine* published in 1842 (Dudgeon, 1921). These principles require in-depth study.

Homeopathy treats the person as a whole and as an individual. The practice of homeopathy convinces the prescriber to view the body as more than the sum of its parts. All symptoms of the expressed complaint or condition, mental, emotional and physical, are regarded as evidence of a natural effort to resolve an inner disturbance and regain the balanced state of health. The aim of homeopathic medicine is to stimulate autoregulation and is chosen in relation to the way the individual reacts.

In acute situations the symptoms are easy to prescribe on because they are clearly defined, such as in earache or measles. Chronic disease is more complicated and so professional homeopathy is advised whereby the root cause of the problem is treated and not just the 'named' disease.

Labour and the birth process is considered to be an 'acute' situation. The similar remedy given will stimulate the concerted effort of the body to promote a physiological and emotional process as best it can. Midwives supporting women through natural childbirth may view homeopathy as yet another intervention. This would be a misconception of a fundamental principle of homeopathy. A remedy is a stimulus only and gives nothing material to the mother nor detracts from her achievement. Midwives and homeopaths aim for a healthy baby to be born to an alert, nurturing and healthy mother whose recovery is speedy. Supporting women to achieve their own physiological potential is part of this. Homeopathy can only work with what is already there, in the person. It adds nothing and can be a great stimulus.

In order to aid communication between families, their midwife and their homeopath the principles of homeopathy are outlined below.

Principles of homeopathy

The law of similars There are natural examples of the law of similars, such as frostbite treated with snow, sadness relieved by hearing of a worse case, phobias treated with facing the object, a cup of tea on a hot day. There are small areas where orthodoxy uses the principle of 'like cures like' without acknowledging it.

Examples include:

- The use of pollen extracts, housedust, etc. to reduce and eliminate sensitivity.
- Nitroglycerine (*Glonoine*) was first introduced by a homeopath for cardiac symptoms and to treat angina. A century later, doctors and homeopaths use it in the management of angina pectoris.
- Metallic gold (*aurum*) was used by homeopaths for rheumatic complaints and was introduced in 1935 to orthodox medicine to treat rheumatoid arthritis.
- Ergot – homeopathic provings revealed circulatory difficulties and so homeopaths used it to treat gangrene and Raynaud's disease. In 1933 doctors successfully used it to treat Raynaud's disease and later intermittent claudication and peripheral vascular disease. The provings revealed headaches and in the nineteenth century homeopaths pioneered its use. Now doctors use it in migraine preparations.

To apply the law of similars, the individual symptoms of the person must be obtained and not a named collective disease concept. The individual clinical picture is matched with the symptoms obtained in drugs tests that are most similar. So 'painful contractions', 'hypertension' and 'failure to progress in labour' are the diagnosis or result of disease and as such are a name for but not the details of the external expression of the internal disease. The 'totality of symptoms' is the sole guide to the selection of a remedy and includes the physical, mental and emotional responses. It need not include every symptom but the principle signs and symptoms, usually mixed together to reveal an essence or style of what is truly going on. It does not ignore useful information obtained from the carers either, including pathology, or the use of conventional drugs or surgery as needed. In fact, the skills of the midwife with her observations and assessment can be crucial in the selection of the most similar and therefore most accurate remedy. The participation of the mother is obviously encouraged although disturbance is avoided, as much information is obtained without asking her a single question, particularly in labour.

The single remedy Only one remedy should be given at a time. This single remedy is the most similar remedy at any one time.

Prescribing the single remedy on the totality of symptoms generates experience of the remedy action and is of further learning value. Giving different remedies for different areas of the mother will confuse this issue and the practitioner will have difficulty evaluating the case. Hahnemann wrote 'It is wrong to employ complex means when simple will suffice' (Dudgeon, 1921). A single remedy is enough to stimulate correction of the whole person.

The minimum dose The smallest dose possible is all that is needed to stimulate a reaction in the self-corrective power of the person. Safety encourages this principle.

Provings (drug tests) The law of similars is a method whereby the medicinal action of the remedy can be verified. So, each time this principle is applied and the remedy works, it is further evidence of the capabilities of medicines and verification of the law of similars. Also, it is not enough to look at 'poisonings' from substances to gain knowledge of the potential remedy's capabilities. 'Provings' need to be carefully done. These are the homeopathic 'drug tests'

A minute dose of the substance is given to a group of healthy people in repeated doses sufficient to elicit symptoms but not damage. In this way, the symptoms can be noted down and a 'symptom picture' of the remedy will appear. No detail is spared but these tests are obviously limited to the sub-toxic range. Symptoms noted are largely subjective and show the changes experienced by each 'prover'. Data are also obtained from toxicology and pharmacology. Organic lesions and profound functional disorders are noted from deliberate and accidental poisoning.

'Provers' today will display exactly the same symptoms as those of the nineteenth century when given the same remedy. So, symptoms in people are unchanging, whilst the modern orthodox medical model of health and disease produces new theories of the causes of disease from year to year and is continually researching ever more complicated pathological and/or biochemical processes. Alongside this continual movement of medical thought and discoveries, there are modern industries always looking for new drugs or medicines to assist in healing the sick.

Homeopathic drug tests, principles and laws are unchanging. Homeopathy applies the law of similars scientifically and systematically, using carefully tested medicines.

The results of provings are published and form the *Materia Medica*. Each remedy's 'symptom picture' is listed. In order to match the symptoms of the patient with a symptom picture of a remedy, often a repertory is used. The

Repertory alphabetically lists symptoms of disease, with the remedy names applying to each symptom. It is thus a cross-reference for the *Materia Medica*. Vast volumes of *Materia Medica* and repertory works are now available on computer.

The law of cure

Homeopaths are able to evaluate their work, especially in chronic cases, through time and observation of the totality of symptoms. This is done anatomically as well as historically. By using the law of cure formulated by Constantine Hering (1800–80) it is possible to assess that healing took place in response to the remedy and not in spite of it.

Natural healing begins by removing the 'disease' away from the vital centres and towards the less vital areas until it is removed. Experience has shown that cure takes place:

- in reverse order of the appearance of symptoms;
- from above to below;
- from within to without;
- from more vital to less vital organs.

The most important of these is the reverse order of appearance.

It can be deduced that onset or exacerbation of an illness will appear as the opposite of the above, with completely new symptoms or more complicated chronic suffering.

The midwife needs to understand this aspect of homeopathy because she may be with a mother who is having professional homeopathic treatment. In this respect, a skin eruption in pregnancy, for example, could be a positive sign of healing from within to without and thus must not be tampered with. It may be an example of how the mother is eliminating, via the skin, a disturbance originally on a deeper level, such as 'wheeziness' of the chest. This eruption will be a passing phase of a curative stimulus. It may also be noted that the skin eruption disappears from above downwards. This is commonly seen in evidence in a measles case, where the spots disappear from the upper body first and then downwards to the extremities.

The homeopath's approach towards disease

The homeopath's approach towards disease is very different to that of the orthodox doctor. For example, doctors view cancer as the disease which needs to be fought. Homeopaths view cancer as the product or result of disease and that it is the underlying disease cause that needs to be cured.

Some obstetricians view birth as normal only in retrospect. Homeopaths, like midwives, view birth as normal until shown not to be.

Aetiology There is a general view of aetiology in orthodox medicine but homeopaths consider every fact, incident or accident, connected with the onset or origin of the presenting ailment. If it is realised that the trouble started after a disappointment, grief, sunstroke, getting wet, over-exertion, loss of sleep, etc., then each factor will give clues to the practitioner as regards the person's susceptibility. This helps in the selection of the remedy because it shows how that person has reacted and may give an accurate description of a remedy. So the first question asked is: 'How did it start?'

In labour, a well-taken case history antenatally would be invaluable but largely the mother's mental and emotional state will show a remedy picture if there is a reason to prescribe. For example, 'since disappointment with her partner or relative she has wanted to be alone and not touched'. In labour, the contractions are erratic, very painful and stop when people or relatives enter the room. The aetiology of disappointment is to be cured – remedy such as *ignatia* may be prescribed to improve the birth process. The emotions may surface during the birth and be productive.

The concept of aetiology in homeopathy is thus not confined to age, sex, race, diet or smoking, for example, nor is the offending microbe searched for and given priority.

How homeopaths prescribe The homeopath is guided by the fixed principles of homeopathy as well as noting the individual susceptibility and energy level. Any symptoms of disease or pain reflect how that person is coping with stress on all levels of the physical, mental and emotional body, as well as the spiritual and sociological.

The 'totality of symptoms', not a disease label, is looked for via observation and questioning at interview. The homeopath will sort through the symptoms to get a picture of the 'whole' individual with the disease. Then, after grading and finding the symptoms in the *Repertory*, an elimination process is begun. This is to use the cross-referencing of symptoms to eliminate certain remedies that do not apply to all symptoms. The remedies left are looked up in the *Materia Medica* to find the one that is most similar. In order to individualise not only the remedy for the person but also its dose and potency, the energy or vitality is assessed to match the energy stimulus of the remedy.

This may at first appear a lengthy process but it is worthwhile when a carefully selected remedy proves later to be the most similar one and thus gives speedy relief. This is especially noticeable in an acute situation.

Case taking Time spent at the initial consultation is not just writing notes or selecting remedies. It can be a powerful healing experience on its own. The mother will be encouraged to tell her story in its entirety without interruption. In order to remind her that the totality of symptoms is being sought the question 'anything else?' can be repeated (Moskowitz, 1992).

The mother's own words, where significant, are noted and objective observations also. The consultation will follow the lines of a medical history, family history and past history. The art of interpersonal skills is essential in the formation of a relationship between midwife and mother. The midwife also needs to be aware of questioning techniques to influence greatly the information obtained in response.

In acute or first aid prescribing, such as during a birth, 'case-taking' is simplified as the mother will be able to describe clearly how she feels and show obvious signs of discomfort in her body language. Her behaviour will show if she is hot or cold, comfortable, coping, tiring rapidly, approaching second stage or becoming distracted too much to be able to surrender to the birth process. The observations of a midwife can be almost intuitive and, through experience, the midwife is an expert at assessing the state of the mother. This is very helpful to a homeopath.

The information needed includes: signs and symptoms; locality; sensations; aetiology; what makes it better or worse, whether there are any symptoms that accompany it; is she crying, shouting, restless, motionless, thirsty or thirstless; nauseous but not relieved by vomiting; is the os uteri rigid; are the contractions too close, too far apart, too strong or too weak?

The midwife could note exactly what the mother says, listening and watching carefully. She should use all her senses to observe and to describe the mother. For example, the midwife's sense of touch is an immensely useful diagnostic tool – used to assess contractions, temperature, sweat and consistency of the cervix – all without asking a question.

It needs to be remembered that at a birth, for example, symptoms must appear exaggerated, unusual or that which is *individual* to the mother in order to prescribe. Pain is normal in birth, therefore there is no remedy for pain, but remedies for exaggerated, individualised expression of that pain. Ineffectual contractions are abnormal and need treatment.

The symptoms point the way to the remedy needed. The aim is not to remove symptoms or 'cover them up'. Symptoms providing the information such as aetiology, location, sensation, concomitants and modalities (see Glossary) are used to find the most similar remedy. This in turn is aimed at the root cause (most commonly on the mental and emotional level) to stimulate self-regulation. Thus, as the *Organon* stated, the aim is 'the rapid, gentle and lasting restoration of health' (Dudgeon, 1921).

MaryAnne, in her forties, was having her third baby at home. She had had influenza for a week before the birth. She felt very tired and congested, when there was spontaneous rupture of the membranes with stale meconium at 6 a.m.

By 11.30 a.m. she was having fair contractions, with slow progress, until the pain increased to 'unbearable'. MaryAnne became irritable and cross, having tried various methods of pain relief. She called out 'I can't bear it'. This was the key to the remedy needed, as the pain appeared to be extreme but the contractions were fair and short. Chamomilla *200c was given and there were no complaints after that.*

MaryAnne had moderate, regular contractions throughout the afternoon but eventually she became indecisive and craved fresh air and there was an obvious lack of thirst. After pulsatilla *200c was given, her contractions became stronger and MaryAnne was coping better. A little later* kali-phos *200c was given and 'a huge surge of energy' was felt. (This remedy is known to work well where any exertion seems a heavy task.)*

At 5.26 p.m. MaryAnne had a spontaneous vaginal delivery of a baby boy in good condition. The stale meconium was not a problem. There was a natural third stage with blood loss of 50 ml.

The three-legged stool A complete symptom is necessary for accurate prescriptions and this involves four areas of enquiry:

- the nature of the sensation;
- the special conditions or modalities of time, temperature, etc. that make it better or worse;
- the aetiology;
- the location.

If the prescriber has at least three of the above and can match the symptoms with those proved in drug testing to be of the nature of a remedy, then a safe prescription can be made. The stool with three legs can stand securely. With four legs, it can stand even more firmly (Koehler, 1986).

Louise suffered with mastitis 7 days postnatally. Breastfeeding advice was expertly given, but the pain and discomfort remained. It started suddenly about 3 p.m.; the right breast was hot, red and throbbing. The skin of the affected area was shiny and taut and the heat was felt even before touching the breast. Louise started to feel feverish. The midwife was aware that not all 'mastitis' cases are infective and whilst the conventional treatment would be in the form of antibiotics or anti-inflammatory drugs, the mother chose homeopathy first. So the complete symptom picture was looked for:

- *the aetiology was unknown;*
- *the location was the right breast;*
- *the sensation was* hot *and throbbing;*
- *the modalities were that it* suddenly *started at 3 p.m.*

A dose of belladonna *30c gave relief whilst addressing the imbalance, to cure and prevent recurrence. The provings of* belladonna *show the sudden onset of symptoms, that the affected parts are burning hot, the pain is throbbing and the right side is often affected.* Belladonna *has been proven to have the time modality of 3 p.m. This observation is relevant because it can be used as a measure for the peaks and troughs of body rhythm that is individually presented and helps differentiate the remedies (see Glossary).*

Practicalities of prescribing   'Dosage' in homeopathy refers to the number of repetitions. This is because it is a stimulus and not a chemical measure. So, if by accident a whole bottle of tablets was ingested, this would still only be one 'dose' or stimulus.

Remedies can be prescribed in different ways. Sometimes they are given as a single dose (probably a high potency) when the homeopath may wait a number of weeks to assess fully the response. A remedy can also be given in a lower potency, singly, or repeated daily or more frequently. The homeopath will choose the method to suit the client and the nature of the condition. Individuals respond better to some methods than others and understanding this is part of the skill of the homeopath. It also explains why self-prescribing may prove ineffective, as it is more difficult to be objective. The medicines are most commonly dispensed as drops, tablets, pills, powders and granules. For babies, powders, granules or crushed soft tablets are useful.

In acute situations such as birth, the remedy stimulus is used up quickly and may need to be repeated a number of times, possibly every 5–30 minutes. This is because the condition calling for it is likely to recur. The prescriber must observe the reaction to the remedy and reduce the number of doses when there is improvement and then stop. It may need to be resumed if the condition worsens again. If after four doses it has not acted, or the picture of what is happening and felt by the mother and baby has changed significantly, then another remedy is chosen. This remedy must be selected on the totality of symptoms as before (Moskowitz, 1992). In the main the general and emotional state of the mother is used to select a remedy. Only one remedy should be given at one time.

The carefully selected and indicated remedy can stimulate reaction and therefore 'act' very fast – 30 seconds to 1 minute in serious situations. Professional homeopaths have successfully treated women and babies in life-threatening situations such as uterine haemorrhage and respiratory distress, respectively.

Correct prescribing during the antenatal period or the labour can readdress an obvious imbalance. This can be a preventative prescription.

Having acquired the necessary skills of the art and science of homeopathy, the midwife may safely and accurately prescribe. She will, of course, remain primarily in attendance as a midwife and is professionally accountable to her UKCC registration (see Chapter 1).

Substances to avoid when under homeopathic treatment

To avoid the possibility of antidoting the beneficial effect of the remedy, some commmonly used substances must be avoided. Coffee, peppermint, menthol, eucalyptus and camphor, and anything containing very strong smells, including essential oils, or flavours, should be avoided. This is because homeopaths have noticed that the remedy action has been interfered with or been arrested in some clients where such substances have been used. It varies from person to person and remedy to substance, so it is worth noting this, if the results of treatment are not as good as expected.

It is also worth considering the fact that aromatherapists are treated by homeopaths with success!. To avoid confusion, individualising this for each client will help, but coffee (in any form), menthol, peppermint, eucalyptus and camphor seem to antidote remedies – no one is sure why. It could be that as the homeopathic remedy is of a dynamic immaterial nature, that stimulates us on an energy level (or vital force), so too is it very sensitive to strong smells. We all know how the aroma of peppermint can make us 'feel fresh' or the smell of coffee can make us 'feel good' and can be uplifting on an energy level . Hence, in some people, there is an effect from these substances that can antidote or overpower the dynamic stimulus of a remedy, because it is a stronger stimulus.

It is perfectly safe to use homeopathic medication whilst being treated by orthodox drugs (British Homeopathic Association leaflet; NAHG, 1992). A homeopathic remedy will not interact with orthodox drugs. However, orthodox drugs sometimes affect the remedy's action and, in order to overcome this, the remedy may need to be repeated more often. Where possible, it is preferable that other medication is avoided.

The expectations of homeopathy

Homeopathy cannot repair irreversible damage, structural or mechanical, and is not a substitute – for emergency surgery or suturing. It can be considered before opting for conventional obstetric treatment, for instance, or when orthodox methods have failed. After taking a remedy, reponses vary from person to person. Some feel an immediate surge of well-being, others may feel tired at first and need to rest before improvement is noticed (Society of Homeopaths, undated). This is notable in pregnancy where energy levels vary during the different trimesters and the mother is very aware of the changes.

Sometimes the original symptoms temporarily worsen, or the mother is made aware of previously felt symptoms that she has had in the past and has not fully recovered from. This indicates that the remedy has stimulated the self-healing or regulating process. These reactions may be subtle and pass unnoticed or, in contrast, quite marked.

Introduction to therapeutics

The midwife will perceive when her client needs more skilled help than she is able to give and so will refer to another practitioner when necessary.

Arnica (*Arnica montana*, 'Leopard's bane') *Arnica* is the most commonly referred-to homeopathic remedy for birth. C.V. Pink, with over 30 years' experience of obstetrics, recognises *arnica* 30c or 200c to be effective in the recovery from birth trauma for mother and baby (Foubister, 1989). Other testimonials to its importance in healing soft tissue bruising include Moskowitz (1992) and Gibson and Gibson (1987).

It is an extremely important first aid remedy and pertains to birth because of the commonly felt sensation of bruising and soreness postnatally. It is excellent where there is trauma from overexertion, tissue damage, bruising, swelling, injury, fear of touch and shock (mental and physical). *Arnica* has an affinity for blood vessels and muscles.

After labour, *arnica* can be given for bruising of the labia or vagina or where the perineum is traumatised after much pushing, an episiotomy or a mechanical delivery. *Arnica* helps prevent bleeding, retained placenta, sepsis and after pains. *Arnica* 30c can be given during a labour as is needed and two to four hourly after birth for a few days, reducing and then stopping when there is improvement.

The midwife is ideally positioned to recognise when *arnica* is indicated and could safely give this on her own accountability. In hospitals, standing orders could be implemented where there is support from the consultants and the pharmacist.

The baby can benefit from *arnica* also, where there is shock, trauma, bruising or cephal haematoma. Here, *arnica* can be given as a crushed tablet or in liquid form one to two hourly to reduce bruising, or in an emergency, repeatedly 15–30 seconds apart.

Caulophyllum (blue cohosh) This remedy has an affinity for the female organs. It is often prescribed for erratic contractions; labour that does not progress; sharp, crampy, spasmodic pains that fly from one place to another; unbearable 'after pains' across lower abdomen extending to groins; and also for rheumatism of the small joints with gynaecological ailments.

The value of *caulophyllum* in labour has been confirmed in research on animals. In a British study of over 200 births, it was shown that *caulophyllum* reduced significantly the numbers of stillbirths in a herd of pigs with a high stillbirth rate (Day, 1984).

Douglas Borland prescribed *caulophyllum* 200c hourly in a labour where progress was slow, the mother was having erratic contractions and was getting exhausted. He considers that it stimulates uterine muscle and brings on the labour. Also it can be used, if there are no individualising symptoms at all, in 'false labours' where the mother is becoming exhausted (Borland, 1982).

Chamomilla (German chamomile) This remedy has an affinity for the nerves and emotions. There is excessive irritability and oversensitivity to pain and external influences. In labour the mother may scream 'I can't bear it' and be very uncivil. There will be a capricious attitude and the mother will be averse to being spoken to or touched. Everything will become worse after anger or vexation. *Chamomilla* prescribed in such a situation will bring calm to the room and the mother will no longer complain of the pain but be able to cope and give birth freely. Here, the potency is of less importance. For instance if 6c is all there is available then this is used. It may need repeating. A 30c may have the desired effect also, after one dose or three. A 200c may be the most similar and so need no repetition.

Chamomilla 6c is used successfully in irritable babies, whether from pain or anger and is found in "teething granules".

Pulsatilla (wind flower) This remedy is most useful in pregnancy. There is a mild, tearful and apprehensive disposition. In labour there is slow progress and the mother tends to get upset. The emotions affect the labour and can lead to faintness, palpitation and poor contractions. A dose of *pulsatilla* will reduce the apprehensions and tearfulness whilst promoting strong, regular contractions and progress.

The homeopathic *Materia Medica* is rich with useful remedies for parturient women, too numerous to include. Within the confines of this chapter, it is impossible to show the full range of *Materia Medica* and its application. Tables 1–12 (reproduced with permission from Barbara Geraghty) show how a given 'problem', diagnosed as a named complaint such as haemorrhoids, ineffectual contractions and mastitis, can be treated homeopathically, using different remedies for the same complaint. This is due to the individualised expression of symptoms that homeopaths need and recognise in order to prescribe. These are by no means an exhaustive comparison of remedies for each complaint, but an introduction to the varying 'scenarios' or indeed the emotion behind the physical complaint.

It is interesting to note the differences, similarities, general symptoms and emotions of each remedy for the same complaint. The midwife will be familiar with the differing emotions and behaviour of labouring women. Where there is, for example, ineffectual contractions, then these observations can be put to good use.

It must be noted that, in all areas, good midwifery advice, support and encouragement in order to achieve a positive change of condition is assumed to have been given. In fact, in some areas, without excellent midwifery care additional treatment may not attain its full potential (Spiby, 1993).

Table 1. Carpal tunnel syndrome

Remedy	Arsenicum	Lycopodium	Sepia
Sensations	Tingling and numbness in fingers	Tingling and numbness in fingers	Tingling and numbness in fingers
With		With or without swelling of wrist and fingers	
Worse	Fingertips on side lain on	Mornings on waking First finger 2nd finger 3rd finger 4th finger	Night
Better for	Warmth		Motion Exercise
Emotionally	Anxious and restless Fear of being alone Wants to be looked after Very demanding	Restless Full of fear and anxiety beneath an exterior of capability	Weighed down by responsibilities, and no longer has the resources to cope Mental and physical 'sag' Better alone
Generally	Marked weakness and prostration Very sensitive to the cold Thirsty for sips	Feeble physique	Ptosis and statis Chilly Worse by becoming heated

Table 2.
Haemorrhoids

Remedy	Arsenicum	Nux-vomica	Pulsatilla	Sepia
Description	Bluish/purple Bleeding Burning	Bleeding Burning		Bleeding
External/ internal	Internal	Internal Protruding Grape-like Large	Internal Blind	Protruding Grape-like
Pain	Extreme	Extreme	Extreme	Extreme
With	Debility	Itching Constipation Large, hard stool Backache Tenesmus	Itching Continually oozing	Constipation Continually oozing
Worse from	Latter months of pregnancy	Latter months of pregnancy	Latter months of pregnancy Childbirth	Latter months of pregnancy
Better from	Bathing in warm water	Bathing in cold water		
Emotionally	Very restless and anxious Fear of being alone Wants to be looked after Difficult and demanding	Nervy, highly sensitive and irritable Impulsive and quarrelsome Irritable when questioned	Gentle, mild, yielding and emotional Clingy, desiring company and consolation	Responds badly to sympathy Torpor from being worn out
Generally	Very sensitive to cold Desires fresh air Tires suddenly	Very chilly Upset by slightest draught	Chilly Dislikes stuffy rooms Thirstless	Chilly Extremely sensitive to cold Sweats easily Run down and exhausted

Other remedies: Ham, Lach, Lil-t, Nit-ac, Mur-ac, Podo, Sab, Staph, Sul, also peony cream to soothe.

Table 3.
Labour

Remedy	Aconite	Arnica	Belladonna
Progress	Failure to progress		Failure to progress
Generally	Fear can stop the contractions Fearful Restless Moaning Anxious expression Parts feel contracted with headache	Denies her suffering Restless Great distress Body feels cold	Vehement Wild Moaning Desires to escape Face flushed, red, hot, eyes glisten Great distress Headache Cramps in hands and legs
Pains	Very severe In rapid succession Ineffectual *Ceasing entirely* from local sensitiveness Great soreness in back	Distressing Too weak Irregular *Ceasing* *False* Ineffectual From local sensitiveness Occur on motion of child	Distressing Severe Too weak *Ceasing* *False* Sudden Spasmodic From nervousness Drawing pain from back to thighs
Fear	That she or the baby will die Remains after the labour		Fearless
Fainting	Fainting	Fainting	Fainting
Nausea/ vomiting			
Exhaustion			Exhaustion
Uterus		Fatigue	
Os	Tender Dry Undilatable		Rigid Thin Hot Tender
Cervix	Undilatable		Fails to soften Hot Very dry
Vulva	Dry		
Vagina	Hot Dry Tender Undilating		Hot
Worse from	Fright Night	Being touched	Jarring
Better from	Repose		

Table 4.
Labour

Remedy	Caulophyllum	Chamomilla	Cimicifuga
Progress	Failure to progress		Failure to progress
Generally	Fretful Too weak to develop pains Fever, thirst Irritability Trembling	'I cannot bear it any more' Rude Nervous Moaning Restless Oversensitive to noise and pain Thirsty Frequent urination	Says she will go crazy Hysterical Melancholy Nervous Complaining Restless Chilliness Twitching Trembling
Pains	Drawing Distressing Spasmodic *Cease from exhaustion* *False* Too short Irregular Ineffectual Sharp, cramping pain in uterine ligaments, bladder or groin flies in all directions	Very severe – unbearable Distressing Too weak Spasmodic *Ceasing* *False* Tearing in abdomen shooting down the leg	Severe Distressing Too weak Ineffectual *Ceasing entirely* The contractions can come if the woman is chilled, and stop when she becomes warmer *False* Tearing, fly around the abdomen With cramps in the hip Talks incessantly, even during a contraction
Fear			Of death Of the birth
Fainting	Fainting	Fainting	Fainting
Nausea/ vomiting	Nausea	Nausea	
Exhaustion	Exhaustion	Exhaustion	
Uterus	Lack of tone		
Os	Rigid Spasmodic contractions	Rigid	Rigid Now dilated, now closed
Cervix	Needle-like pains	Fails to soften	Fails to soften
Vulva			
Vagina	Profuse secretion of mucus	Dark coagulated blood	
Worse from	Cold	Oversensitive to noise and pain Anger	Oversensitive to noise and pain Anger
Better from	Cool, fresh air	Cool, fresh air	

Table 5.
Labour

Remedy	Gelsemium	Kali carbonicum	Kali phosphoricum	Natrum mur
Progress	Failure to progress	Failure to progress		Failure to progress
Generally	Dreads the confinement Chatters during the first stage Headache Dark flushed face Trembling Exhausted, even at start of labour	Obstinate Oversensitive Restless Chilly after contraction Anxiety felt in the stomach Flatulence and bloated abdomen	Exhausted Mental tiredness Cannot concentrate on her breathing	Does not want to go through with the labour Desires privacy Melancholy Thirsty for cold gulps
Pains	Distressing Too weak Ineffectual *Cease entirely* *False* Cramps in abdomen go through to and up the back, then extend to the hips	Distressing Too weak Ineffectual Light touch can stop the contractions *Ceasing* Sharp, bearing-down pain from back to pelvis Cutting in lumbar region Linger and pass down to buttocks	Too weak Slow – every 15–30 min Ineffectual	Too weak *Ceasing*, from interruption or emotions Spasmodic drawing in back descending to thigh Headache at beginning of labour
Fear	Anticipatory fear	Imaginations in general Being alone		
Fainting				
Nausea/ vomiting	Nausea in early labour			
Exhaustion	Exhaustion	Exhaustion	Exhaustion	Exhaustion
Uterus	Uterine inertia			
Os	Rigid Thick			
Cervix		Fails to dilate		Fails to soften Constrictive pain
Vulva				
Vagina				
Worse from	Ordeals Emotions	Light touch		Sympathy
Better from	Urination Bending forward Movement	Back being pressed hard		

Table 6.
Labour

Remedy	Pulsatilla	Secale	Sepia
Progress	Failure to progress	Failure to progress	Failure to progress
Generally	Apologetic Changeable – laughing, then weeping Face pale Wants sympathy Great distress Thirstless with dry mouth	Stupor Parts open and loose without action Trembling when contractions cease Refuses to be covered	Snappy, irritable and indifferent Resentful if left 'I've had enough' Sensitive to tobacco smell Cold extremities and flushes of heat
Pains	Distressing Too short Too weak Irregular Ineffectual *Ceasing* *False* On motion of child Cutting Pressing spasmodic in back	Distressing Too short Too weak Irregular Ineffectual *Ceasing* *False*	Severe Too weak *Ceasing* *False* Spasmodic shooting pains extend upwards Felt in the back Sensation of weight in the anus
Fear	Being alone		
Fainting	Faintness	Fainting	Fainting
Nausea/ vomiting	Nausea and vomiting		
Exhaustion	Exhaustion		
Uterus	Uterine inertia	Uterine inertia	
Os		Rigid	
Cervix	Fails to dilate	Fails to soften	Indurated
Vulva			
Vagina			
Worse from			
Better from	Company Fresh air	Cool, fresh air	Covered

Table 7.
Recovering
from operative
procedures in
obstetrics

Remedy	Arnica	Bellis perennis	Calendula	Causticum	Chamomilla
Procedure	Caesarian Forceps Episiotomy	Caesarian	Forceps Episiotomy	Episiotomy	Caesarian
For	Wounds Pain Prevents swelling and bruising of soft tissue Anti-sepsis	Bumps Lumps Old injuries Abdominal wounds or trauma	Where skin is broken Aids regeneration Anti-sepsis To bring torn labia or perineum together	Rawness and soreness	Anger Pain
With	Shock Sore/bruised feeling Bad dreams Does not wish to be touched Denies her suffering – 'I'm all right'	Bruised soreness not helped by arnica Where lump remains	Offensive discharge Pain is more severe than the wound warrants	Pain makes it almost impossible to walk Sadness and fright	Unbearable pain The woman is so sensitive to the pain that she becomes enraged by it Snaps, snarls and demands relief
Worse from	Trauma Shock overexertion	Abdominal surgery	Cuts	Coffee Change of weather	Evening Fresh air Coffee Wind
Better from				Cold drinks Heat	Uncovering
Notes	Useful before hypericum for intense pain Do not apply externally to broken skin	Can be considered as a 'deeper acting' arnica in respect of the bruising and soreness	Alternate with other remedies, e.g. arnica or bellis perennis/as required Taken in tablet form Can be used as lotion (diluted) externally		

Table 8.
Recovering
from operative
procedures in
obstetrics

Remedy	Hypericum	Phosphorus	Secale	Staphysagria
Procedure	Caesarian	Caesarian Forceps	Caesarian	Caesarian Forceps Episiotomy
For	Injury to nerve-rich parts of the body Wounds slow to heal Inflammation	Wounds bleed freely with bright red blood, slow to clot Burning pains		Knife wounds Following unpleasant examination
With	Intense pains, shooting along the course of the nerves, more severe than wound warrants Shock from injury Severe headache after forceps delivery	Need for sympathy Despite being fearful and irritable when tired or upset, she is easily comforted and reassured	A state of stupor with anxiety May be anguish, fear of death, or laughing mania	Feelings of humiliation, anger and indignation, especially if the operative procedure was more than expected
Worse from	Cold Pressure Touch	Cold During evening During morning Fears	Heat	Exertion Catheterisaion Fasting Touch Tobacco Incision
Better from		After sleep Massage Cold drinks Reassurance	Cold bathing	
Notes	Also available in 'hypercal', a blend of hypericum and calendula mother tinctures Add 5 drops hypercal to a glass of water and bathe affected area several times daily	Helps eliminate anaesthetic and reduce postoperative nausea	This is a remedy made from ergot	

Table 9.
Breastfeeding
and breast
problems

Remedy	Belladonna	Bryonia	Calcarea carbonica	Chamomilla
Mastitis	Mastitis	Mastitis	Mastitis	Mastitis
Nipples	Acute swelling		Hot swelling	Cracked sore
Breasts	Red-streaked face from centre circumference Inflamed Engorged Tender Hot	Pale Inflamed Engorged Tender Hot Hard	Distended swollen glands	Hard glands
Pains	Throbbing	On slightest movement	As of excoriation and ulceration of nipples	Can hardly bear the pain of nursing
With	High fever Dry burning heat Flushed face Dilated pupils		Debility Fever Head sweat at night	Fever
Generally/ emotionally	Excited Possible delirium	Nausea on sitting up in bed Dryness and thirst Lips begin to crack	Fear that something might happen, e.g. death	Irritable, 'cannot bear it'
Worse from	Jarring	Movement	Cold air	Evening
Better from	Lying down	Alone		Uncovering
Milk supply	Low Over-abundant Galactorrhoea	Retarded Over-abundant Galactorrhoea	Low Over-abundant Galactorrhoea	
Milk			Watery, refused by child	Cheesy, + blood and pus
After weaning	Erysipelatous inflammation			
NB Where no other symptoms are present use *Castor Equi* for sore/cracked nipples	To dry up milk			

Table 10. Breastfeeding and breast problems

Remedy	Phytolacca	Pulsatilla	Silica
Mastitis	Mastitis	Mastitis	Mastitis
Nipples	Cracled Sore Swollen Mammary abscesses and pus	Cracked	Cracked Sore Inverted
Breasts	Inflamed 'like a brick' Lumpy Stony hard		Inflamed Burning pain Lumpy Deep red in the centre, with rose- coloured periphery Swollen
Pains	Unbeasrable while nursing Radiates over the entire body	Weeps while nursing Pain extends to chest, neck and down the back Changes from place to place	Worse in left breast While nursing Cutting in breasts and uterus
With	Raised temperature, As in flu Suppressed lochia Bad breath	Scanty lochia Milky white lochia	Head sweat at night Constipation No power to expel stool
Generally/ emotionally		Mild Tearful	Excited Yielding Anxious
Worse from			
Better from			
Milk supply	Low Galactorrhoea	Low Used to increase the flow Galactorrhoea in those not nursing	Suppressed Galactorrhoea
Milk	With blood	Thin, watering, acrid	Refused by child (blood)
Weaning		Breast swollen tense	
After weaning		To dry up milk	

NB Where no other symptoms are present, use castor equi for sore/cracked nipples.

Table 11.
Ophthalamia
neonatorum

Remedy	Aconite	Argentum nitricum	Calcarea carbonica	Lycopodium	Pulsatilla
Discharge		Purulent Offensive Yellow	Purulent Possibly smelly	Purulent	Purulent Offensive Thick Yellow
Eyelids	Hard Swollen Red	Glued together Red	Glued together Gritty Itchy	Glued together Ulcerated Red	Glued together Itching
Eyes	Aching Burning Red Sensitive to light Watering profusely	Corners of eye red and inflamed Red Sensitive to light	Gritty Sensitive to light Watering	Sensitive to light Watering	Aching Burning Itching Watering
Worse from	Cold, dry wind	Heat	For cold	Warm applications	Evening Warm room
Better from		Cold Cold compress	Heat Lying down		Cold Cold bathing Fresh air
Generally	In a state of great fear Restless Anxious	Fidgety Desires company	Happy when well Lethargic and obstinate when ill	May sleep well at night and cry all day	Want to be carried around gently Clingy and dependent

Table 12.
Colic

Remedy	Chamomilla	Colocynthis	Nux vomica	Secale
Abdomen	Bloated	Bloated		Bloated Tight like a drum
Pains	Unbearable	Cutting Griping Violent In waves	Cramping Griping Pressing Sore/bruised	
Cause	Anger	Anger Excitement Eating fruit	Breastfeeding mother eating spicy food or drinking too much tea, coffee or cola	Syntometrine
With	Diarrhoea with green stool Baby cries out while passing stool	Diarrhoea with pasty or green stool Nausea Vomiting		Diarrhoea Watery, olive-green stool
Worse from	Evening	After drinking Drinking cold drink when overheated	Morning After eating Coughing During fever Tight clothing	
Better from	Uncovering Sweating	Bending double Passing stool Pressure, being held over the knees	Warmth of bed Hot drinks Passing stool Passing wind	Baby better with nappy off
Emotionally/ generally	Angry, tolerates nothing and nobody	Restless Anxious Irritable from the pains	Irritable if chilled or tired	Anxious Stupor

Conclusions

- Informed choice must be offered to women (House of Commons Health Committee, 1992).
- Women and midwives need information on, and access to, homeopathy, amongst other therapies.
- Homeopathy offers swift correction to many of the common problems for which midwives call medical aid.
- Homeopathy can work for emergency obstetric situations and minimise trauma whilst promoting healing.
- Women and babies would benefit from homeopathic preventative medicine – an area in which orthodoxy is relatively unfamiliar.
- Homeopathy can improve the health of the neediest women efficiently, cheaply and safely.

Most obstetricians have ignored evidence that is at variance with their accepted practice and abstain from trials to test the effectiveness of alternatives (Tew, 1990). Midwives are in a position to meet the needs of a woman using or wanting to use homeopathy. The midwifery profession should look to undertake research into the effectiveness of homeopathy in midwifery care. Midwives are experts at observing the progress of pregnancy and birth and their skills could be invaluable in the application of high quality homeopathic care. Those attending mothers and babies can look to homeopathy as an effective system of medicine without risk.

Training   **Homeopathic practitioners**   The Faculty of Homeopathy is authorised by Act of Parliament to train medically qualified doctors (as well as dentists, pharmacists and vets) in homeopathic medicine. The Faculty offers short diploma courses for doctors at educational centres in Britain. The examinations lead to membership of the Faculty of Homeopathy (M F Hom). This is recognised in medical circles and appropriately trained general practitioners will have these letters after their name. Names of trained general practitioners can be obtained from the Family Health Service Associations (FHSA). General practitioners offering such specialisation may now publicise it. The local pharmacy will also know of general practitioners in the area offering homeopathy. The NHS prescription form can be dispensed by those chemists registered in the NHS. Notices will be obvious in the pharmacies, stating that they have homeopathic medicines available.

The term 'lay homeopath' usually means non-professional homeopath, i.e. someone using homeopathy without a qualification. There is no all-encompassing register of professional homeopaths. Those registered with the Society of Homeopaths are professional homeopaths who have been fully examined according to the principles and practice established by Samuel Hahnemann. They have a proper understanding and knowledge of homeopathic *Materia Medica* and *Repertory*. They have been adequately trained in the essential medical sciences and skills and have had suitable clinical training and experience. They agree by the Society's Code of Ethics. Practitioners are issued with a Certificate of Registration and may use the initials RSHom. Some will use FSHom. This denotes Fellowship of the Society of Homeopaths, awarded for contribution to homeopathy or the work of the Society.

The Society has a Professional Conduct Director and a complaints procedure. Litigation against homeopathic practitioners is virtually unheard of. Members include midwives, doctors, nurses, pharmacists, physiotherapists and health visitors.

The Society has a list of recognised Colleges of Homeopathy, each of which will have their own awards for graduates to receive a diploma or licentiate, after completion of a 3–4 year course. The Society also has a list of graduates gaining experience prior to registration or who have chosen not to register with the Society of Homeopaths.

Insurance cover is obtainable from other sources outside the Society. Members of the Royal College of Midwives using homeopathy in their midwifery care have insurance cover for this, but only this, type of practice.

Further information on homeopathy

For more information about homeopathy and homeopathic training contact:

The Society of Homeopaths
2 Artizan Road, Northampton NN1 4HU, UK
Tel: 0604 21400
For the register of Homeopaths and recommended colleges

The Institute of Complementary Medicine
21 Portland Place, London W1 3AF, UK
Tel: 071 636 9543

The Hahnemann Society
Humane Education Centre,
Bounds Green Road, London N22 4EU, UK

The Faculty of Homeopathy
The Royal Homeopathic Hospital,
Great Ormond Street, London
WC1N 3HR, UK

The College of Homeopathy
Regents College,
Inner Circle, Regents Park, London
NW1 4NS, UK
Tel: 071 487 7416

The Foundation for Homeopathic Education and Research
5916 Chaot Crest,
Oakland, CA 94618, USA
(for current research available)

Ainsworths Pharmacy
38 New Cavendish Street, London
W1M 7LH, UK
Tel: 071 935 5330

Helios Pharmacy
97 Camden Road, Tunbridge Wells, Kent
TN1 2QP, UK
Tel: 0892 536393/537254

References

Borland D. (1982) *Homeopathy in Practice.* Beaconsfield Press, British Homeopathic Association (undated) Leaflet.

Choudhury (1988) *Indications of Miasm.* B. Jain Publishers, Put Ltd, New Delhi.

Close S. (reprinted 1981) *The Genius of Homeopathy*, p. 213. B. Jain Publishers, New Delhi.

Coulter H.L. (1981) *Homeopathic Science and Modern Medicine*, pp. 88, 97. North Atlantic Books, Berkeley, California.

Cullen W. (1789) *A Treatise of the Materia Medica.* Edinburgh.

Day C.E.I. (1984) Control of stillbirth in pigs using homeopathy. *British Homeopathic Journal*, **73**, 142–143.

Dhunny J. (1993) Professional issues relating to the use of homeopathy within midwifery practice. Unpublished professional development assignment.

Dudgeon R.E. (1921) *Samuel Hahnemann: Organon of Medicine,* 6th edition, 1842, pp. 31, 40–41, 139. B. Jain Publishers (P) Ltd, New Delhi.

Enkin M., Keirse M. and Chalmers I. *A Guide to Effective Care in Pregnancy and Childbirth.* Oxford University Press, Oxford.

Foubister D. (1989) *Tutorials on Homeopathy*, pp. 5, 68. Beaconsfield Press.

Furnham A. and Smith C. (1988) Choosing alternative medicine: a comparison of the beliefs of patients visiting a GP and a Homeopath. *Social Science in Medicine*, **26(7)**, 685–689.

Geraghty B. (1993) Homeopathy for Midwives. Unpublished final thesis for graduation of The London College of Classical Homeopathy at Morley College, London.

Gibson S. and Gibson R. (1987) *Homeopathy for Everyone.* Penguin, London.

Goodliffe H. (1990) Therapies under threat. *Nursing Times* **(86)26**, 48–49.

Hahnemann S. (1828, reprinted 1987) *The Chronic Diseases*, p. 17. B. Jain Publishers (P) Ltd, New Delhi.

Handley R. (1990) *A Homeopathic Love Story.* North Atlantic Books, Berkeley, California.

House of Commons Health Committee (1992) Second Report: Maternity Services, Vol. 1. HMSO, London.

Kleijam J., Knipschild P. and Riet G. (1991) Clinical trials of homeopathy. *British Medical Journal*, **302**, 316–323.

Koehler G. (1986) *The Handbook of Homeopathy.* Thorsons.

Moskowitz R. (1992) *Homeopathic Medicines for Pregnancy and Childbirth*, pp. 12, 13, 19, 60. North Atlantic Books, Berkeley, California.

National Association of Homeopathic Groups (NAHG) (Summer 1992) National Health Service Homeopathy Newsletter.

Patel M.S. (1987a) Evaluation of holistic medicine. *Social Science in Medicine*, **24(2)**, 169–175.

Patel M.S. (1987b) Problems in the evaluation of alternative medicine. *Social Science in Medicine*, **25(6)**, 669–678.

Rankin-Box D. (1991) Proceed with caution. *Nursing Times*, **87**, 34–36.

Royal College of Midwives (1993) Julie Dhunny to RCM, personal correspondence.

Society of Homeopaths (undated) *Homeopathy: the past, present and future medicine* (leaflet). Northampton.

Society of Homeopaths (1993) *Register of Homeopaths.*

Spiby H. (1993) Giving complementary therapy within midwifery care for the 1990s. *Midwives Chronicle*, **106(1261)**, 38–40.

Tew M. (1990) *Safer Childbirth?* pp. 35, 209, 294. Chapman & Hall.

Ullman D. (1991) *Discovering Homeopathy: Medicine for the Twenty-first Century.* Thorsons.

UKCC (1989) *Exercising Accountability.*

UKCC (1992a) *Code of Professional Conduct.*

UKCC (1992b) *Standards for the Administration of Medicines.*

UKCC (1992c) *The Scope of Professional Practice.*

UKCC (1993) *Midwives' Rules.*

UKCC (1994) *The Midwife's Code of Practice.*

Vithoulkas G. (1986) *The Science of Homeopathy*, Ch. 5. Thorsons.

Further reading

Castro M. (1992) *Homeopathy for Mother and Baby.* Macmillan.

Coulter L. (1981) *Homeopathic Science and Modern Medicine. The Physics of Healing with Microdoses.* North Atlantic Books.

Koehler G. (1986) *The Handbook of Homeopathy. Its Principles and Practice.* Thorsons.

Moskowitz R. (1992) *Homeopathic Medicines for Pregnancy and Childbirth.* North Atlantic Books.

Ullman D. (1991) *Discovering Homeopathy: Medicine for the Twenty-first Century.* Thorsons.

**APPENDIX 1
Homeopathy –
the more
'scientific'
medicine**

The criticism of homeopathy is theoretical. In order to judge whether it works or not, the homeopathic method needs to be applied to see if sick or 'diseased' persons get well.

Homeopaths do not follow the orthodox method of defining a disorder and then prescribing a remedy to counteract the process. Nor do they justify their method in terms of cause and effect, or 'explain' in physiological terms as does orthodox medicine. Practice is justified by practice and the drug tests are pure experiments. The selection of a homeopathic remedy is based on the symptoms in the provings. Homeopathic practice has not changed for nearly 200 years and is based on fixed principles and laws. The orthodox 'reductionist' view of explaining disease and drug actions at the cellular, microbiological or biochemical level will always be beyond the grasp of the researcher. This is because the living human being is more that the sum of its parts, or just a collection of specialised cells.

Coulter (1981) writes how the reductionist view was accepted in all sciences in the early nineteenth century and has now been discarded by everyone except 'orthodox' physicians. 'Orthodox' medicine lacks a precisely structured doctrine. Coulter suggests that homeopathy is the more 'scientific' method of medicine due to its rigour and precision of its principles. The laws of application and the principles can be seen as a unified hypothesis. Homeopathic treatment tests this hypothesis and the noted successes give the hypothesis validity.

The outdated cause and effect relations of orthodox medicine have not been formulated into an operational theory governed by principles.

This is where the difficulty lies, in that orthodox medicine condemns homeopathy because it does not conform to their views of what is 'scientific'. The main requirement for a clinical trial from an orthodox point of view is to assemble homogeneous groups of people with the same 'named disease'. The treated and untreated cases are then matched.

Homeopathy has always maintained that there are no diseases but diseased individuals and that each person is different so group homogenity is almost impossible. Despite having to observe inappropriate 'orthodox' protocols for clinical trials, homeopathic remedies have been shown to be effective in such trials. In 1980 a group of doctors and homeopathic physicians in Glasgow treated 46 patients with rheumatoid arthritis. Half were treated with conventional anti-inflammatory medications, together with placebo. The other half were treated with the same anti-inflammatory medications together with the indicated homeopathic remedies. The patients on homeopathic remedies showed significant improvement over those on placebo.

The research evidence supporting homeopathy seldom elicits a response from orthodox medicine, despite its publication. Dr Foubister quotes Dr Charles Wheeler in an address to the British Medical Association:

> To say that the vast body of medical opinion for a hundred years has rejected homeopathy is true, but to imply that it has rejected it after trial and investigation is a gross fallacy. Each successive decade has handed its prejudice and ignorance onto the next and the simple tests which would have settled the matter once and for all have never been made, save by the few, who, in consequence, have maintained the heresy.

The midwife can make herself familiar with the published research and consider conducting a trial within the maternity unit. In recent years there have been positive research findings published but not, as yet, relating to homeopathy within midwifery practice (Kleijam *et al.*, 1991). This author knows of one trial being conducted by midwives with regard to the use of arnica for perineal trauma.

The public are well informed and are disappointed with what 'science' has to offer. The holistic perspective of homeopathy is attractive as it has a more comprehensive approach to promote and improve health rather than eradicate disease or ailment (Patel, 1987a). Patel also suggests that there is a need for other ways of evaluating homeopathy. He recommends that emphasis be placed on value for money, that is the improvement of health in an effective and low cost manner (Patel, 1987b).

Sarah Budd

Chapter 10 **Acupuncture**

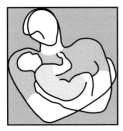

Introduction
In presenting acupuncture as it is used today in midwifery, in a Western hospital, it is necessary to review the history of acupuncture. It is also helpful to have an understanding not only of the theory of Traditional Chinese Medicine, but also the underlying philosophical framework of Chinese thought. Modern Western ideas on acupuncture will then be outlined.

The term 'acupuncture' comes from the Latin *acus*, meaning a needle, and *punctura*, to puncture. In China, thousands of years ago, it was noted that soldiers wounded by arrows sometimes recovered from illnesses which had affected them for many years. The idea evolved that, by penetrating the skin at certain points, diseases were apparently cured. The Chinese began to copy the effects of the arrow, by puncturing the skin with needles. Acupuncture is an important part of Traditional Chinese Medicine, which includes other techniques such as 'cupping', 'moxibustion', massage ('Tuina'), and Chinese herbal medicine. Over the past 2500 years, medical scholars in every age have contributed to the refinement and development of the art of acupuncture in China. Over the last 20 years acupuncture has dramatically increased in popularity in many parts of the world. There is an increasing interest in the use of it in midwifery practice. The World Health Organization states that there is sufficient evidence supporting the therapeutic effects of acupuncture for it to be considered as an important part of primary health care and that it should be fully integrated with conventional medicine.

Acupuncture is a technique of initiating, controlling or accelerating physiological functions of the body. Acupuncture theory incorporates a complete scientific model that permits the precise calculation of which acupuncture points to use, when and how to combine them, and which points to combine together – all based on observations of the signs and symptoms of the patient (Bensoussan, 1991).

Details of therapy

Needles are inserted into the skin at the acupuncture points. There are over two thousand points on the body, although only approximately two hundred are commonly used in everyday practice. The earliest recorded acupuncture needles were made of stone. In early times, they would also have been made of bone, slivers of bamboo and later bronze, iron, silver and gold. They are now made of stainless steel, are of hair-like thinness, and produce relatively little pain when inserted. The length and gauge refer to the needle body, the part between the handle and the tip. The length ranges from 1.25 centimetres (cm) to 12.5 cm. The gauge ranges from 0.45 cm (26 gauge) to 0.22 cm (34 gauge). In this country, 30 to 34 gauge would be most commonly used. The length of needle and depth of needling depends on factors such as the location of the point and the size of the person being treated. For example, to treat sciatica, a needle may be inserted into the buttock to a depth of at least 3 cm and the needle would therefore need to be at least 4 cm long, whereas to treat sinusitis, a needle may be inserted alongside the nostril where there is much less flesh; this needle need only be 1.25 cm long and inserted to a depth of 0.5 cm. Figure 1 shows acupuncture needles.

Fig. 1. Acupuncture needles. (Photo: Nik Screen).

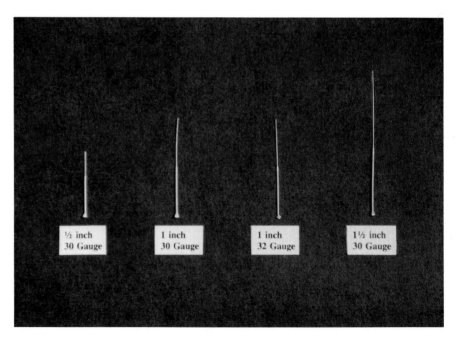

½ inch
30 Gauge

1 inch
30 Gauge

1 inch
32 Gauge

1½ inch
30 Gauge

After insertion, needles are manipulated by rotation according to the condition being treated. This leads to a feeling of warmth and distension around the needle, sometimes also described as a tingling or electric sensation. This is how the practitioner knows that the needle is in the right place. The needles are usually retained for approximately 20 minutes, although this may vary. During treatment, there is often a pleasant feeling of deep relaxation and some people fall asleep. The effect may last for some hours and it is wise to reassure the client that this is normal. In the case of pregnant women, it is often a much needed rest.

Another way of stimulating the needles is by the use of electro-acupuncture. This was first used in China in the 1930s and is now widely employed. Light leads are attached to the handle of the needle by a small clip and a mild electric current passed through the needle. The amount of stimulation can be objectively measured and regulated by adjusting the current, amplitude and frequency. This can produce a higher and more continuous level of stimulation than manual manipulation which is often needed in acupuncture analgesia and anaesthesia. For pain relief in labour, the woman can select the frequency and intensity of the stimulation for maximum analgesic effect. Figure 2 shows an electro-acupuncture machine.

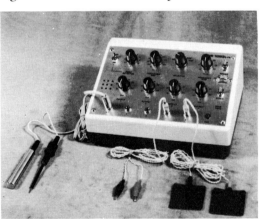

Fig. 2. Electro-acupuncture machine.

Another technique used in Traditional Chinese Medicine alongside acupuncture is 'moxibustion'. This has many applications in general treatment, but in obstetrics, tends to be used for encouraging version in breech presentation. This will be discussed in the section on treatments during pregnancy. A moxa stick is shown in Figure 3.

Acupuncture needles are manufactured in this country now as well as being imported from China and Japan. There are several suppliers who provide many different types of equipment which may be used by the acupuncturist. Needles may be disposable or reusable and the choice made by the practitioner may depend on access to safe sterilisation methods. Registered practitioners are required by their local authority to prove they have adequate sterilisation equipment, or means of sterilisation at a local hospital, as well as safe facilities

Fig. 3. Moxa stick.
(Photo: Nik Screen).

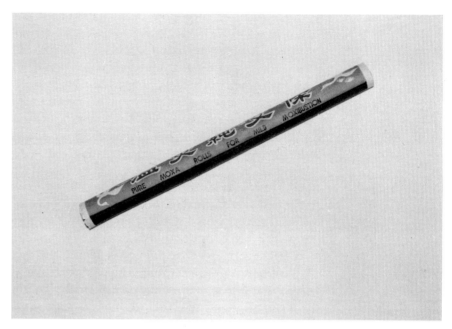

for the disposal of both single-use and reusable needles. This is to reassure those coming for treatment that the needles will not be a source of infections such as hepatitis and human immunodeficiency virus (HIV).

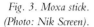

Diagnosis   In determining the pattern of disharmony, the acupuncturist needs a detailed understanding of the person's lifestyle, diet, work, medical history, emotional states etc. The diagnosis is made by questioning, observation, and examination of the pulse and tongue. The practitioner is looking at a whole pattern rather than symptoms in isolation. Tongue and pulse diagnosis are highly refined in Chinese Medicine. The pulse is felt at the wrists on the radial artery and its strength, rhythm and quality indicate the balance of energy and state of the disease. The tongue, through its shape, colour, movement and coating, indicates the progression and degree of the illness.

Just as there are those who do not respond to drugs, so there are those who do not respond to acupuncture. Some diseases are very difficult to cure, particularly if they have progressed to the point where the person is very weak. There are no restrictions on who may have treatment. Babies can be treated, although finger pressure, 'Shiatsu', is usually preferable to needles. Women can be treated for complications of pregnancy without causing harm to the mother or baby, though certain points must be avoided if there is any likelihood of miscarriage. Acupuncture can be combined with Western drug therapy, or can be used to eliminate dependence on drugs for chronic conditions.

An appointment for acupuncture treatment may be anything from 30 minutes to 1 hour duration. The first appointment is longer as a detailed case history is taken. The number of treatments needed varies tremendously according to the condition and the person being treated. Women treated for sickness in pregnancy sometimes recover fully after just one treatment, although three or four are usually needed. Some benefit is usually felt after each treatment. Backache in pregnancy tends to take longer, usually needing five or six treatments.

Traditional Chinese medicine

Traditional Chinese Medicine is a system of medicine which uses not only acupuncture but herbs, diet, massage ('Tuina') and exercise for the prevention and treatment of disease. Acupuncture theory is drawn from an ancient Chinese text, *The Yellow Emperor's Classic of Internal Medicine (The Nei Jing)* compiled between 300 and 100 BC (Kaptchuk, 1983). The theories of medicine it contains are still regarded as the most authoritative guide to Traditional Chinese Medicine.

The Chinese medical system stems from a philosophy very different to that of Western medicine. Acupuncture is a method of using fine needles to stimulate channels of energy running beneath the surface of the skin. This affects a change in the energy balance of the body and works to restore health. The Chinese call this energy or life force 'Qi', pronounced 'chee'. Qi pervades all things and in humans, is derived partly from heredity and partly from the food we eat and air we breathe. It keeps the blood circulating, warms the body and fights disease. Qi flows through channels or meridians which form a network in the body and link all parts and functions together so that they work as one unit. There are 12 main channels, each connected to an internal organ and each named after that organ (Fig. 4A). As well as this, there are eight extra channels, which also follow a set pathway in the body. The auricle of the ear has a complete set of acupuncture points corresponding to different parts and systems of the body (Fig. 4B). If the ear is likened to the flexed fetus with the lobe representing the fetal head, the acupuncture points correspond approximately with the anatomy of the body. Ear acupuncture originated in China, but was greatly developed in France in the 1950s by Dr Nogier, who added pragmatic points to the traditional ones. It is symptomatic and relatively easy to learn. Short acupuncture needles, usually half an inch in length, may be used at the time of a treatment. Another method is to use stud-like or embedded needles or seeds which may be left *in situ* for several days. The seeds are usually mustard seeds which are very hard, and when pressed, strongly stimulate the point. The advantage of seeds over needles is that they do not break the skin, and therefore are less likely to cause infection when left *in situ* for several days.

In health, the Qi moves smoothly through the channels, but if for some reason it becomes blocked, or too weak or too strong, then illness occurs. The aim of the acupuncturist is to correct the flow of Qi by inserting thin needles into particular points on the channels and so affect a change in a part or function of the body. The logic underlying Chinese medical theory assumes that a part can only be understood in its relation to the whole. The Chinese identify

Fig. 4(A). Illustration of acupuncture channels and points.

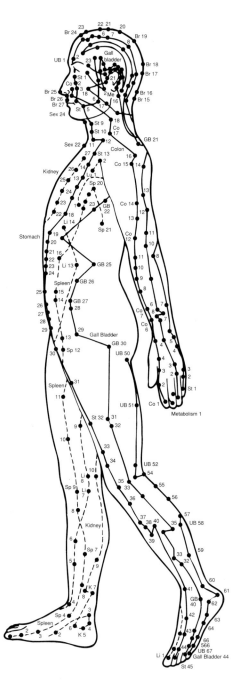

the relationships between phenomena by the theory of Yin and Yang, two opposing forces. Yin, originally signifying the northern side of the mountain, implies coldness, darkness, the interior, passiveness, and the negative. Yang, the Southern side, implies warmth, light, activity, expressiveness, and the positive. If either Yin or Yang become out of balance, then health disorders result. An

Fig. 4(B). Distribution of auricular points

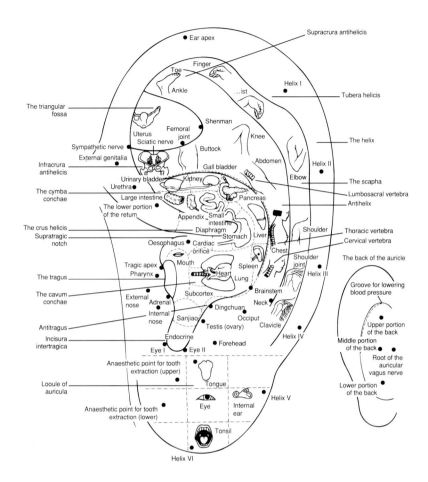

organ that is too Yin is too sluggish, static and accumulates waste. An organ that is too Yang is overactive, out of control, and may generate heat. As well as the principles of Yin and Yang, traditional Chinese medicine uses other polarities by which all diseases and disharmonies can be described. Together, they are called the 'eight principles'. They include empty–full, hot–cold, and excess–deficient, and are used to group symptoms. An example would be red face, rapid pulse, fever, dark urine and pain made worse by heat are hot, Yang symptoms, while slow movements, slow pulse, pale tongue, thin clear urine and pain improved by warmth would be symptoms of a cold, Yin condition. This classification of disease suggests suitable methods of treatment; for the patient diagnosed as having a hot condition, the treatment will aim to disperse the heat. If the diagnosis is too weak and cold it will aim to build strength and warm up by using moxibustion. Traditional Chinese medicine takes into account not only the disease symptoms, but also the age, habits, physical and emotional traits and all other aspects of the individual, looking at the whole person, as an inextricable part of the environment. Internal causes of disease may be constitutional, of an emotional nature or as a result of habits such as overindulgence. Emotional problems may be traced to a physical origin, and physical symptoms may be emotionally induced. An example would be excess anger, causing the energy to rush up to the head causing a red face, bloodshot eyes, headache, stiff shoulders etc. Disharmony of the liver may cause irritability, anger, sighing, and depression.

External causes of disease are mostly associated with the environment, especially weather conditions such as cold, damp, heat etc. and particularly sudden changes in weather; exercise and rest, too much or too little of either can harm the balance of energy; trauma, such as accidents, falls, operations etc. In China, the emphasis is on prevention of disease. Every morning, one can observe hundreds of ordinary people of all ages practising their Tai Chi or Qi-Gong exercises in the parks or outside their homes, to encourage the free flow of Qi.

Picture a peasant working in the fields in the Han dynasty, 154 BC in northern China. A bitterly cold north wind blows, and in the evening she has an itchy throat, runny nose, cough, severe stiff neck and headache. The local acupuncturist diagnoses 'Exterior invasion of Wind-Cold'. Treatment is given, and after a few hours, there is a marked improvement.

A businessman in the city of London suffers from anxiety, insomnia and headaches. He is under considerable pressure at work, with heavy responsibility and long hours. A friend recommends an acupuncturist, who diagnoses 'Liver Qi stagnation' caused by the pressure at work. After a few weekly treatments, there is much improvement.

Such is the awesome power of Chinese medicine, that although it originated thousands of years ago, it can still successfully diagnose and treat

Fig. 5. Diagram of Chong and Ren channels.

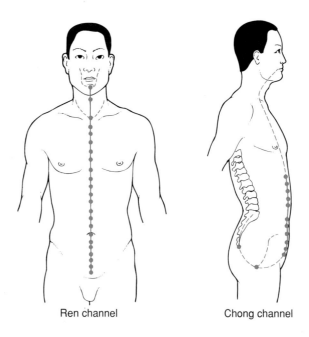

Ren channel   Chong channel

twentieth century health problems brought about by a lifestyle very different to that of the peasant.

Traditional Chinese Medicine theory and obstetrics

Several of the eight extra meridians referred to in the previous section are very much concerned with women's physiology and with childbirth, particularly the '*Ren*' and '*Chong*' channels (Fig. 5). The Chinese character for *Ren* means 'pregnancy and nourishment'. If the *Ren* channel is working well, then one is able to conceive and nourish the fetus. The channel starts in the uterus, emerges at the perineum and ascends the anterior midline of the body. The *Chong* channel is known as the 'Sea of Blood'. It also starts in the uterus, emerges at the perineum and travels up the trunk bilaterally. It is very much concerned with healthy menstruation and conception. In traditional Chinese medicine it is really the ability to conceive that indicates that the *Ren* and *Chong* channels are functioning. Acupuncture has apparently been used successfully in some cases of infertility. Great emphasis is placed on the blood. Nourishment of the fetus during pregnancy via the placenta, and after the baby is born in the milk, are both considered to make great demands on the woman's blood. In China, great emphasis is placed on the woman's diet during pregnancy as well as observing other lifestyle modifications.

Some of the 12 regular channels are also involved in reproduction, particularly the Kidney, Liver, Spleen and Heart meridians. The Kidney is said to control physical growth, development, maturation, and reproduction. It is also the ultimate control for the other organs and for Qi and blood. The Chinese include the adrenal glands when talking about the kidney, and in Western terms, this importance of the kidney can be understood in terms of steroidal and hormone production. Certain acupuncture points should be avoided during pregnancy as they may cause miscarriage. In particular, points 'Sanyinjiao or Spleen 6' located on the lower leg and 'Hegu or Large Intestine 4' located on the hand (Fig. 6). Of course these points may be advantageous in the post-mature woman who is heading for induction of labour.

Fig. 6. Diagram of points 'Hegu' and 'Sanyinjiao'.

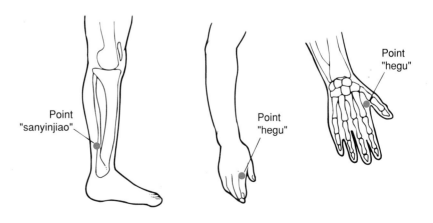

There are a number of studies on induction of labour with acupuncture (see 'Application to midwifery practice', p. 233).

As the *Nei Jing* is compiled of numerous texts with many revisions and refinements, it will be easy to understand that further details of traditional Chinese medicine theory are beyond the scope of this chapter.

The western explanation . . . and research

There are now both theories and experimental evidence to explain some aspects of acupuncture, particularly its effect in pain relief. A tremendous amount of research has been carried out which attempts to legitimise its use in terms of Western science. To researchers, acupuncture presents a specific problem in that it is a different scientific model from Western medicine and adopts distinct terminology such as 'energy' and 'channels'. The methodology used is extremely variable, both this has resulted in many papers which are of poor quality and of little value. It is important that an agreed and satisfactory methodology be established for the evaluation of acupuncture.

The popularisation of acupuncture in the West came about through observation of operations under acupuncture analgesia in China. This led to more research in the field, and in the West and in China where they could see that more scientific research would promote acupuncture analgesia in the West.

A number of physiological changes have been reported following acupuncture treatment. Functional changes include:

* controlling peristaltic activity in the digestive process, smooth muscle influence in the control of urination and childbirth;
* altering haemodynamics, such as blood pressure, cardiac output and microcirculation;
* the modification of body or blood chemistry as evidenced by production of enzymes and hormones, changes in cellular and humoral immunity, and alterations of blood cell counts, e.g. white blood cells and platelets.

The following trials illustrate some of the above findings. They are not at this stage directly concerned with obstetrics, such trials being included in a separate section, but as pregnancy involves so many physiological changes and a number of patients develop medical complications, they are of some relevance.

Takishima *et al.* (1982) and Yu and Lee (1976) demonstrated that acupuncture generally improved bronchoconstriction and pulmonary function during clinical attacks of asthma. Altering haemodynamics, Omura (1975) demonstrated that acupuncture had a prolonged effect on microcirculation in the brain and peripheral tissue. Wu (1982) and several other researchers monitored changes in electrocardiograms (ECGs) and cardiac echoes after needling the point 'Neiguan' (or Pericardium 6).

Biochemical alterations include for example restoring levels of stomach acidity, free stomach acids, pepsin and gastric lipase from needling three specific points (Shanghai College of Traditional Chinese Medicine, 1983).

Numerous clinical surveys illustrate that viral, bacterial and protozoal infections may be effectively treated with acupuncture. Qiu (1985) discusses the effect of acupuncture on raising the immunity of the body. The possible changes in the immune system brought about by acupuncture include:

- changes in the cellular immune ability of the body – white blood cells, sensitised T-lymphocytes and their phagocytic activity;
- changes in the humoral immune ability – production of immunoglobulins by B-lymphocytes;
- changes in the reticuloendothelial sysytem – macrophages in the liver, lymph nodes, spleen, and bone marrow;
- the anti-allergic effect of needling (suppressing hypersensitivity).

Bresler and Kroening (1976) comment that 'When an area of the skin anywhere on the body is stimulated, the immune/ inflammatory system is mobilised. This reaction to acupuncture may involve histamine, bradykinin, cyclic AMP, serotonin, prostaglandins, and a variety of substances yet to be discovered.'

Trials carried out on patients with a whole range of psychological and emotional disorders show mixed results. Some concluded that it was a cheaper and safer method of treatment than others currently in use (Schaub and Fazal Haq, 1977). Others were more disappointed with their results (Fischer *et al.*, 1984), but it has been pointed out by Bensoussan (1991) that no attempt was made at a differential diagnosis in Chinese terms, which augured badly for their experimental outcome.

In summary, research into what mediates the acupuncture effect focuses on three main areas:

- Neural mediation, which incorporates the concept that nerve fibres transmit and carry the acupuncture effect, and this is confirmed by experiments which test the acupuncture influence after denervation in the region of needling, interference with neural transmission of the acupuncture impulse, or following nerve section.
- Humoral mediation, which includes communication of the acupuncture effect via the circulation of neurotransmittors and other hormones in the bloodstream and cerebrospinal fluid.
- Bioelectric mediation, which maintains that the meridians are electrically distinct and that changes in them act as precursors to humoral and neurological responses.

Acupuncture today in Britain

The recent British Medical Association report on complementary medicine (BMA, 1993) states that one in four of the 28 000 members surveyed by the

Consumers Association in 1991 had consulted a practitioner of complementary medicine in the preceding 12 months. They included the practices of acupuncture, chiropractic, herbalism, homoeopathy, osteopathy, aromatherapy and reflexology. The register of acupuncturists published by the Council for Acupuncture at the time of writing has 1114 members. Most are in private practice, but there are a growing number of practitioners working in the National Health Service, some in pain clinics, working alongside anaesthetists, some in general practitioners' surgeries, some in maternity units. Physiotherapists with an interest in acupuncture often combine it with their routine work. There is also a growing number of general practitioners who incorporate acupuncture into their practice.

Application to midwifery practice

Acupuncture is ideal for childbirth. It offers a safe, easy to administer, inexpensive treatment to women during the antenatal, intrapartum, and postpartum period. Women have always been cautious about taking drugs in pregnancy, and since the thalidomide disaster so have their doctors. The so-called 'minor disorders' of pregnancy are anything but minor if you are the one suffering from them, and for years midwives and general practitioners have felt the frustration of not being able to offer much in the way of remedies for these problems. Now there is an answer. It has been around for 2000 years, but has not been readily available to us here in the West until recently.

More midwives around the country are becoming interested in acupuncture as the mothers under their care report the great relief it has given them. There has also been a vast amount of media interest with many articles in journals such as the *Midwives Chronicle* and *Nursing Times*. Several maternity units in England have one or more midwives who offer acupuncture to their patients. Others have shown an interest, and are encouraging midwives to train, in some cases with funding as well. One maternity unit in Plymouth has two midwives trained in acupuncture, and together they have treated over 2000 women with pregnancy-related problems. The service has been available since 1988 and has had tremendous support from both management and medical staff (Budd, 1992).

Uses in pregnancy

There are many conditions which may be helped by acupuncture during pregnancy. In the Plymouth maternity unit, the most common are backache, sciatica and sickness/nausea. The success rate for these is very high. Women are referred for treatment with all sorts of conditions, as illustrated in the table below, but we will look at some of the more common in detail.

Sickness. Hyperemesis.	Nausea. Heartburn.
Carpal tunnel syndrome	Headaches. Migraines.
Varicose veins.	Constipation.
Vulval varices.	Haemorrhoids.

Abdominal pain.   Backache. Sciatica.
Drug addiction.   Smoking.
Breech presentation.   Induction of labour.
Skin rashes.   Sinusitis.

It is not the purpose of this chapter to discuss all the different treatments for various disorders, but a few examples will be given for the most common of these, illustrated by some case histories. There will be reference made to research where available, although the majority of papers are on the use of acupuncture for analgesia in labour or the induction of labour.

Sickness, nausea and hypermesis

These can cause absolute misery in early pregnancy, and in the unfortunate few can last the whole duration! Women who have severe hyperemesis needing hospitalisation may be separated from other children causing much heartache and inconvenience in the home, with partners taking time off work, etc. They can be treated with acupuncture as inpatients, and when well enough to go home again, may continue treatment on an outpatient basis if necessary. The number of treatments needed varies greatly according to the individual and severity. Some women notice an immediate improvement and even cancel their second appointment! This is unusual though, and three treatments is the average. Needles are inserted into the wrists at the point 'Neiguan' (Pericardium 6) and 'Zhongwan' (Ren 12) in most cases, with other points being added if indicated. As mentioned previously, each treatment is adapted according to the individual. Research into the actions of the point 'Neiguan' has been carried out by Professor Dundee amongst others (Dundee *et al.*, 1988). He has published papers on the use of the point on patients suffering chemotherapy-induced sickness, but also has a paper on the use of acupressure with positive results (Dundee *et al.*, 1988, 1989; see also Chapter 7).

Helen had a history of vomiting until term in her first pregnancy. She presented in her second pregnancy at 12 weeks' gestation, having been referred by her general practitioner. She had nausea and vomiting every day, which was worse in the evenings. She worked full time as a teacher. She was also constipated, having her bowels open only once per week. Otherwise she was well. After the first acupuncture treatment, she noticed less nausea, and a reduction in the frequency of vomiting, which was just beginning to return when she came for her second treatment. She had had her bowels open twice in 5 days. After three more treatments, the nausea had gone completely, and she had not been sick . By mutual agreement, she stopped treatment, with the understanding that she could return if necessary.

Tina B. had suffered from sickness in her first pregnancy until the 17th week. She presented in her second pregnancy at 10 weeks' gestation having been referred by her community midwife. She worked 4 days per week as a midwife (and was also studying for a degree). She complained of constant nausea, and was sick several times per day, morning and evening. She had no appetite or energy. When a full history had been taken, a traditional Chinese medicine diagnosis of Stomach/Spleen deficiency was made. After one treatment, she improved immediately, the nausea had gone, and she had only vomited once in 4 days. Treatment was repeated once, and she decided she did not need to continue. She admitted to having felt sceptical before she started treatment. She was delighted with the results, having expected the pattern to be repeated from last time.

Backache and sciatica This is another common complaint in pregnancy. In many women, it is fortunately just a problem during pregnancy, but there are also those who have had back trouble for a long time, which is often exacerbated by the hormonal influences as well as the postural changes which come about as the pregnancy advances. Physiotherapy is sometimes more appropriate, and with a good relationship between the two departments, referrals may go back and forth. Some women do not have any relief from physiotherapy, and try acupuncture, and vice versa.

In the early stages, it may be possible to carry out the treatment with the woman lying prone, but as the 'bump' grows, she needs to lie on her side with a pillow between her knees. Needles are inserted locally around the area of pain as well as lower down the legs. Points are used which tonify the Kidney Qi, responsible for the health of the lower back area and for bones in general in Traditional Chinese Medicine. The first treatment may well aggravate the situation as the 'stagnant Qi' starts moving, and it is important to warn her of this. After the second treatment, there usually follows a progressive improvement. Again, the number of treatments needed varies from person to person, but is usually around five or six.

Victoria presented at 25 weeks' gestation in her first pregnancy, having been referred by her general practitioner. She worked full time as a state registered nurse. Five years previously, she had suffered from sciatic nerve entrapment from lifting a patient at work. She had been treated with physiotherapy and three epidurals. She now had low back pain, radiating down her right leg. The first acupuncture treatment stirred up her backache, as she had been warned, but then it had eased. After four visits, it had improved enough for her to stop treatment. She needed one 'top-up' treatment 2 months later, but was otherwise delighted with the results.

Constipation   Most women notice a change in bowel habit during pregnancy, and again, we can probably blame the hormones for this, particularly the relaxation of plain muscle by progesterone. In those who have a problem anyway, it can become a major discomfort and cause great distress. Acupuncture points are chosen according to the individual case, but are usually in the arm, just above the wrist, and in the leg, just below the knee. Results are usually quite dramatic as illustrated in the following case history.

Tania had a history of irritable bowel syndrome and constipation, with painful bowel movements every 2 or 3 days. She was taking isphaghula husk (Fybogel), senna and lactulose (20 ml three times daily). Like most women, she was keen to stop her medication during pregnancy. Her general practitioner referred her for acupuncture at 19 weeks' gestation in her first pregnancy. Her constipation had started 4 years previously after having glandular fever, with an enlarged spleen. At this time, she had been bedridden for 3 months. After a full case history and examination of her pulse and tongue, the traditional Chinese medicine picture was one of 'heat retention', probably due to the glandular fever. After the first acupuncture treatment, she opened her bowels 1 hour later. At her second treatment 10 days later, her bowel movements were noticeably easier, with no bleeding. She had stopped the lactulose. After the second treatment, she was having daily bowel movements, and had stopped all medication.

Breech presentation   This area of Traditional Chinese Medicine application to midwifery practice has attracted much attention. The technique used to encourage version of the fetus is called 'moxibustion', which means the burning of the herb 'moxa', the Chinese name for mugwort (*Artemesia vulgaris* or St John's Herb). The technique involves heating an acupuncture point on both feet for 15 minutes, up to 10 times, on a daily basis. This seems to increase fetal activity, hopefully enough to turn the fetus from breech to cephalic presentation. Studies conducted in China on this technique report varying success rates ranging from 80.9% to 90.3% (Wei Wen, 1979; Co-operative Research Group of Moxibustion Version of Jangxi Province, 1984). A study conducted in Italy in 1990 (Cardini *et al.*, 1991) reported 66.6% success rate on a group of 33 women of gestational ages ranging from 30 to 38 weeks. Most research papers on moxibustion show that the 34th week of gestation is the optimum time to carry out the technique giving a higher success rate. A trial conducted by the author is in progress which hopes to demonstrate further the effect of this technique on the mother and fetus. Regarding the mechanism of action, a trial carried out by the Co-operative Research Group of Moxibustion Version of Jangxi

Province (1984) postulates that the increase in corticoadrenal secretion, through the resulting increase in placental oestrogens and changes in prostaglandin levels which they measured, raises basal tone and enhances uterine contractility, stimulating fetal motility, and thus making version more likely. This increase in fetal motility is one of the more striking features of moxibustion, perceived by almost all the women during the second half of the 15 minute treatment, and persisting even after the end of stimulation.

Figure 7 shows the hypothetical mechanism of action of moxa stimulation of the 'zhiyin', point (Co-operative Research Group Of Moxibustion Version, 1984) A second study by the same authors presents the results of

Fig. 7. Diagram showing hypothetical mechanism of action of moxa stimulation of the 'zhiyin' point.

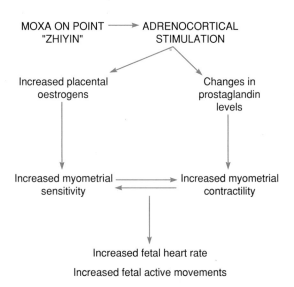

1 week's treatment with moxa in 241 pregnant women of gestational age ranging from 28 to 34 weeks in comparison with 264 control subjects. In the moxa treated women, there were 195 versions (81%) as against 130 (49%) in the control group, the difference being statistically significant ($P < 0.05$). When moxa treatment was continued for a further 7 days, the overall success rate was 87%.

Cardini's trial confirmed findings in the Chinese trials that the success rate is higher in multigravidae, as would probably be expected, owing to the reduced tone of the abdominal muscles.

As this technique does not involve any needles, and needs daily application for up to 10 days, the woman's partner or a friend can be instructed in its application, and they can continue treatment at home. This has the advantage not only of convenience, but also gives them a sense of control over the situation, and when successful, a tremendous feeling of having sorted out the problem for themselves.

With further research to prove the efficacy of this technique, it may be possible for it to become a routine treatment in the management of breech presentation. Midwives could easily be trained in its application. The obvious advantages are a decrease in the number of breech births and their complications, as well as a potential reduction in the Caesarean section rate in primigravid breech presentation (routine in many units) It is also extremely cheap, with moxa sticks currently costing 20 pence each! Most mothers only need two sticks per course of treatment, with some needing four.

Induction of labour This application of acupuncture in obstetrics has stimulated a number of clinical studies in various countries. In the *Jia Yi Jing* (dated 282 AD), a Chinese Jin dynasty classic, it is stated: 'In prolonged labour and retained placenta use *Kunlun*', an acupuncture point behind the medial malleolus. Studies have explored acupuncture's ability to initiate contractions prior to rupture of the membranes, and prior to the woman experiencing any labour pains (Kubista *et al.*, 1975; Ying *et al.*, 1985; Dunn *et al.*, 1989). Other investigators noted that with acupuncture, 'the relation between the force of contraction and the degree of dilation of the cervix differed from that in spontaneous and oxytocin induced labours' (Tsuei and Lai, 1974). The implication here is that different physiological pathways are possibly involved in acupuncture-induced labour. The accumulated results of hundreds of studies have shown that virtually any hormone or neurotransmitter may be affected by appropriate acupuncture stimulation (Bensoussan, 1991). This may explain the difference between the two methods of induction of labour.

In approximately 12 separate clinical studies on the induction of labour with acupuncture, negative side effects have still to be reported or identified. This is in contrast to the possible side effects of Syntocinon, such as abnormally strong or prolonged contractions or rupture of the uterus, as well as other responses (Wren, 1985). However, some researchers found a disadvantage in that the strength and frequency of contractions cannot be controlled, although the contractions stimulated by acupuncture resembled those of spontaneous labour (Kubista *et al.*, 1975; Yip *et al.*, 1976). Another disadvantage may be that the period of acupuncture necessary to stimulate contractions can be as long as 5 hours in some cases, which may not be practical or acceptable to the woman. It is the experience of this author that when attempting induction around term, often by maternal request, several treatments are needed, each lasting 1 hour, on a daily basis. However, in the case of a typical para two, whose third labour is slow to establish, or in cases where the membranes have already ruptured, acupuncture stimulation is far easier and has a much higher success rate. This can often negate the need for augmentation with Syntocinon, and the accompanying monitoring by fetal scalp electrode and lack of mobility that go with it.

The acupuncture points most commonly used to stimulate contractions are 'Hegu' or Large Intestine 4, and 'Sanyinjiao' or Spleen 6, needled together, bilaterally. They are often stimulated by an electro-acupuncture unit for maximum effect. They are located on the hand, between the thumb and index finger, and on the leg, just above the medial malleolus. In traditional Chinese medicine terms, they have a very strong effect on the energy of the uterus, causing it to descend, and it is for this reason that both these points are amongst those listed as being forbidden for use earlier in the pregnancy. In some cases, firm pressure to these points may be enough when needles are unavailable, to bring back contractions that have weakened during an established labour.

Analgesia in labour Again, this application of acupuncture in obstetrics has aroused much interest, and a certain amount of research. In some cases, it has been the reason for the introduction of acupuncture into maternity units by midwives (Skelton, 1988; Budd, 1992).

The results of studies on acupuncture analgesia in labour vary tremendously. One of the main problems in assessing analgesia is the subjectivity of pain perception. The methods of assessing this also vary tremendously, making comparisons between trials difficult.

The first reported acupuncture deliveries in Europe were done by Dr Christman Ehrstroem in Stockholm, Sweden, in 1972. In 1974, Darras, in France, reported 20 electro-acupuncture deliveries. They were primiparae and multiparae, all non-operative deliveries without episiotomy or forceps. He reported 16 successful, three partially successful, and one failure.

More recently, Martoudis and Christofides (1990) conducted a trial in Cyprus using an interesting combination of an auricular point with a point on the hand, on 186 parturients. The time of acupuncture stimulation varied from 20 to 30 minutes, and the analgesic effect began to be effective at a mean time of 40 minutes. The duration of the analgesic effect was a mean time of 6 hours. In all the parturients who delivered during this period of time, no analgesic drugs were necessary. In 24 cases, electro–acupuncture had no effect, and these received analgesic drugs. The average Apgar score was 9.60 at 1 minute, a very high average which speaks well for the safety of the method. In order to evaluate the results of the treatment as objectively as possible, questionnaires were given to the parturients themselves, as well as to the midwife in charge of the delivery room and to the delivering doctor.

The recordings taken before the insertion of needles show clearly that pain was felt at the beginning of the contraction, and went at the end of the contraction (Fig. 8). Recordings taken when the effect of the electro-acupuncture was maximal show that pain was felt at a much later stage of the contraction, and ended much earlier than the end of the contraction. The authors concluded that their method produced slight to very good results in 87.5% of the cases.

Fig. 8. 'CTG' recording from trial. Top: before acupuncture; bottom: after/with acupuncture.

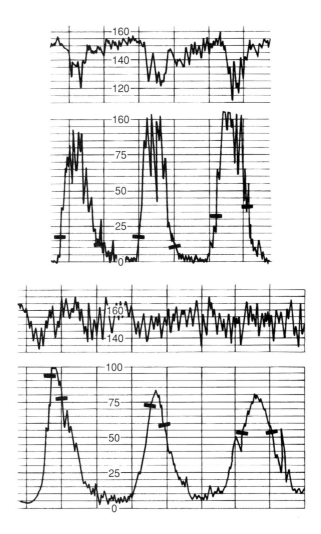

The methods used in other trials on acupuncture analgesia in labour were quite different to the above, and produced just as variable results. One contrasting report is that of Wallis *et al.* (1974), who studied 21 women in labour with acupuncture analgesia. They concluded that 19 of the 21 regarded the acupuncture treatment as unsuccessful in providing analgesia for labour and delivery. The points used were selected on an individual basis, and were taken from a selection of 17! These points were located on the abdomen, back, legs and ear. It is the opinion of this author that the restriction in the mobility of the woman during acupuncture may have had a very negative influence on the effect of the treatment. However, other studies which also used 'body points' showed much higher success rates, such as Perera (1979), so other factors must be involved.

Irene Skelton was the first midwife in Britain to carry out a study on acupuncture and labour, reported in 1988. It was a 2 year study involving 170 births in Glasgow, investigating the comparative effectiveness of conventional analgesics and acupuncture. She concluded that 'Acupuncture has a significant part to play in the control of labour pain . . . Women who received acupuncture felt more in control of their labour and delivery and were generally more satisfied with the "birth experience" than the control group.'

In the Plymouth unit, acupuncture analgesia for labour has been offered since 1988. The women hear about it from their community midwives, during parentcraft talks, from the hospital tours, their general practitioners, hospital midwives and doctors, and of course, by the powerful 'word of mouth'. They are then advised to contact the midwife/acupuncturist during the third trimester and then to meet them and see the equipment. A demonstration is often given of the needling of an ear point so they know what to expect, as many have never had acupuncture treatment before. It is pointed out that there are only two midwives trained to provide acupuncture at the moment and it is therefore not a 24 hour service, so they should not rely on it totally. It is made as available as possible within the limitations of running a busy outpatient clinic. There is often the flexibility to stay with the woman in labour and hopefully deliver her, as well as providing the acupuncture. This is extremely satisfying for both parties, and ties in well with the 'Know your midwife' scheme.

The method of application of ear acupuncture for labour has been altered with experience. In the early days, points on the hand and leg were chosen, according to the ancient texts, and methods used more recently by researchers, but these were found to restrict mobility too much. Ear points are now used, usually with electro-stimulation (Fig. 9). Half-inch needles are inserted into the chosen points and taped down. The cartilage of the ear is tough enough to hold the needles in place quite firmly. Light leads from the electro-acupuncture machine are attached to two of the needles and the woman is instructed in the use of the stimulator. She is in control of the intensity of the stimulation, but the frequency is determined, and pre-set by the practitioner. Once in place, the woman is free to mobilise or assume any position she finds comfortable. If she decides she would like a bath, the electricity is discontinued, but the needles may be left in place. The effect usually takes around 10–20 minutes to build up, and the labouring woman becomes noticeably more calm and relaxed – able to cope with the contractions, even though she can still feel them. Some start to fall asleep in between contractions and wake up half way through the next one. This sleepy, very relaxed state may well be due to the stimulation of serotonin. The degree of analgesia obtained varies tremendously, as it does with other methods, and is of course subjective. In some cases, the acupuncture is not enough, especially when nearing transition into the second stage of labour. This is when Entonox can be a great help, and is usually enough to see her through until pushing commences. Of course in a very long and tiring labour, possibly with complications, epidural anaesthesia may become necessary and it is

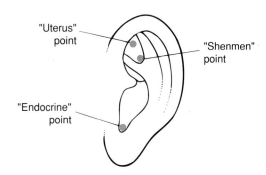

Fig. 9. Diagram of ear points used for analgesia in labour.

important that the woman feels able to ask for this without feeling she has failed by not coping with acupuncture alone. This is pointed out to her when she comes to discuss acupuncture analgesia during the antenatal period.

The points used for analgesia are 'Uterus', 'Shenmen' and 'Endocrine'. The first is chosen for obvious reasons as the organ being targeted. The second point is used for general analgesia and relaxation in the whole body, and the third to stimulate contractions. There is no research available at the time of writing which looks at the use of ear points alone in labour. The clinical trials conducted so far have mainly used body points, although Martoudis and Christofides (1990) used a combination of ear and body points.

In a review of eight clinical trials on acupuncture analgesia for labour, six showed favourable or successful results (Darras, 1974; Ledergerber, 1976; Hyodo and Gega, 1977; Perera, 1979; Skelton, 1988; Martoudis and Christofides, 1990) and two were negative (Wallis, 1974; Abouleish, 1975). Most of these studies were carried out on small numbers of women. They were of differing design, only some using controls, and using varying methods of assessment. As is often the case, further research needs to be carried out in a standardised manner on large numbers of women. One of the problems with this is of course the funding for such research. Another is the availability of suitably trained practitioners to carry it out. As a majority of medical research is funded by pharmaceutical companies, finding money for research into a complementary therapy which may negate the need for medication can be a problem.

Postnatal Problems

Haemorrhoids Haemorrhoids are an extremely common complaint in pregnancy and the immediate postnatal period, causing much discomfort and distress, and may often lead to problems with breast feeding due to poor positioning. There is an 'empirical' point for haemorrhoids called 'Chengshan' or UB 57, which is located on the back of the calf. It is on the urinary bladder meridian which passes around the anus, and even when used on its own, this point can give tremendous relief within hours, reducing the swelling, pain and discomfort in the area. Often one treatment is enough, but if not, and the mother and baby are still in hospital, it can be repeated on a daily basis, which is convenient before the busy times start at home. If necessary, she may return as an outpatient.

Retention of urine This is fortunately not that common, but when it happens can have serious implications, and apart from the distress of repeated catheterisation, causes great unhappiness from being kept in hospital when looking forward to, and having planned to go home soon after the birth. It is often associated with traumatic forceps deliveries, oedematous perinei and sometimes epidural anaesthesia. In traditional Chinese medicine terms, the acupuncture can tonify the bladder and draw energy to the area, causing the sensation of needing to pass urine, which is often absent in these cases. Needles are usually inserted into points on the lower leg as well as locally, above the symphysis pubis, and strong stimulation is used. Even when she has already tried for several days without success to begin to empty her bladder, one treatment may well be enough to stimulate the urge to pass a good volume of urine within an hour. Repeated treatments may be necessary.

Insufficient lactation Acupuncture can be particularly useful in the situation where a mother is under a lot of stress, and despite a strong desire to breast feed her baby, finds that her milk production is reducing. This is often the case with premature births, where the baby is still being cared for in the special care baby unit, and particularly when he or she is unwell and struggling. Part of the physiology of lactation involves the neurohormonal reflex set up by stimulation of the nipple leading to the release of oxytocin from the posterior pituitary. This reflex can be suppressed by the higher centres in the brain, causing stress and anxiety to affect the 'let down' reflex.

Acupuncture treatment can be aimed at strong relaxation as well as providing a 'tonic' to build the mother up, and increase the flow of energy or 'Qi' to the breast. It is known that acupuncture has a strong influence on hormone levels, and there are suggestions of its influence on the higher centres, so it is reasonable to speculate that its success in promoting lactation is due to an increase in levels of oxytocin and prolactin.

The use of acupuncture by midwives

Training, registers, how to find an acupuncturist There are several acupuncture training schools in this country which are listed below. These are all recognised by the Council for Acupuncture, the governing body for the acupuncture profession. Training in some of these schools leads to automatic admission to one of the acupuncture registers. Admission to a register for those who have trained elsewhere is by interview and occasionally examination. The Council for Acupuncture publish an annual directory of practitioners in the country which is a recommended method of choosing a practitioner. The Royal College of Midwives are aware of midwives who are also trained acupuncturists, especially those practising in the NHS.

Acupuncture training The minimum training period in this country is 3 years (full/part-time) and the British College of Acupuncture is the only one to require students to have some medical, paramedic or other practising qualification prior to entry. Prospectuses and full details of courses can be obtained from the colleges by sending a stamped addressed envelope.

An alternative and quicker training can be found in China! There are many international training colleges in China, a list of which can be found with the above. My colleague trained in Nanjing on their 3 month course, which can be followed by another 3 month advanced course. It is an extremely intensive course, and some knowledge of basic theory and acupuncture point location before departure is highly recommended. Interpreters are provided! Funding may be available, but it takes much patience and many application forms to find it. There are several midwives who have been successful in this though and have had their whole training paid for by awards or charitable means. The author has been contacted (for advice) by several midwives in different parts of the country whose health authorities have encouraged them to train as acupuncturists, with sponsorship offered.

Acupuncture colleges in England
British College of Acupuncture (BAAR)
8 Hunter Street, London WC1, UK
Tel: 071 833 8164

Chung San Acupuncture School (CSAS)
15 Porchester Gardens, London W2 4DB, UK
Tel: 071 727 6778

College of Traditional Acupuncture UK (TAS)
Tao House, Queensway, Royal Leamington Spa, Warwickshire, CV31 3LZ, UK
Tel: 0926 422121

International College of Oriental Medicine UK (IROM)
Green Hedges House, Green Hedges Avenue, East Grinstead, West Sussex, RH19 1DZ, UK
Tel: 0342 313106

London School of Acupuncture and Traditional Chinese Medicine (RTCM)

4th Floor, 60 Bunhill Row, London EC1Y 8QD, UK
Tel: 071 490 0513.

Northern College of Acupuncture (RTCM)
124 Acomb Road, York YO2 4EY, UK
Tel: 0904 785120/784828

Professional associations represented in brackets after name of college are as follows:

British Acupuncture Association and Register (BAAR)
Chung San Acupuncture Society (CSAS)
Traditional Acupuncture Society (TAS)
International Register of Oriental Medicine (UK) (IROM)
Register of Traditional Chinese Medicine (RTCM)

Governing Body for all the above is:
The Council For Acupuncture
179 Gloucester Place, London NW1 6DX, UK
Tel: 071 724 5756, Fax: 071 724 5330

International training colleges in China
Beijing Association of Traditional Chinese Medicine
7a Dongdan Santiao, Beijing 100005, China
Tel: (1) 550 460

Beijing College of Traditional Chinese Medicine
11 Heping Jie Beikou, Beijing 100029, China
Tel: (1) 4225–566

Chengdu College of Traditional Chinese Medicine
15 Shierqiao Jie, Chengdu, Sichuan 610075, China
Tel: (28) 669241

Guangzhou Institute of Traditional Chinese Medicine
10 Jichang Road, Sanyuanli, Guangzhou, Guangdong., China

Nanjing College of Traditional Chinese Medicine
282 Hanzhong Lu, Nanjing, 210029, Jiangsu, China
Tel: (25) 649-121, Fax: (25) 741-323

Shanghai College of Traditional Chinese Medicine
23 Lingling Road, Shanghai 200032, China
Tel: (21) 438 5400, Fax: (21) 439 8290

References

Abouleish E.B. (1975) Acupuncture in Obstetrics. *Anaesthesia and Analgesia*, **54(1)**, 83.

Bensoussan A. (1991), *The Vital Meridian*. Churchill Livingstone.

Bresler D. and Kroening R. (1976). Three essential factors in effective acupuncture therapy. *American Journal of Chinese Medicine*, **4(1)**, 81.

British Medical Association (BMA) (1993) *Complementary Medicine, New Approaches to Good Practice*. Oxford University Press, Oxford.

Budd S. (1992) Traditional Chinese medicine in obstetrics. *Midwives Chronicle and Nursing Notes*, **105**, 140.

Cardini F., Basevi V., Valentini A. and Martellato A. (1991) Moxibustion and breech presentation: preliminary results. *American Journal of Chinese Medicine*, **XIX(2)**, 105.

Co-operative Research Group of Moxibustion Version of Jangxi Province (1984). Clinical observation on the effects of version by moxibustion. *Abstracts from the Second National Symposium on Acupuncture and Moxibustion and Acupuncture Anaesthesia. Beijing, China*, p. 150. All China Society of Acupuncture and Moxibustion.

Darras J.C. (1974) Acupuncture update. *Symposium, held in New York, by National Acupuncture Research Society*, October.

Dundee J., Sourial F., Ghaly R. and Bell P. (1988) Acupressure reduces morning sickness. *Journal of the Royal Society of Medicine*, **81**, 456.

Dundee J., Ghaly R., Fitzpatrick K. *et.al.* (1989) Acupuncture prophylaxis of cancer chemotherapy-induced sickness. *Journal of the Royal Society of Medicine*, **82**, 268.

Dunn P., Rogers D. and Halford K. (1989) Transcutaneous electric nerve stimulation at acupuncture points in the induction of uterine contractions. *Obstetrics and Gynaecology*, **73**, 286.

Fischer M., Behr A. and v. Reumont J. (1984) Acupuncture – a therapeutic concept in the treatment of painful conditions and functional disorders. *Acupuncture and Electrotherapeutics Research*, **9**, 11.

Hyodo M. and Gega O. (1977) The use of acupuncture analgesia for normal delivery. *American Journal of Chinese Medicine*, **5(1)**, 63.

Kaptchuk T. (1983) *Chinese Medicine, The Web That Has No Weaver*. Rider.

Kubista E., Kucera H. and Muller-Tyl. (1975) Initiating contractions of the gravid uterus through electroacupuncture. *American Journal of Chinese Medicine*, **3(4)**, 343.

Ledergerber C.P. (1976) Electroacupuncture in obstetrics. *Acupuncture and Electrotherapeutics Research*, **2**, 105.

Martoudis S. and Christofides K. (1990) Electroacupuncture for pain relief in labour. *Acupuncture in Medicine*, **8(2)**, 51.

Omura Y. (1975) Pathophysiology of acupuncture treatment; effects of acupuncture on cardiovascular and nervous systems. *Acupuncture and Electrotherapeutics Research*, **1**, 511.

Perera W. (1979) Acupuncture in childbirth. *British Journal of Acupuncture*, **2(1)**, 12.

Qiu M. (1985) Lecture Presented on the Occasion of the Fourth International Advanced Studies Program in Acupuncture, Nanjing.

Schaub M. and Fazal Haq M. (1977) Electro-acupuncture treatment in psychiatry. *American Journal of Chinese Medicine*, **5(1)**, 85.

Shanghai College of Traditional Chinese Medicine. (1981) *Acupuncture: A Comprehensive Text* (Eds O'Connor and Bensky). Eastland Press.

Skelton I. (1988) Acupuncture and labour – a summary of results. *Midwives Chronicle and Nursing Notes*, May, 134.

Takishima T., Suetsugu M., Gen T., Ishihara T. and Watanabe K. (1982) The bronchodilating effect of acupuncture in patients with acute asthma. *Annals of Allergy*, **48(1)**, 44.

Tsuei J. and Lai Y. (1974) Induction of labour by acupuncture and electrical stimulation. *Obstetrics and Gynaecology*, **43(3)**, 337.

Wallis L., Shnider S., Palahniuk R. and Spivey H. (1974) An evaluation of acupuncture analgesia in obstetrics. *Anesthesiology*, **41(6)**, 596.

Wei Wen (1979) Correcting abnormal fetal positions with moxibustion. *Midwives Chronicle and Nursing Notes*, **92(1),** 103, 432.

Wren B.G. (Ed.) (1985) *Handbook of Obstetrics and Gynaecology*, 2nd Edn. Chapman and Hall.

Wu Y. (1982) Therapeutic effect and mechanism of acupuncture at neiguan (Per 6) in chronic rheumatic heart disease. *Journal of Traditional Chinese Medicine*, **2(1)**, 51.

Ying Y., Lin J. and Robins J. (1985) Acupuncture for the induction of cervical dilatation in preparation for first trimester abortion and its influence on HCG. *Journal of Reproductive Medicine*, **30(7)**, 530.

Yip S., Pang J. and Sung M. (1976) Induction of labour by acupuncture electro-stimulation. *American Journal of Chinese Medicine*, **4(3)**, 257.

Yu D. Y. and Lee S. P. Effect of acupuncture on bronchial asthma. *Clinical Science and Molecular Medicine*, **51(5)**, 503.

Further reading

Bensoussan A. (1991) *The Vital Meridian*. Churchill Livingstone.
This book explores the biomedical and scientific aspects of acupuncture. It presents a thorough, easily accessible review of research conducted in China and in the West.

Kaptchuk T. (1985) *Chinese Medicine. The Web That Has No Weaver*. Rider.
An interesting approach to the principles of Chinese medical thought, which develops an interaction between modern Western medicine and traditional Chinese medicine

Lewith G. and Aldridge D. (Eds) (1993) *Clinical Research Methodology For Complementary Therapies*. Hodder and Stoughton.
This book lays out the fundamentals required for clinical research within a range of complementary therapies and brings together some innovative ideas.

Low R. (1990) *Acupuncture in Gynaecology And Obstetrics*. Thorsons.
A textbook for practitioners and students of Chinese medicine on the application of acupuncture in this important area.

Maciocia G. (1989) *The Foundations of Chinese Medicine*. Churchill Livingstone.
An excellent textbook on the theory of Chinese Medicine which draws on modern and ancient classical Chinese texts. It explains the application of the theory of Chinese medicine to a Western medical practice, emphasising Western types of diseases and patients.

Penelope L. Conway

Chapter 11 Osteopathy During Pregnancy

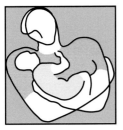

The aim of this chapter is to explain how osteopathy can assist midwives to provide optimum care to the women they look after during the various stages of pregnancy, labour and the puerperium.

There is no shortcut to osteopathic diagnosis and treatment, and a 4 year full-time course cannot be condensed into one chapter of a book. Because of this, osteopathy is not suitable for the midwife to incorporate in her practice, but rather for her to appreciate when a woman could benefit from referral. Osteopathic treatment is safe, gentle and non-invasive and therefore eminently appropriate for pregnant women.

There are few side effects and few contraindications to treatment. The main side effects may be feeling tired after treatment, and a possible increase in symptoms for 24 hours. Contraindications to osteopathic treatment could include

- any history of or threatened miscarriage;
- active pathology;
- inflammatory conditions;
- some cases of joint hypermobility.

In all these cases the osteopath would discuss the difficulty with the woman concerned, and if necessary with her midwife and general practitioner as well.

Osteopathy is a safe method of treatment even during the early stages of pregnancy. There are no recorded, or even anecdotal cases of miscarriage or abortion being brought on by osteopathic treatment. However, it is usual practice to avoid strong treatments during the twelfth week and the sixteenth week of pregnancy, when miscarriage is more likely to occur naturally.

This author has not encountered any osteopaths who treat only pregnant women, but naturally there are some practitioners who by virtue of their interest and experience see many more than others. All osteopaths should be willing and able to treat pregnant women.

Historical context

Osteopathy was first conceived over 100 years ago by a physician called Andrew Taylor Still. Still was a country doctor in the Midwest of America who became disenchanted with the medical and surgical knowledge and practice at that time. He spent many years experimenting and developing a new theory of drugless medicine which he called osteopathy. His approach to health care was based on the unity of the body and the proper alignment and function of the musculoskeletal system. He envisaged osteopathy as a complete system of medicine which would employ only manipulative and adjustive techniques which would return to the body the power to heal itself.

Still founded the first School of Osteopathy in Kirksville, Missouri, in 1892. A few American-trained osteopaths came to practise in Britain, and in 1917 the British School of Osteopathy was set up by James Martin Littlejohn who had travelled to America to study. The number of practising osteopaths grew slowly but steadily and in 1934 the profession had progressed sufficiently for a Private Members Bill to be presented to Parliament calling for state registration for osteopaths Unfortunately, due to the opposition of the medical establishment, the Bill failed. However at the suggestion of the then Minister of Health, a voluntary Register of Osteopaths was set up to oversee training and provide guarantees of standards and ethics to the public. The Register gave accreditation to osteopathic schools and accepted their graduates as members able to use the designation MRO (Member of the Register of Osteopaths) after their name.

The profession still grew slowly and by 1979 there were only 354 registered osteopaths. Because osteopaths practised under Common Law, anyone could call themselves an osteopath even if they had received little or no training. The Register was therefore vitally important as a safeguard for patients.

Throughout the 1980s public recognition of osteopathy increased, as did acceptance by the medical profession, with many patients being referred by their general practitioner or consultant. State recognition still seemed a long way off, unless as a Profession Supplementary to Medicine, which was not an option many registered osteopaths would consider. Then in 1990 the

King's Fund set up a working party to consider the status of osteopathy. Their report incorporated a model bill for statutory registration. A much larger and better organised osteopathic profession was able to find a sponsor for a Private Member's Bill which enjoyed all-party support, and the Osteopaths Act received Royal Assent on 1 July 1993.

Within the next 2 years a General Osteopathic Council (GOsC) will be set up to regulate osteopaths and osteopathy. At this early stage no one can foresee what effects this momentous change in status will eventually involve.

What is osteopathy?

Osteopathy is concerned with restoring and maintaining balance in the neuro-musculoskeletal systems of the body. This fine balance may have been disturbed by alterations in soft tissues through misuse, or change of use, through trauma to bones or joints, or by modification to the innervation of any of these structures. Therefore it is necessary to look at the patient as a whole, not just the area causing symptoms, so that the interaction of the different systems, and the effects they have on each other, can be included in the diagnostic process. Osteopathy is concerned with the biomechanics of the body and the maintenance of appropriate mechanical function.

The osteopath aims to preserve the balance between muscles, joints, ligamentous structures and nerves which allow the body to function effectively. During pregnancy this balance is constantly under attack from alterations in weight and weight bearing, hormonal changes and fluctuations in fluid balance. In addition there are the 'normal' influences of injury, overuse and physical or mental stress.

The osteopath will attempt to minimise the impact of all these changes by a carefully considered treatment plan formulated for that particular woman. Osteopaths treat people not conditions.

Osteopathy today

Until the implementation of the Osteopaths Act and statutory registration procedures osteopaths practise under Common Law which allows anyone to heal the sick as long as they do not offer to treat certain named conditions. Anyone can self-refer to an osteopath, it is not necessary to have a letter from a medical practitioner, although this is always most welcome. All osteopaths are private practitioners and the cost of treatment varies considerably, with most osteopaths operating a sliding scale of fees for those in financial need. Most private health insurance schemes will cover the cost of osteopathic treatment. Fund-holding general practices are now able to employ osteopaths directly, or pay for their patients to have treatment. This trend will inevitably increase over the next few years. Several National Health Service trust hospitals are exploring the feasibility of employing osteopaths.

When people hear the word 'osteopath' most of them immediately think of low back pain, but osteopaths are much more than spinal manipulators.

Originally osteopaths treated any and all conditions, but advances in surgery and drug therapies rendered osteopathy obsolete for many complaints. Osteopaths specialised in, and became very proficient at treating minor orthopaedic disorders. More recently, as people have become disenchanted with drugs and invasive procedures, osteopaths have returned to treating a much wider range of problems. Most now treat asthma, dysmenorrhoea, indigestion and migraine as well as the more common musculoskeletal conditions.

Going to the osteopath

There are registered osteopaths practising in most areas of the British Isles, and a recommendation to a particular Practitioner is often forthcoming from friends or local health professionals. Alternatively the General Council and Register of Osteopaths will supply a list. Osteopaths can also be found through Yellow Pages or Thompson local directories. Some osteopaths practise on their own, others in group practices often incorporating several different disciplines.

Most osteopaths will treat pregnant women, but no osteopath will accept a woman for treatment if she is not receiving medical antenatal care as well. During pregnancy osteopathy is truly complementary, not alternative.

Having selected a practitioner and made an appointment the first part of the initial consultation will involve the osteopath taking a detailed and comprehensive case history. This will include details of occupation and lifestyle as well as information about the problem. For pregnant women obstetric information will also be required, such as estimated date of delivery, home or hospital delivery, any previous pregnancies, and any problems associated with previous deliveries. The next part of the record taking will address past and present medical history including details of diet, genitourinary system, gastrointestinal system and any cardiovascular problems.

Not all pregnant women who consult an osteopath are in pain; some attend just for advice or reassurance, or as part of a 'well woman' approach to pregnancy. They are anxious to be examined for any problems that may arise later so that they can go into labour as well prepared as possible.

The woman would then be asked to undress to her underwear and remove her shoes before the next part of the examination which is the osteopathic evaluation.

The osteopath will observe the woman standing – checking spinal curves in both antero-posterior and lateral planes, and also areas of weight bearing. They would also consider the way in which weight was transferred through the lower extremities, whether this was equally distributed and if the knees were held fully extended and locked, thereby allowing the glutei and hamstrings to relax. They would also check whether the ankles were inverted or everted, and if there was flattening of the medial arch of the foot with associated spreading of the toes to provide a wider base. Medial arch flatten-

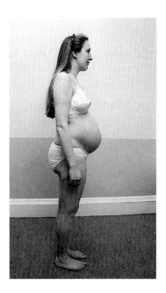
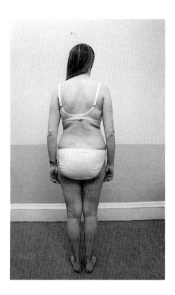

Fig. 11.1. Lateral view of woman, 32 weeks pregnant.

Fig. 11.2. Posterior view of woman, 32 weeks pregnant, to show lateral curves.

ing is common in the later stages of pregnancy to accommodate increased weight bearing.

Only by looking at the woman as a whole, not just investigating the area giving symptoms, can the osteopath assess how the body is adapting to the pregnancy.

The osteopath will then palpate the vertebral column and spinal muscles (still with the woman standing) to pick up any areas of increased or reduced tone. They will also be looking for any evidence of localised spinal scoliosis or rotation.

The woman will be asked to perform a range of active spinal movements which the osteopath will observe for;

- range of movement;
- equality of movement throughout the spine;
- any limitation by pain.

The osteopath will ask the woman to sit on the treatment table and her sitting posture and range of movement will be observed. This may also include rib mobility, important for easier breathing, particularly in the later stages of pregnancy when the fundus of the uterus presses on the diaphragm. Active movements of the cervical spine will be checked as a guide to general spinal mobility.

The woman would then be asked to lie supine so that if necessary her reflexes could be checked, and her hip joint mobility tested. Many women with limited spinal mobility overuse their hip joints in order to adapt their

Fig. 11.3. Checking mobility of lower ribcage.

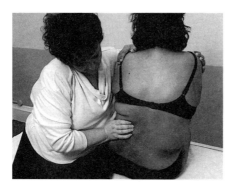

Fig. 11.4. Assessing hip joint mobility.

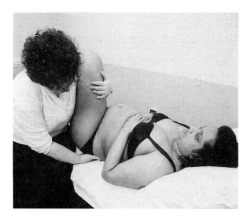

posture whilst pregnant, and a good range of movement in the hip joints also increases the options for birth positions. The osteopath would also compare leg lengths and pelvic levels. Most pregnant women are not very comfortable and may become hypotensive lying supine, particularly during the later stages of pregnancy, so other lower extremity joints would only be checked if they were causing problems.

Then the osteopath would make a more detailed assessment of the main area causing symptoms by moving the joints passively and palpating for alterations in local muscle tone and ligamentous stretch. This applies to both spinal and peripheral joints.

If necessary this may be followed by neurological and/or other system examinations. This would usually be carried out if the woman was complaining of any parasthesia (pins and needles or numbness) or referred pain. Any unexpected breathlessness or palpitations would warrant a cardiovascular system examination.

The osteopath now has all the information from the history and examination and can evaluate the findings in order to reach a diagnosis and formulate a treatment plan. Because pregnancy is a time of so much postural change

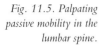
Fig. 11.5. Palpating passive mobility in the lumbar spine.

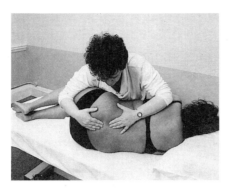

and adaptation, the diagnosis should be regarded more as an evaluation at that moment in time. There is an immense variation in the rate of growth of every fetus which necessitates a continuous and continuing reassessment of the woman's stance and mobility. Two weeks later her osteopathic profile could have changed dramatically.

When the diagnosis has been established the osteopath will explain the findings and discuss the aims of treatment. For most people the paramount factor is relief of symptoms, but this may necessitate a change in lifestyle or working practice, as well as osteopathic treatment.

The treatment plan may include:

- Soft tissue techniques to relax and stretch shortened musculature. These are specialised massage techniques which aim to release tension in the muscle fibres which often limit mobility.
- Articulatory techniques to stretch muscles and ligamentous structures rhythmically. These techniques take an area, usually in the spine, through a small range of movement in a repetitive manner, with the osteopath applying a little more force as necessary.
- Friction to improve local circulation. This is usually applied by steady pressure with the thumbs to a particular area of very shortened muscle.
- High velocity thrust – putting one apophyseal joint through a very specific range of movement. This is the classic osteopathic technique which produces the 'crack' from the joint concerned. Osteopaths limit the movement of surrounding spinal joints by a combination of flexion and rotation so that when a gentle force is applied locally only one joint will separate causing the sound.

Pregnant women are not comfortable with excessive lumbar spinal rotation and relax more readily if techniques are adapted to allow for more flexion than is usual. Treatment is usually weekly or biweekly until symptoms improve, and then every 2 weeks. Women are encouraged to attend until delivery if possible as changes in weight bearing make them vulnerable to recurring problems during pregnancy. They will be advised to return about

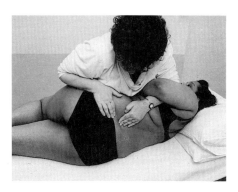

Fig. 11.6. Applying a 'high velocity thrust' technique in the lumbar spine.

6 weeks after delivery so that their posture and mobility can be assessed again. Many women return sooner, particularly if the delivery has been accompanied by backache.

Most of the treatment will be given with the woman lying on her side with the abdomen supported on a small pillow. This position is often the most comfortable for the mother and all osteopathic techniques can be adapted to take account of this factor. Some of the treatment may be given with the woman sitting. Particularly in the later stages of pregnancy when changing position is difficult, the treatment should be organised to allow the woman to change her position as little as possible. The comfort of the woman is of paramount importance.

When the woman is about 34 weeks' gestation, partners or anyone who will be present at the delivery are invited to attend the treatment to be shown some simple pain-relieving techniques that can be used during labour. These are useful for midwives to learn as well and are described in detail later. However, as these techniques are very successful, anyone who starts using them should be prepared to continue until delivery.

Stages of pregnancy

Pre-conception care Pre-conception care is a relatively new area of concern and interest for the medical profession, encouraging women to improve their nutrition and general lifestyle before becoming pregnant. For many years however osteopaths have been advising young women to improve their posture and spinal mobility before attempting to become pregnant. This was due to treating so many older women who could trace the onset of their low back symptoms to a pregnancy many years earlier. Low back pain during pregnancy may be common, but that does not make it inevitable.

There is also some anecdotal evidence that osteopathic treatment is helpful in cases of unexplained infertility. To date there has not been any formal research into this subject, but hopefully collaborative endeavours of this type will become easier after statutory registration. The innervation of the reproductive organs arises from the lumbar spine, so it would not seem too unconventional to treat this area in both partners.

The extra weight and changes in weight bearing that occur during pregnancy require good spinal and peripheral joint mobility, so it would seem prudent to deal with any problems in the lumbar or thoracic spine before becoming pregnant. A full range of movement in both hip joints is also important if the woman wishes to have a wide range of options for positions at delivery.

First trimester During the early stages of pregnancy problems often arise in the thoracic spine due to a rapid increase in the size and sensitivity of the breasts. This can lead to flexion of the thoracic spine and internal rotation of the shoulders as a protective mechanism. This can result in muscle shortening and fatigue.

Nausea and vomiting can adversely effect the ribs and thoracic spine as the woman holds on to the basin or lavatory bowl and retches constantly. Gentle osteopathic treatment aimed at releasing the intercostal muscles and diaphragm is usually very helpful, and work to improve the mobility of the thoracic spine and adjacent soft tissues often relieves the feelings of nausea.

The lumbar spine does not have to undergo much adaptation in the first weeks as the uterus has not risen above the pubic symphysis. However this author has seen women with severe ligamentous low backache which started at 6 weeks' gestation and could only be hormonally induced, as no other changes were discernible.

Jenny came for advice and treatment after the birth of her second child. She had developed severe backache when only 16 weeks pregnant, and had been confined to bed, some of the time in hospital, for the remainder of the pregnancy. A diagnosis was made of ligamentous backache, but no treatment was offered other than bed rest and limiting the size of her family to the two children she had already. Jenny and her husband had planned a much larger family and their religious beliefs did not allow for contraception.

Fig. 11.7. Technique for stretching intercostal muscles.

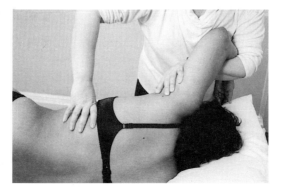

On examination it was found that her lumbar erector spinae and interspinous ligaments were overstretched causing increased mobility in her lumbar spine and at the thoraco-lumbar junction. During her second pregnancy the increased weight and change in centre of gravity caused further stretch of the spinal muscles and ligaments leading to early fatigue on any sustained sitting or standing.

Treatment was aimed at encouraging the ligaments to shorten, and increasing the mobility of the underlying lumbar and thoracic spinal joints. Treatment continued for some time, but it was not possible to assess fully a final outcome until Jenny became pregnant again.

After 1 year Jenny was pregnant and continued with treatment. She remained pain free until 36 weeks' gestation and has had two subsequent pain-free pregnancies, only requiring treatment during the pregnancies and not in between.

Second trimester As the pregnancy progresses and the uterus rises out of the pelvic cavity many of the problems encountered are postural – or rather they are caused by the inability of the woman to adapt to her changing centre of gravity. This may be due to an old injury to the lumbar spine several years earlier, perhaps following a fall, or to an immobile thoraco-lumbar area as a consequence of osteochondrosis. The lumbo-sacral and thoraco-lumbar regions of the spine are the main adaptive areas for weight bearing, and therefore bear the impact of the changes taking place.

Fig. 11.8. Diagram to show possible changes in weight bearing.

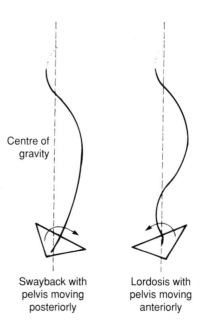

Centre of gravity

Swayback with pelvis moving posteriorly

Lordosis with pelvis moving anteriorly

Whatever the underlying cause, the effect is to prevent the woman from developing a 'pregnant posture'. This normally involves either increasing the lumbar lordosis and tilting the pelvis anteriorly, or flattening the lumbar curve and rotating the pelvis posteriorly. The upper part of the spine adapts accordingly so that a centre of gravity is maintained while standing. The increased weight is thus carried through spinal muscles and apophyseal joints which were not designed for this task. The result is often discomfort and pain. The tone of the abdominal muscles can also affect the way in which the postural changes develop. A woman who has strong abdominal muscles and is a primigravida will develop a very different posture to a multipara with poor abdominal tone.

The other factor which has to be considered is the rising level of circulating relaxin, and the effect it has on ligamentous tissue, allowing it to lengthen whilst retaining its stretch.

Adaptation is also occurring at the hip joint, knee and ankle joints, symphysis pubis and abdominal musculature at this time. These are all areas of potential discomfort and pain and all structures which respond well to osteopathic treatment. This may just involve soft tissue relaxation techniques, or articulatory techniques where joints are taken through a range of passive movement in a repetitive manner to encourage ligamentous stretch.

Many women who already have a child carry their toddler on one or other hip. This requires rotation of one side of the pelvis often resulting in sacro-iliac problems which as well as causing local pain often lead to referred pain in the hip or groin, and changes in the lateral spinal curves. Any of these problems, which can be both tiring and debilitating for the woman, can be eased with appropriate osteopathic intervention. Symptomatic relief, particularly from sacro-iliac lesions, can be very dramatic and most welcome. However the woman must also be discouraged from carrying the toddler on her hip in the future, and advised on how to cope with the conflicting demands of her small child and her lumbar spine.

At this stage of pregnancy many women will still be working. This can cause problems if chairs or desks are not adjustable. For anyone working at a keyboard it becomes increasingly difficult to sit really close to the desk. A lower chair may make sitting for long periods more comfortable, and a footrest (it could even be two telephone directories) rotates the pelvis posteriorly so that the lumbar spine is supported by the chair. The osteopath can often suggest such simple alterations to a working environment which make life more comfortable. Allowing the woman to continue working for as long as possible is an important consideration nowadays.

Third trimester In the later stages of pregnancy, as the fundus of the uterus rises and presses on the diaphragm, breathing becomes more difficult, particularly taking a deep breath. The lower ribs are splayed, and upper rib breathing predominates. Gentle rib stretching and relaxation of the diaphragm can improve this situation.

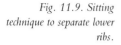

Fig. 11.9. Sitting technique to separate lower ribs.

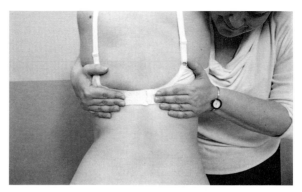

When contracted the diaphragm may also constrict the oesophageal opening causing difficulty with swallowing and allowing reflux to occur. Direct treatment to the diaphragm and mid-thoracic spine will ease the discomfort rapidly.

Excessive weight gain at this time will make the simplest everyday tasks difficult to perform. Unfortunately osteopathic treatment does not aid weight loss, but may help the woman to move more easily. Treatment to the feet and knees can assist lymphatic drainage and make walking more comfortable. Advice can be offered on the most suitable positions for sitting and sleeping, and the easiest way of changing position from upright to recumbent.

At this stage of the pregnancy the osteopath may discuss with the woman which birth position would be most suitable for her, taking into consideration her pattern of mobility and any factors which could aggravate a previous injury.

The final pre-delivery treatment should be given as near to the estimated date of delivery as the woman feels comfortable. Osteopathic treatment is safe at any time during pregnancy and some practitioners have been able to treat women during labour as well.

It must not be overlooked that at any time during her pregnancy a woman may develop a musculoskeletal problem which is totally unrelated to the pregnancy. Pregnant women are more vulnerable to injury because of their increased ligamentous laxity, but any pre-existing condition can continue to be treated.

Can osteopathy help?

Sciatica Irritation of the sciatic nerve can occur anywhere along its path causing pain and or paraesthesia in the lower extremity. The cause of the nerve compression can range from protrusion of an intervertebral disc to spasm in the piriformis muscle. Accurate diagnosis of the level of the nerve root involved and the cause of the irritation is necessary and most are amenable to osteopathic treatment.

Carpal tunnel syndrome Oedema in the later stages of pregnancy can lead to compression of the median nerve as it passes through the flexor retinaculum at the wrist. The symptoms are tingling and numbness in the hands, particularly in the morning. Osteopathic treatment to the forearm and wrist can help by aiding drainage and improving the mobility of the joints of the wrist. An improvement is seen after only one or two treatments.

Meralgia parasthetica This is an area of reduced sensation and possibly soreness over the distribution of the lateral cutaneous nerve of the thigh. This corresponds to the antero-lateral portion of the upper half of the thigh. The symptoms often appear at about 20 weeks. Treatment is directed at stretching the nerve root within its fascial sheath, and releasing any compressive tension around the inguinal canal. This involves articulating the hip joint into extension to stretch the tissues of the anterior compartment of the thigh.

Diabetes Diabetes is not usually treated osteopathically, although there are some practitioners who would attempt direct treatment to the pancreas. However it is important to note that any diabetics who have osteopathic treatment for other problems should always check their insulin levels after treatment. Osteopathic treatment has a similar effect to exercise and can noticeably alter insulin requirements.

Symphysis pubis pain This can be very difficult to treat and does not always respond. This is often the case when excessive separation of the symphysis pubis renders it unstable. Treatment to the sacro-iliac joints may help by encouraging posterior rotation of the pelvis which takes some of the strain off the anterior structures. Local friction techniques may encourage ligamentous shortening. The woman should be advised to wear some form of support (preferably a maternity panty-girdle) and to sit on a wedge cushion, again to influence posterior rotation. Placing the feet on a box or stool also helps. Pelvic rocking exercises should be suggested.

If the pain is due to lack of mobility at the symphysis pubis or a shearing movement of the joint, this will usually respond much better to osteopathic treatment.

Coccydinia Localised pain in the region of the coccyx often following a fall or previous difficult delivery can be treated successfully but it may be necessary for the manipulation to be performed per rectum. A chaperone would always be provided if necessary.

Oedematous ankles If the oedema did not require the use of diuretics and was purely gravitational the osteopath may try to improve the lymphatic drainage by releasing any restrictions at the ankle, knee and hip joints and applying longitudinal stretch techniques to the posterior muscle groups. Soft tissue techniques should never be used because of the risk of a deep vein thrombosis.

Indigestion and heartburn These both respond well to relaxation of the diaphragm and techniques to improve the mobility of the ribcage and thoracic spine.

Round ligament pain Pain in the groin is sometimes due to pressure on the round ligament as it passes through the inguinal canal. Local soft tissue and stretching techniques are often helpful in this condition.

Pain relief during labour

Simple massage techniques used to relax the erector spinae muscles during the early stages of labour can be very effective for pain relief. They can be performed by the midwife or anyone present at the delivery. The woman can be in any position except supine, but it is easier for the operator if she is lying on her side or sitting astride a chair. The lumbar musculature is then more readily accessible. The lateral border of the thumb and thenar eminence are used to apply pressure with one or both hands. The technique involves cross fibre stretching of the muscles. Baby oil or talcum powder can be applied to the skin to improve contact and lessen friction. The applicator hand is placed on the back in the sulcus (groove) between the spinous processes of the lumbar vertebrae and the muscle belly of the erecter spinae. By maintaining skin contact and attempting to move the muscle belly away from the centre line the muscle is bowed and stretched. When the limit of the muscle stretch is reached, the pressure is released but not the skin contact. The hand is moved smoothly up or down the spine 2 or 3 cm and the movement is repeated. The pressure should be firm and consistent and the whole manoeuvre slow and rhythmic. The intention is to stretch and relax the muscle belly.

This technique is most effective in the lumbar spine and sacral area, but can be used as far up as the cervico-thoracic junction.

When contractions become more intense, firm pressure can be applied over the sacrum, using the palm of the hand with the fingers pointing downwards. If possible pressure is maintained throughout a contraction, and is applied as if the sacrum formed part of the circumference of a circle, and was being moved round the arc caudally. This technique is most useful if the woman is on all fours, as it can be combined with circumduction of the pelvis.

Maintaining firm pressure can be very tiring for the practitioner and she should attempt to use her body weight to apply the force by locking her elbow against her side and leaning on her arm.

During the second stage of labour, between the mother's pushes, it is useful for any of her attendants to massage her neck and shoulders which take much of the strain along with the accessory muscles of respiration.

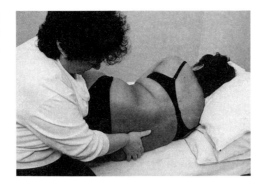

Fig. 11.10. Stretching lumbar erector spinae muscles.

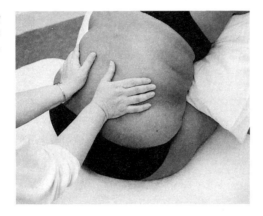

Fig. 11.11. Stretching lumbar erector spinae with woman sitting.

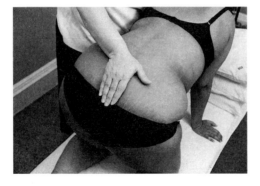

Fig. 11.12. Maintaining firm pressure over sacrum.

After delivery

Women who require an assisted delivery either by forceps or ventouse, or need stitches, are invariably placed in the lithotomy position while these manoeuvres are carried out. At this time their relaxin levels are very high and they are often fatigued. This position results in flattening of the lumbar spine and rotation of the ilia posteriorly. Maintaining this position for any length of time is a source of real concern, due to the excess strain placed on the hip joints and lumbar spine when they are at their most vulnerable.

The situation can be improved by placing a small pillow or even a rolled up towel under the lumbar spine to support the extension curve. This has

Fig. 11.13. Diagram to
show forces acting on
lumbar spine in lithotomy
position.

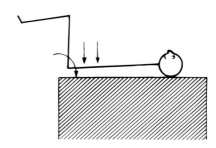

the effect of balancing some of the downward and rotational forces, thus
minimising ligamentous stretch.

Many women experience low backache for the first time in the immediate postpartum period, and this author feels that the lithotomy position is
often the cause. Prevention is always preferable to treatment. Some women
who have epidural anaesthesia complain of ongoing low back pain. As these
are often the same women who require assisted delivery and extensive
perineal suturing, with the added disadvantage of loss of proprioceptive
control of the lower extremities, the positional factor could be the aetiology
in these cases.

Postnatal period

Most antenatal education ends with the birth of the baby, and many new
mothers are unprepared for the changes that a baby will bring to their lives.
These are occurring at a time when the woman is vulnerable both physically
and psychologically.

With more home deliveries and 'domino' schemes taking place, and even
women who have delivered in hospital being transferred after 24 hours, the
transition time from pregnant woman to responsible mother has been considerably shortened. The new mother may not be prepared for the extra
bending and lifting involved in caring for a baby, and the fatigue brought on
by an altered sleep pattern. This combination can lead to a recurrence of
back pain usually at a junctional area. This is the reason for the osteopath
asking all pregnant women to return after delivery for an osteopathic examination. This will involve their posture and mobility being reassessed, and the
osteopath giving advice on the necessity for further treatment, or possibly
just suggestions regarding the height of the changing mat for the baby.

The other major cause of postnatal back problems is the position adopted
for feeding, whether breast or bottle. Because of inexperience, and often discomfort from sutures as well, new mothers sit unsatisfactorily when feeding.
Breastfeeding mothers bend over the baby rather than raising the baby to the
breast. This can lead to mid-thoracic and cervico-thoracic discomfort as well

as muscular problems in the shoulder and arm supporting the baby. The woman often fears that if she moves, or even takes a deep breath once feeding is established, the baby will stop sucking and never 'latch on' again. The baby may be being held in an uncomfortable and unsuitable position, which can contribute to sore nipples as well as musculoskeletal problems.

Bottle feeding can also lead to back and shoulder pain, particularly if the baby feeds very slowly and the same unsuitable position is maintained for a long time.

The only alteration required usually involves raising the baby to the breast or bottle by placing pillows on the woman's lap so she no longer has to bend forward. Any treatment to the thoracic spine will have little long-term effect without some adaptation of the causative factors.

Treatment to this area often effects milk production, and many women produce copious amounts of milk during and after treatment.

Aziza developed severe subscapular pain when her first child was 3 weeks old. The pain radiated anteriorly underneath both breasts, and was aggravated by inspiration and rotation. She was given an electrocardiogram and lung function tests and sent to a respiratory consultant because the pain led to panic attacks and hyperventilation. Diolofenac was prescribed and Aziza had to give up breastfeeding. As she could not lift her baby her mother had to take over the care of the baby.

Four years later she became pregnant again and at 26 weeks' gestation the pain returned and Aziza came for treatment. On examination her dorsal spine and ribs had very restricted mobility. Her breathing was mainly upper rib cage and this was aggravated by the fundus of the uterus pressing on the underside of the diaphragm. Treatment was instituted to relax the intercostal muscles and increase the mobility and separation of her ribs and thoracic vertebrae. Over a period of weeks the pains decreased, and with the reduction in symptoms the panic attacks disappeared. It was also recommended that Aziza wore a well-fitting supportive bra as her breasts were very large. She delivered a healthy girl after a 45 minute second stage without any anaesthesia.

The neonate   The postnatal visit is also a useful opportunity to examine the baby osteopathically. This would involve checking the limbs for equal development and full range of mobility, and if the osteopath had specialised training, checking the cranium for equal rhythmic movement. Until recently, cranial osteopathy was not part of the undergraduate course, and had to be studied by choice after qualification. Any osteopath who is not proficient in cranial work will recommend a colleague who is, if this is required.

The difference between osteopathy and chiropractic

Chiropractic also started in America at the turn of the century, but developed from a very different philosophical basis to osteopathy. This however was of little concern to those people receiving treatment. There is only one college of chiropractic in Britain, and until it opened in 1965 all chiropractors trained in America or Europe.

Chiropractors are more concerned with the relative position of joints, particularly vertebral joints, than their relative mobility, and often take X-rays before and after treatment to illustrate the changes brought about by their manipulation. They are also more interested in spinal joints than peripheral joints, and the treatment does not involve much soft tissue or articulation technique.

The main difference noticed by the patient is a different approach to manipulative techniques. Osteopaths usually use long leverage techniques to release a particular joint. This involves locking the joints above and below, using rotation and flexion or extension, so that when a high velocity thrust is applied to the area only one specific apophyseal joint will be released. Chiropractors, being more concerned with positional factors than mobility, apply a very high velocity thrust locally to the joint they wish to move. Many of their techniques require the recipient to be prone during treatment.

The difference between osteopathy and physiotherapy

The practice of physiotherapy has changed considerably during the past 20 years, and many physiotherapists now include massage and manipulation in their treatment regime. However, many people still visit their general practitioner for a diagnosis, with referral to a physiotherapist being just for treatment. While the osteopath is primarily concerned with biomechanical problems, and consideration of the person as a whole, the physiotherapist looks mainly at the area giving symptoms. Osteopaths use just manual treatment, but physiotherapists place significant importance on the use of electrical equipment as well.

Specially trained obstetric physiotherapists are available in some hospitals, but their work is usually restricted to ante- and postnatal exercise classes, and advising women after Caesarian section.

Osteopathy in other countries

In most of Europe, which functions under Napoleonic rather than Common Law, osteopathy is technically illegal because it is not state registered. This situation will obviously have to change, at least in the European Community following the passing of the Osteopaths Act. At the moment osteopaths practising in Europe have to work under the direction of a medical practitioner, or have another qualification themselves such as physiotherapy which does have state recognition.

There are osteopaths practising in Australia and New Zealand most of whom trained in Britain. Both countries now have their own licensing boards and anyone wanting to practise there may have to take their qualifying examinations.

In America, osteopathy developed in a very different manner to Britain. In the 1960s the American colleges of osteopathy joined the medical establishment with the result that an American DO is a Doctor of Osteopathy, and in every way the equal of an MD a Doctor of Medicine. Unfortunately this has had the consequence of American osteopaths doing very little osteopathy as we understand the term. Osteopathic techniques are just one of a whole range of medical and surgical procedures the American DO can employ, and osteopathic hospitals are very similar to general hospitals. Because of the different training in America, and the licensing laws peculiar to each State, it is impossible for a British-trained osteopath to practise in America without undergoing most of their training again.

An American text book of *Osteopathic Obstetrics* by O.P. Grow DO published in 1933 contains very little about osteopathic treatment as we recognise it today. However he does recommend direct pressure on the lumbar spine for pain relief, as well as: pressure applied above the symphysis pubis to assist engagement; direct pressure on the clitoris to effect 'osteopathic anaesthesia' before any internal examinations; a sharp tug on the pubic hair to stimulate the uterus to clamp down and prevent excessive haemorrhage; and lumbar extension immediately following delivery to stop haemorrhaging.

Many of Grow's other ideas such as allowing the woman to walk about during labour, and to put the baby to the breast immediately after delivery seem very modern, but he also advocated bed rest for 14 days after the birth, which returns the book to its own era.

Research

Research into osteopathy and the outcome of treatment has historically been difficult because of the individuality of the practitioners and their preferred methods of treatment. This renders any trial fraught with complications and inaccuracies. In the past osteopaths attempted to follow the medical model for trials of treatment, but this was always unsuccessful because it proved impossible to treat all volunteers in exactly the same way. The very nature of the treatment made this impractical. Also introducing more than one practitioner into the trial made uniformity of diagnosis and treatment a difficult goal. It is also difficult to quantify the results of a therapy where so much depends on the interaction between practitioner and patient. Obviously some research was carried out, but this was often of a more information gathering type – what was the most common area for symptoms? or, how far were people prepared to travel to visit an osteopath?, which provided useful statistics but did not add to the body of osteopathic knowledge.

A *Which* report in 1986 suggested that osteopathy was the most widely used complementary therapy, and that 90% of patients claimed to have been cured or improved by treatment. This could not be considered as research although the findings were most welcome. The dearth of research on pregnant women is even greater, as each practice may have only a few pregnant women attending at any given time, and they could all be at different stages of pregnancy. Even in America virtually no research of a purely osteopathic nature has been carried out on pregnant women. In this country collaborative research has often been hampered by lack of funding or cooperation. Hopefully these problems are all in the past and several research initiatives are presently under way, or in the planning stage. In the interim doubting medical professionals will have to rely on the testimony of thousands of women who have obtained lasting relief from the unnecessary aches and discomforts of pregnancy following osteopathic treatment. There is a large number of small-scale trials which have been carried out by students as part of their degree submissions. While some relate to the increased joint mobility of pregnant women, none so far has resulted in a change to the treatment rationale.

The story so far

The stated aim of this chapter is to inform midwives and other health professionals of the usefulness of osteopathy as an adjunctive treatment for pregnant women. As already stated, osteopathic treatment is safe, non-invasive, usually painless, but primarily effective for pregnant women, and should always be considered a feasible option when offering optimum care. The future of antenatal care must lie in a partnership between allopathic and complementary practitioners working for the better health and well-being of mother and baby.

Training

There are three main schools of osteopathy in Britain which together produce about 150 graduates each year. There is also one school which provides a 1 year postgraduate course for medical practitioners. All of the schools provide 4 year full-time degree courses, with one offering a 5 year option with a mixed mode of attendance as well.

All the schools require 'A' levels or their equivalent for entry, and many students present with a previous degree. Different criteria exist for mature students who may comprise up to 50% of any given cohort.

Each school has its own syllabus but they follow broadly similar lines. The early part of the course includes the detailed anatomy and physiology required, alongside psychology, pathology, clinical medicine and osteopathic studies. All the schools have large outpatient clinics where students spend hundreds of hours later in the course evaluating, diagnosing and treating patients under supervision. The aim is not just to train osteopaths but to provide the skills which allow students to become competent practitioners.

Although all of the courses are degree courses, all the schools are private institutions and do not attract any funding from central government. This means they have to charge students full cost fees, and the mandatory grant from the local education authority only covers 15% of the cost. It remains to be seen if statutory registration will alter this situation. It is however one of the reasons why there is such a high proportion of mature students – often people who have worked for a few years in order to fund their studies.

Useful addresses

General Council and Register of Osteopaths Ltd
56 London Street, Reading, Berkshire RG1 4SQ, UK
Tel: 0734 576585

British School of Osteopathy
1–4 Suffolk Street, London SW1Y 4HG, UK
Tel: 071 930 0254, Fax: 071 839 1098

British College of Osteopathy and Naturopathy
6 Netherhall Gardens, London NW3 5RR, UK
Tel: 071 435 6464, Fax: 071 431 3630

European School of Osteopathy
104 Tonbridge Road, Maidstone, Kent ME16 8SL, UK
Tel: 0622 671558, Fax: 0622 662165

London College of Osteopathic Medicine
8–10 Boston Place, London NW1 6QH, UK
Tel: 071 262 5250

All the schools have outpatient clinics which are open to the public for self-referral, and some run specialist clinics including expectant mothers' clinics.

Osteopathic Information Service
P.O. Box 2074
Reading,
Berkshire RG1 4YR
Tel: 0734 512051

The OIS acts as an information service for the press and public, representing all facets of the profession.

References

Grow O.P. (1933) *Osteopathic Obstetrics*. Journal Printing Co., Missouri.

Which? (October 1986) Consumers Association.

Report of a working Party on Osteopathy (1991) Kings Fund. King Edwards Hospital Fund for London.

Further reading

Sandler S. (1987) *Osteopathy (Alternative Health)*. Macdonald Optima,

Hartman (1985) *Handbook of Osteopathic Technique*. Hutchinson.

Sue Mack

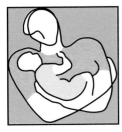

Chapter 12 ## Attitudes to Complementary Therapy

'One of the main reasons for the current upsurge of "official" interest in non-conventional medicine is the rapidly increasing number of patients who are seeking help from such practitioners' (British Medical Association, 1993).

Whilst there are no precise figures available there does seem to be a strong consumer-led movement towards the use of non-conventional therapy. One in five of the population are now thought to consult a non-conventional health practitioner: as a business it is estimated to be worth £450 million per year; increasing numbers of health professionals are now training or have trained in complementary therapies; the press regularly carries articles informing readers of the use of alternative therapies by the rich and famous or warning or informing the general public about the treatments available.

The terms 'alternative', 'non-conventional' and 'complementary' are often used interchangeably. Here alternative therapies are seen as those given in place of orthodox medicine, complementary as those given alongside, and non-conventional as those not generally taught as part of medical, nursing or midwifery training and considered essential knowledge for practitioners.

The fact that increasing numbers of people are consulting an increasing number of non-conventional therapists is undisputed, the reasons are less clear and the way that people make that choice is also uncertain. This chapter is not intended to be a researched study into the use of complementary therapy in pregnancy and childbearing but is based on interviews with consumers, pregnant women and new mothers, midwives, GPs and obstetricians. These were conducted in various parts of England, including an inner city area, a London suburb, and a semi-rural district. These are necessarily self-selected individuals as they all agreed to be interviewed, anonymity being assured. This is about thoughts, feelings, expectations and experiences of current practice in non-conventional medicine as expressed by 65 individuals.

The consumers   A study by Fulder and Munro in 1985 suggested that nationally there were 12 non-conventional practitioners per 100 000 population. The British Holistic Medical Association estimates a growth in the number of therapists of about 11% per year. The BMA survey in 1991 showed a membership of 3000 for the representative bodies for acupuncture and osteopathy alone. The Consumers Association survey (1992) showed a consultation rate among their members of 1:4, with osteopathy, chiropractic, homeopathy and acupuncture in order of popularity. A study by Thomas (1991) suggested that 70 600 patients were seen nationally for osteopathy, acupuncture, chiropractic, homeopathy and naturopathy. Those attending non-conventional therapists are mainly drawn from social classes I and II and two-thirds are women. There is a weighting to consultations in London and the south-east (Office of Population Studies, 1991).

Many of those consulting a non-conventional therapist were also seeing an orthodox practitioner. The study by Thomas (1991) showed that 64% had received previous care from a GP or hospital, and 22% had consulted their GP in the 2 weeks before seeing another therapist. Twenty-four per cent of those in their study were also receiving orthodox treatment. This was then clearly being seen by many of the consumers as a 'complementary therapy'. Fulder and Munro in 1985 also found that 33.4% were simultaneously receiving conventional medical treatment.

The interviews   In discussion, those women who had consulted a non-conventional practitioner had done so for a variety of reasons. Behind many of them was the feeling or experience that they would be treated 'holistically', that they would receive attention as a whole person and 'not just as a condition'. It is the difference in philosophy and focus as well as the felt need that affects women's choice of a healer. As doctors over the last century have had more effective drugs and surgical procedures they have had to rely less on counselling, knowledge of the family and psychosocial support to heal the person. Buckman and Sabbagh (1993) describe this as the change from patient–centred medicine to disease control medicine and of 'conventional medicine pursuing the goal of science and the mechanistic cure of the curable disease and complementary medicine adhering faithfully to the traditions of the healer patient relationship'. It was this philosophy that was particularly important to some women in childbearing, when they did not consider themselves to be ill and were not seeking diagnosis or cure, but information, advice, support and care. The focus of the complementary therapist was seen to be the enhancement of health as well as the treatment of particular conditions. Most of those women who had consulted a non-conventional practitioner were also attending antenatal appointments regularly and were intending to deliver or had delivered in hospital. The women fell into three main groups: those who had consulted complementary practitioners in the past and were pleased with the attention and treatment they had received and were therefore well disposed towards non-conventional therapies; those who felt they wanted extra support or care during childbearing and had asked advice about who to consult either for general health enhancement or for a specific problem; and thirdly those women who did not feel certain that orthodox medicine offered the choice of care they wanted during pregnancy and labour and chose to find a practitioner who would offer that care, often selecting an independent midwife.

For those who had already consulted a non-conventional therapist there seemed to be a generalising effect, that is, they were prepared to consult therapists in other branches of complementary medicine, having had experience of one. They had mostly sought help in the past concerning a specific problem but also regarded some therapies as offering pro-active or preventive treatment.

One woman had been particularly keen to seek nutritional advice.

I had not led a particularly healthy lifestyle before the pregnancy, snatching meals or missing them completely and not ever bothering to cook properly during the week. My partner was more concerned with diet and encouraged me to consider it a bit more carefully when we decided to try for a family. I stopped smoking, although this had not been very much and reduced the drinking to a glass or two of wine at the weekends, except for the occasional party. When I spoke to the GP before conception, she was quite helpful but it was all very general, eat more fruit that sort of thing. I felt that because of the bad diet in the past I needed something a bit more geared to my needs. I consulted a nutritionalist and then a herbalist and both were really helpful, giving advice and support throughout the pregnancy as well. The midwives that I told about it were very interested and were asking me for more information about it. I was worried that they would object in some way but in fact they were really interested and supportive.

Some women did not discuss the complementary care they were receiving with their doctors or midwives; the reasons given for this were that the doctor or midwife would object or feel in some way slighted, and the women did not want to upset their health professional as they wanted their support particularly at the time of delivery.

Roisin, a 35 year old professional woman, had never consulted non-conventional therapists in the past nor had any other members of her family. After delivery she suffered a great deal of soreness in the perineum and this was affecting her ability to care as well as she wanted for her new baby. She was reluctant to consult her GP as he had been very judgemental about her being pregnant outside marriage and she felt he may 'give her another lecture' and wanted to find help elsewhere. She asked other women and then her health visitor who suggested a local herbalist. This treatment was successful but Roisin did not feel able to tell her doctor about it although the health visitor encouraged her to do so.

Other women were happy to discuss their non-conventional treatment and had no objection to information being passed between anyone who was treating them.

Some women asked for referral to complementary practitioners from their GP or midwife. In each case that was discussed with the author, this had been for a particular problem during the pregnancy or that she had suffered beforehand. In several cases these were musculoskeletal problems, and they had been referred to chiropractors or osteopaths. Some had experienced some reluctance from the GP or felt there was a lack of information about local practitioners or their qualifications. They had felt there was no objection from the health professionals but a lack of support or straightforward information. Many of these women were professionals who had no difficulty in researching the subject and making an informed choice. They were also in a position to pay for the service. Some women had received help through their NHS hospital, where massage was offered as a way of treating pain from tense muscles and general anxiety. This was given by a midwife but had to be fitted into her free time. The treatment was greatly appreciated by the women who received it but several mentioned feeling unsure about accepting it as 'she seemed so busy'. This group were very keen to explore other therapies, particularly the non-invasive forms, such as reflexology and aromatherapy. They were not looking for treatment for a specific condition but rather a way of improving their general sense of well-being and dealing with what they considered to be the more minor problems of childbearing, such as aches and pains, breast tenderness and nausea. They were well informed in general terms about the more popular therapies. Some women mentioned anxieties about the safety of acupuncture with the danger of the transmission of AIDS, and others were not sure about using homeopathic medicines, feeling that they may be dangerous or poisonous. These women thought they would probably discuss this with a doctor first before approaching a therapist, and if their doctor expressed doubts then they would not use the therapy. Most of this group of mothers believed they could discuss complementary therapies with the midwife but were not sure how much she would know about them. Only one woman remembered being asked about complementary therapies at her first antenatal appointment and only those who had attended a hospital where they were offered massage and relaxation by the midwives remembered seeing any information in posters or handbooks about any complementary therapy. The majority of women said that they would prefer to be offered therapy through their GP or antenatal unit and would like it to be seen as part of the general care. They mostly referred to reflexology, massage, aromatherapy and relaxation in this context, feeling that osteopathy, acupuncture and homeopathy were specialist treatments. They recognised that this may cause problems with time and availability but as one woman said 'it would be a lot more useful than all that weighing and blood-taking'.

The women who had decided to avoid all orthodox medicine as far as possible during their pregnancy had generally been committed to the use of alternative medicine in the time before conception or had experienced what they felt to be inappropriate or ineffective care in the past. One expressed her disappointment at the way her hospital had promised a named midwife to care for her during her first pregnancy, but this had often not been possible as the midwife was away or not on that shift. Whilst she realised this could happen she felt that her expectations had been raised wrongly. Many of this group of women felt that childbearing did not require medicine and preferred to choose the way they were treated and by whom. This measure of control was very important to most of them. They wanted to develop a relationship with the person or people who were going to deliver the baby, and to be seen as a 'whole person, not just a womb' for the whole of the pregnancy and afterwards. Not all were disappointed or angry with orthodox treatment, but they wanted to be treated in a different way and not to have the experience medicalised. One felt strongly that she wanted to be attended and supported by women who would be more understanding of her feelings and needs. Most of this group of women were able to pay the costs of non-NHS care although some were making considerable sacrifices to do so. All were conscious they were privileged to be able to make a choice.

The women interviewed who had not consulted any non-conventional therapists either did not know anything about the therapies or had been put off in some way. Those who had no information expressed interest in some things that they felt would be a good experience and not likely to be uncomfortable or embarrassing. They had positive responses to aromatherapy and massage of all kinds. There was uncertainty for some at the idea of acupuncture or osteopathy, unless there was a specific reason, although several knew someone who had consulted an osteopath with good results. Acupuncture was more associated with stopping smoking than pregnancy.

Hypnotherapy was not regarded very seriously by many women, although again it was positively associated with stopping smoking. Homeopathy was quite well regarded, especially as some larger high street chemists now sold homeopathic preparations. Some women were anxious about using these in pregnancy for fear they might harm the baby and did not feel they would be able to judge from the literature available.

A majority of the women who had not considered complementary therapies said that they would do so if recommended by the doctor or midwife, particularly if they were assured of both the safety of the practice and the reliability of the therapist. Many would like to be offered therapies through their antenatal clinic or GP surgery. They felt that this would ensure good practice and safety. For some, cost was the overriding factor. If the treatment could be offered free or at a very low rate they would be keen to try some therapies. Several women felt that complementary therapies might have something to offer in problems such as nausea and vomiting and back pain. They felt the amount of distress this caused them was marginalised by the health professionals and that being recommended to rest more was no help when you had other children and a home and sometimes a job to organise.

Sources of information about non-conventional therapies were for many women hit and miss. For those who had felt confident about researching information and making judgements about it, the greatest complaint was the difficulty in assessing the qualifications and experience of the therapist without asking direct questions. Some felt they should look for someone who was medically trained or qualified as a midwife; this would offer a certain basis of knowledge and expertise. Others felt confident to approach the practitioner directly and ask about training and areas of interest. The lack of a general accreditation to practise caused some women concern. Many chose a practitioner by recommendation and did not check qualifications or training. The fact that someone else had a good experience was enough. Several women said that they would have liked access to a database of approved practitioners either through the GP or the clinic.

General information came mostly through word of mouth or articles in newspapers or magazines. Some of the women who were concerned about using alternative therapies had read articles that had put them off in some way. These included stories about unqualified practitioners and missed serious illnesses; none had related directly to pregnancy. Other mothers felt that stories of the use of therapies by the rich and famous, or by people they saw as 'cranks and weirdos', meant that they did not have a great deal to offer to them.

Many felt that lack of information, written or verbal, was the main reason for not considering any alternative to orthodox medicine and that information from someone they trusted would help them to assess its usefulness. This included friends and family as well as health professionals.

The midwives   The UKCC and the Royal College of Midwives both accept that there is growing interest among midwives in the use of complementary therapies in their practice. The UKCC publishes a leaflet giving guidelines for midwives. This states that the midwife is responsible for judging her competency in any therapy she is using with a patient. It also advises her to check her insurance cover and to be aware of local policies. Consideration is also to be given to the consent of the patient and the role of the doctor (see Chapter 1).

The Royal College of Midwives has experienced increasing interest from midwives in study days and training information about complementary therapies. They feel that the interest is often coming from the consumers who regard complementary medicine as sometimes safer and giving them more control. They are able to choose the therapy and the therapist, and not be regarded as patients.

Midwifery journals are also increasingly carrying articles concerning the use of various therapies and assessing their value, and the universities are beginning to offer courses for health professionals in complementary therapies.

The interviews   Whilst the guidelines from the UKCC are clear about the role of the midwife in the practice of complementary therapies, many of the midwives did not feel so clear about what they were 'allowed' to do. Some were concerned about judging their competency to give advice about such things as dietary supplements or over-the-counter homeopathic and herbal treatments for common ailments in pregnancy.

The greatest observable difference in the groups of midwives interviewed was the knowledge they had of complementary therapies. Whilst very few had no interest the level of interest varied tremendously. Where there was a midwife or midwifery tutor with an interest or qualification in some form of non-conventional therapy the general interest increased enormously. This seemed to have a generalising effect, so that an interest in and the use of one therapy easily became an openness to other therapies and their value to the women. Many of the midwives practising complementary therapies were doing so with only minimal support, in that they were having to provide this in their own time or with the help of colleagues to cover their other duties. In some places, once the value of a therapy became established then it was more acceptable and in some cases institutionalised. Lack of time was one of the major problems identified by the midwives. Many could not see how they could include therapies such as massage, aromatherapy or reflexology into their routine practice. A few community midwives felt that it did fit well into postnatal visits where the mother and baby were not experiencing major difficulties that required her attention.

The majority of midwives with some interest in complementary therapies wanted much more teaching about them in their normal training. They believed that if they had more information they could give much more guidance to the women in their care, make some choices about pursuing training for themselves and support those women already receiving therapy outside the hospital system. Some had felt embarrassed by their lack of knowledge when women asked about non-conventional treatments for frequently occurring problems of pregnancy. They were particularly interested in being able to suggest alternative treatments for such problems as nausea and vomiting, breastpain, backache, sleeplessness and appetite disturbance. They also wanted to be able to help the women who were expressing anxiety and depression. One group of midwives in an area where a number of their clients sought their own complementary therapies, felt they should have more information when a woman came in to deliver, particularly if they were to be accompanied by a therapist. They were generally positive about this but felt concern at their own lack of knowledge. They did not expect to be experts but to have some understanding of the place of unfamiliar therapies.

Several midwives were aware of practitioners in their area and some had consulted them personally. They were very uncertain however of whether they were covered by insurance for giving advice to their clients. Some would like to have had a list of practitioners and the costs available to women. They were concerned about the qualifications of complementary therapists and some expressed doubts about referring to anyone who was not medically qualified or had midwifery training. Some midwives, and this did not seem to follow any geographical pattern, were not aware of the use of many therapies in childbearing. They did not ask clients about their own use of complementary therapies and assumed that they were not being practised. They had no knowledge of any use in their own hospitals, although some were aware of discussion and information in the professional press. Most felt that there was no time or opportunity to learn or practise new skills and did not see a role for informing their mothers.

A few midwives interviewed had a full training in a branch of non-conventional therapy and were trying to integrate this into their practice. Others who were trained and committed to a therapy had opted to work outside the hospital/GP system for philosophical as well as practical reasons.

Sarah Budd, who writes the acupuncture chapter, works at Freedom Fields Hospital, Plymouth, and here gives the story of her move to acupuncture.

The acupuncture service in our maternity unit came about following the increase in demand from mothers for less intervention and a wish for methods to help them cope during labour that did not involve the use of strong drugs. This was around 1985 and when an acupuncturist brought his wife in during her first labour, and administered acupuncture, we looked on with interest. She had a calm, controlled labour which was of average duration. This was either coincidence, or acupuncture did indeed have something to offer.

I approached my manager with the view that if women in labour were to have acupuncture, then it should be the midwife who administered it as part of her total care. I pointed out that I was keen to train, and had investigated the various schools and costing. I was granted study leave, but had to fund the course myself. Through the Midwives Chronicle, *I applied for various awards and was successful in all 3 years of my training. I studied part time for 3 years at the London School of Acupuncture and Traditional Chinese Medicine. Having qualified, I still did not feel confident enough to set up the service in our unit, as I did not feel I had sufficient practical experience, so courtesy of the Johnson and Johnson Travel Award, a bursary from the hospital and a personal bank loan, I set off for China. I went for the 1 month clinical course in Nanjing, South East China. Working 6 days a week, seeing up to 40 patients each day, of all ages and with a tremendous range of conditions to be treated, I soon felt more competent. I returned to the unit, and contacted our consultant obstetricians with my objectives. They were supportive and happy for me to treat the women under their care without referring back to them. I joined the Register of Traditional Chinese Medicine, which, amongst other things, gave me insurance cover. I informed the Royal College of Midwives and the local Health Authority of my intentions, and started using my acupuncture skills. I was based on the labour ward at the time, so initially was just using acupuncture to augment contractions or as analgesia for labour. Gradually I was being asked to help with problems such as backache and sickness. These numbers grew at a tremendous rate, and I was soon doing two jobs at once. Eventually the demand was so great that I was taken off the labour ward, and given a new post as Midwifery Sister/Acupuncturist. The typical week involves treating outpatients most of the time, seeing inpatients on the wards and of course, looking after women in labour with acupuncture as a priority. This often means rearranging outpatients. There is administration, research, talks and computer work to be fitted in, as well as attending meetings, keeping up to date with activities in the unit, and sorting out a waiting list for those wanting appointments. The midwifery skills are very much called on, as the majority of women coming for treatment have queries about their pregnancy, or may even have developed a problem or two since last seen by their own midwife and which can be sorted out for them. I am sure that most of them feel much happier about having treatment during pregnancy from someone qualified as a midwife. From our side, to offer relief from so many discomforts and worries is a most rewarding and fulfilling experience.*

Another of the contributors to this book, Helen Stapleton, works as an herbalist and independent midwife and explains her philosophy thus.

The practice of medicine has a deeply entrenched political perspective which is often ignored or deliberately omitted from historical accounts. It is surely no accident that the history of both herbal medicine and the midwifery profession rarely draws on material from the archives of our predecessors whose vast repository of knowledge has been so thoroughly dismissed in a short space of time. The current climate, whereby a revival of interest is gaining ground for finding more gentle ways of doing things, provides us with a pertinent opportunity for exploring and reaffirming women's history. It is a sobering realisation that these same women/witch/midwife healers were often the only general medical practitioners available for the majority of the population, who had access neither to doctors nor hospitals and whose constitutional health was seriously undermined by the pernicious effects of poverty with repercussions associated with maternal and child ill-health. In singling out these women and labelling them as charlatans and criminals, the underlying misogyny of the (Catholic) church was confirmed. Its particularly venomous attitude towards midwives was illustrated by the Reverends Kramer and Sprenger, fifteenth century Dominican priests who wrote: 'no one does more harm to the Catholic Church than Midwives' (Ehrenreich and English, 1973).

According to the Church, the vital healing force lay not in the earth, but in the power of a (male) God. As disease, sickness and even labour pains were perceived as God given, so only Church-approved individuals could initiate any remedial action. Needless to say, those designated for the job were not women. The suppression of female healers in Western cultures by both the Church and latterly by the medical establishment reflects a wider political context, which incorporates class and gender struggles. Within this arena, the status of women healers has periodically risen and fallen, more in accordance with the degree of tolerance shown to them by the ruling patriarchy, rather than a reflection of the efficacy of their practice.

This story of woman as healer is woven like a subtle but complex tapestry which honours the sacredness and balance of the natural world rather than supporting the current Western view which sees it as a limitless resource for exploitation and appropriation. The current ontological shift in the search for an ecologically sustained future has much to gain from an examination of the world views of ancient civilisations. They saw the created world and the creative force not as separate and distinct, but rather as dynamic and interrelated impulses. There is evidence of a new cosmology emerging in which the purpose and value of human life assumes a radically different emphasis. This newly emerging paradigm, based on the need to add meaning to human existence, honours the feminine principle and consciously espouses a reordering of priorities, while simultaneously inviting a sense of the divine into our everyday lives. Perhaps it is this impulse which has generated the tremendous interest in complementary and alternative medicine as indicated by the increasing numbers visiting practitioners. The writing of this book, with so much of the material contributed by practising midwives, similarly reflects a reuniting of the art of healing with the skill of midwifery.

Most of the midwives interviewed were open to and interested in the use of complementary therapies in childbearing. They felt that the general philosophies of most of the therapies were sympathetic and belonged in midwifery practice. They were, however, often uncertain about whether they were in a legal position to offer advice or information and were keen to be better informed. In units where there was a midwife practising a therapy, and the interest had become general, there was sometimes a great deal of support from colleagues. It seemed to be in these units that other midwives were talking about learning new skills themselves and were enthusiastic about the benefits to the mothers, not just in terms of treatment but also in the improved communication between staff and clients that emerged from the use of some treatments. There was very little concern expressed about how this would be received by the doctors. Most midwives thought that they would inform them but that they would not necessarily need their approval or agreement, particularly for therapies such as aromatherapy, reflexology and massage. Where midwives did feel that there would be negative reactions from consultants it was mainly about the relevance of the treatments, not an outright objection.

Some hospitals are developing policies for the use of complementary therapies throughout the hospital including the maternity unit. St Bartholomews Hospital, London, has suggested guidelines for nurses and midwives wishing to practise a range of therapies, all non-invasive: aromatherapy, reflexology, shiatsu, acupressure and holistic massage. It refers to Competent Nurse/Therapists (CNT), who are registered nurses who have also undertaken a recognised training in a therapy and been awarded a qualification by a professional body which meets their criteria for each therapy. Their work is to be supervised by a Nurse Manager. The CNT is responsible for deciding if a client is suitable for therapy, but anyone currently under medical care should only be treated if the consent of the medical personnel is first obtained. This may be consent 'in principle'. They are also required to gain the informed consent of the patient. Evaluation is to be monitored at unit/ward level and to include the opinions of the clients.

This system of clear policy guidelines helps the staff to feel more certain of the boundaries not just in a negative way, of what they may not do, but in a positive framework of what practices are possible and indeed welcomed.

Another maternity unit that has developed the use of complementary therapies is at Queen Mary's Hospital, Sidcup, Kent, where midwives offer aromatherapy and reflexology to mothers. Here, a working party of midwives, midwifery managers, and a midwifery educationalist have developed guidelines for the use of the therapies and have arranged appropriate training for those midwives who are not already qualified. Initially they have only dealt with labouring and postnatal women for conditions which are normally the province of the midwife. Reflexology is offered on an 'on call' basis by qualified midwives. Pharmacy staff provide the bottles and labels and blend the oils needed for aromatherapy. Funding has come from offering massage and reflexology sessions to staff for a small fee. This covers the cost of buying essential oils augmented by the fees from the loan of TENS machines. Records are kept in the case notes as a way of collecting data for a proposed retrospective study. They have also established a maternity and gynaecology staff interest group offering education, lectures, a journal club and case discussion. It is hoped this will encourage staff to develop their skills and enable them to expand the services offered to the mothers.

The general practitioners

Several studies have shown increasing interest in and support for non-conventional medicine among GPs. Wharton and Lewith in 1986 in a study of 200 GPs in Avon found that 76% had referred for acupuncture, herbal medicine, spinal manipulation, homeopathy, faith healing and hypnosis to medically qualified practitioners and 72% to non-medically qualified therapists during the previous year. Only 9% thought that the techniques were not useful to patients. However at this time the authors considered that from their assessment of the doctors' comments concerning the use of such therapies, their overall knowledge of the techniques was poor. Anderson and Anderson, in a study in Oxfordshire in 1986, found that 59% had referred patients for some form of complementary medicine, and 41% felt that such therapies were valid. They also found that 31% of GPs said they had a working knowledge of a technique; 27% of those were in spinal manipulation and 14% in acupuncture. Many were responding to interest expressed by their patients. In the study by Anderson and Anderson 95% of the GPs asked said that one or more patients had discussed alternative therapies with them during the past year.

Training of doctors in most branches of complementary medicine has increased over the last decade. Anderson and Anderson found that 41% of the GPs in their study had attended lectures and 12% were fully trained in some technique. Forty-two per cent expressed an interest in further training.

Of the 16% (35) actually practising non-conventional techniques, 13 were using manipulation and nine hypnotherapy. Perhaps giving some cause for concern, nine were practising without any training, including acupuncture, manipulation, hypnotherapy, transcendental meditation and faith healing. Wharton and Lewith found that 38% of GPs in their study had some training, although as they say 'instruction was usually limited to weekend courses or informal sessions during their trainee year. No respondent gave a specific qualification' (Wharton and Lewith, 1986).

Of those in the studies expressing concern about the use of complementary therapies, 3% in the Avon study felt that non-medical practitioners should be banned, and 21% felt that they should be licensed and recognised as 'supplementary to medicine'. The Oxfordshire study showed that 16% objected to non-conventional medicine on the grounds that it is 'unscientific'.

The interviews None of the GPs interviewed from various parts of the country expressed any outright objection to the use of complementary therapies in childbearing. One inner city GP said that his role was to ensure as far as possible the best outcome, 'a healthy baby and a happy mother', and he was prepared to consider any treatment that would lead to this end. Some did make clear that they did not have any real knowledge of any of the techniques but this did not prevent them referring patients to practitioners if they thought this would be of some help.

Those with the least knowledge rarely suggested complementary therapies to their patients but were prepared to respond to a request. The number of enquiries from patients varied very much around the country. A GP in a semi-rural and one in the inner city remarked on how few patients discussed alternatives with them. Those who did report suggesting complementary therapies in childbearing found a good response in their clients. Most felt that they would be happy to offer some therapies within the practice if that could be arranged practically and financially. The cost of the treatments was an issue that was discussed by every GP. Most thought that their patients would not want to or be able to pay and would like to see many of the treatments being offered on the NHS. Some were beginning to provide this within their own surgeries. One practice in the Home Counties has given over part of their surgery to a multi-therapy practice of non-conventional therapists. They do not control the work of the therapists but aim to establish good relationships that allow them to refer appropriate clients to them and receive good feedback about treatment, progress and future needs. This is bought in by the practice as a service to their patients. Patients wanting further care are at liberty to pay for this themselves.

The advantage most frequently mentioned by GPs for women in pregnancy and childbearing was for the treatment of symptoms that they felt powerless to do anything about. These included, nausea, sleep disturbance, indigestion and backache. Many felt that these could be well treated by complementary practitioners or that at least the women would have more support and understanding about the conditions. There was some anxiety expressed among the GPs about the suitability of alternative treatments in pregnancy and most had one 'horror story' to tell of someone taking an inappropriate substance or being treated wrongly. These were enough to discourage some practitioners from referring to anyone but a qualified medical practitioner. In most of the interviews, doctors expressed some concern about the training and qualifications of practitioners and several mentioned the need for some regulatory body, to oversee the practice of those who were not medically qualified. Some GPs did not express any doubts about those who were doctors practising any form of non-conventional therapy regardless of their training in that therapy. Others were concerned that a doctor might use acupuncture or hypnotherapy with only minimal experience and training, and thought they would prefer to refer to a trained non-medical therapist.

The issue of referrals was addressed by most of the GPs. There was no pattern of how, when or whom to refer to. Most used personal knowledge or word of mouth as a guide to referral. Whilst expressing doubts about qualifications and training many had no idea of either when they referred to a therapist they knew, trusted or had good reports about. It was this personal information that informed decisions if not opinions.

GPs who were themselves trained in some branch of non-conventional therapy were the most interested to use other forms of therapy and were also affecting attitudes within their practices. Just as midwives with an interest in an alternative therapy were found to influence the whole unit, the same was true of GPs in general. In some cases the doctor had chosen a particular practice or group of partners because of a willingness to try non-conventional therapies where appropriate. Where this was the case the doctor would suggest alternative therapies to childbearing women as a better choice of treatment or support.

Where GPs objected to or did not consider alternative or complementary therapies they mostly cited lack of time to train in or practise the therapy. A few felt they only had a placebo affect to offer. Some thought there was no research to support the therapy, although admitted that they did not look for research outside the standard medical press.

Younger doctors were on the whole more open to alternative medicine. Some had received some lectures during training but most felt these only equipped them to know about the major therapies and when to refer patients. Some felt the teaching had come too early in their medical training and that it was only when you were in practice that you really became aware of the needs of the patients and where they might be met. Several doctors expressed an interest in training in a non-conventional therapy but felt that it would be extremely difficult to do this properly whilst running a busy practice. One had chosen to train in acupuncture whilst on maternity leave and working part-time with young children. She felt this had been arduous but worthwhile and she was able to offer acupuncture to some patients. She had not received much support from colleagues but no outright hostility.

Most of the GPs had some interest in non-conventional therapies but very few had direct knowledge or experience. The majority felt that it could usefully be used in childbearing although thought that it would be difficult to implement in a general practice. Several were beginning to explore their greater freedom to employ other non-medical practitioners and thought they might extend their input to antenatal sessions. If there was a nurse, health visitor or midwife interested in training or already qualified most GPs thought this would offer the best kind of help to the patients.

The consultants At this time there is no written policy statement concerning complementary therapy from the Royal College of Obstetricians and Gynaecologists. There does not seem to be any research available on consultants' attitudes to and use of non-conventional medicine.

The interviews Most of the consultants felt that obstetric practice had altered considerably in attitudes and that there was much more openness to change and that alternative therapy was included in that change. Few had any knowledge of or training in any non-conventional treatments or knew other gynaecologists or obstetricians who did. The most positive attitudes seemed to be from those who had themselves consulted or experienced some member of their family receiving treatment from a non-conventional practitioner.

The most commonly expressed anxieties were concerning the training and qualifications of therapists. They did not have any worries about doctors practising as alternative therapists nor any great concern about midwives as long as they were using non-invasive techniques. They were not very well informed about the kind of training available and the regulating bodies already existing for the whole range of therapies. They also discussed concern about the lack of research in most areas of non-conventional therapy but agreed that they did not consult journals concerned with the alternatives. Lack of research in osteopathy, for example, did not raise concern as they felt that osteopaths were well trained and regulated. Information appeared to haphazard and anecdotal.

Most felt that the limitations of time and facilities would prevent midwives in their units from using complementary therapies, although they generally had no objection to them initiating their use. Where complementary therapies were being offered in a unit, it was felt that this was usually midwife led and that there was little interest from clients. Asked if they ever discussed clients' use of complementary therapies most said that they did not and assumed that the woman would mention it if appropriate. When patients did express an interest in or a request for alternative treatment most felt that they would be happy with this if it did not threaten the safety of the woman. One consultant said that he felt that most women considered the complementary therapies to be safer than conventional medicine, whereas doctors felt that on balance it is the other way round. Where midwives had initiated the use of therapies such as massage, reflexology and aromatherapy, the consultants were pleased with the reactions of women and anxiety about their use lessened until it became seen as a normal part of treatment. The influence of midwives in this area was very clear. A midwife who was competent and confident in her use of a particular treatment was respected and well regarded and the therapy seen as advantageous to patients. Personal contact with a non-conventional therapy or therapist was again the key to influencing either positively or negatively attitudes of medical practitioners to that therapy.

The purchasers

A recent publication by the National Association of Health Authorities and Trusts with Yorkshire region and Bradford District Health Authority (DHA) (NAHAT, 1993) felt that the division between purchaser and provider and the emphasis on patient choice may affect the use of complementary therapies. Their survey was intended to discover purchasers' attitudes to the availability of complementary therapies in the NHS and their approach to purchasing such therapies. Of the replies received 39 authorities/fundholders stated that complementary therapies should not be available on the NHS. Seventy per cent of Family Health Services Authority (FHSA) and General Practitioner Fund Holders (GPFH) and 65% of DHAs were in favour of all or some being free at the point of contact. Those most favourably viewed for NHS provision were homeopathy, acupuncture, osteopathy and chiropractic. As far as policy is concerned 15% of FHSAs and 31% of DHAs had agreed a policy about complementary therapies. Some of these were specific but others only outlined an approach.

Decisions were declared to be most affected by evidence of effectiveness. There is very little agreement on this as the report says 'It would seem that purchasers are either not basing their decisions on the same evidence or the available evidence is open to wide interpretation.' The lack of randomised trials is again mentioned here as a reason for some authorities not encouraging non-conventional treatments. The report highlights the fact that much of the scientific work associated with the therapies is not available in those journals most often available in local, medical hospital or university libraries.

The report mentions particularly the lack of consistency in purchasers' decisions with regard to funding therapies, based largely it suggests on a lack of agreement about the effectiveness and not on any negative attitude in general. The report suggests that a research and development strategy should be agreed and action should include 'additional research into the effectiveness, evaluation of complementary medicine services currently available, research into the cost/benefits and the development of standards for training and qualification.' There is no suggestion overall that there is major reluctance to make some complementary therapies free at the point of contact, in fact NAHAT found that there was considerable interest in and support for some treatments. This would overcome some of the difficulties that patients encounter over payment for treatment.

The media   Interest from the media in complementary therapies varies considerably in tone and content. The popular press and magazines carry regular articles on various aspects of alternative medicine. Some of these are prompted by the public 'admission' by someone well known or a member of the Royal family that they use alternative therapists. The articles that follow this are usually information giving about some kinds of therapy but not usually detailed enough to help people decide about its use. Some GPs remarked about increased interest from patients when a particular treatment had been highlighted in the press. Women's magazines and the 'quality' press also carry articles outlining the various therapies and suggesting some of the counterindications for their use. Very few of these articles refer directly to childbearing women but where they do it is mostly to emphasise the dangers of the unsupervised use of homeopathic or herbal medicines available over the counter.

Attitudes to alternative therapies are discussed in most articles on the subject in both the popular and the medical press. An article in the *Independent on Sunday* (4 July 1993) referring to the Osteopaths Bill and its passage through Parliament gives this as an example of 'how far yesterdays "quacks" are becoming today's establishment and how fringe ideas are being transformed into modern orthodoxy'. The article goes on to describe how the previous BMA report of 1986 referred to alternative therapies as 'a return to primitive beliefs and outmoded practices'. Whilst countering this in the article with a balanced view of the 1993 BMA report, the very fact of introducing such powerful words again links them with complementary therapies. Very few articles in either the press or medical journals are free of loaded, emotive words. An item on a radio phone in regarding attitudes to alternative treatments began 'useless, witch doctory or harmful, is this how we should regard alternative medicine?'; the fact that the speaker was then supportive to most of the therapies discussed may not have wholly balanced the emotive language of this introduction.

Until recently the advertising of complementary therapies was barely in evidence. The entry into the marketplace and the powerful advertising of an increasing range of herbal and homeopathic remedies and food supplements has increased the market by 50% in 5 years (*Independent*, 2 June 1993). Sales at present are fairly small and represent about 21 pence per head in Britain compared with over £5 per head in Holland, however it is seen by the manufacturers and suppliers as potentially highly profitable. It also reflects the attitudes of the public and their increasing willingness to consider remedies that offer something different to conventional medicine either in terms of safety, perceived therapeutic value, ease of access or philosophy.

Another area explored in many articles, especially in the popular and non-scientific medical press, is the reason for the accepted increase in interest in complementary medicine. A London GP quoted in *Hospital Doctor* (4 March 1993) believes that 'it is important to ascertain whether a patient turning to alternative medicine is doing so out of desperation and disillusionment with orthodox medicine or because it is an approach that suits an individual's beliefs and tastes'. Prof. V. Marks in the same article believes that the growth of interest is due in part to 'a lack of confidence in mainstream treatment. There are communication problems and the role of the doctor as confidante to the patient is disappearing, alternative therapists have the time to listen.' A surgeon suggests that the medical profession is singularly bad at communication, 'failing to deal with the patient as well as the disease'.

The psychiatrist Professor Anthony Clare, writing in the *Daily Mail* (5 May 1993) believes that 'part of the appeal of unorthodox therapies is to be found in the challenge they pose to orthodox arrogance, orthodox control, orthodox rationality. Many disillusioned people have come to distrust reason preferring instead to flirt with colourful varieties of unreason.' Whilst Professor Clare then goes on to suggest that acupuncture, massage, chiropractic and homeopathy have been subjected to scientific study and have now crossed the divide between orthodox and alternative medicine, he also asserts that 'much of what is termed "alternative" has never been subjected to proper scientific assessment and never shown to be superior to a placebo or sugar pill in the treatment of whatever ailment it claims to cure.'

It is this area of criticism from established medicine and some members of the general public and the media which is most often used as a stick with which to beat complementary therapies, and it is incumbent on the therapists who practise and are conscious of the benefits to clients, to regulate their profession. The public deserves protection in all forms of medical practice. We always take a risk when we allow someone to affect our bodies, that risk can be and must be minimised. We cannot expect the client to be scientifically informed, therefore we must take responsibility, as practitioners, for informing, supporting and protecting clients or potential clients, as well as promoting the choices and control that complementary therapies can offer.

Conclusion

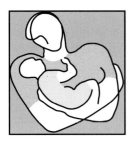

This book is intended to be an introduction to complementary medicine for the pregnant and childbearing woman and those who care for her. It is not intended as 'how to' guide but as an overview of those therapies commonly available and their application in midwifery. There are books available that contain more detailed information, many of them noted at the end of the chapters, as well as training courses for those who seek to extend their practice. The editors hope that this book may widen the debate about the value of complementary therapies, and encourage women, midwives and doctors to seek out more information about the treatments outlined here or to explore others that may offer the pregnant and childbearing woman care, support and choice.

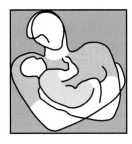

Glossary

abortifacient induces abortion

carminative a property of certain essential oils or herbal remedies causing expulsion of gas from the intestines

caudal literally towards the tail

chi see Ki.

concomitants the principle complaint is accompanied by another sensation or a pain/disorder is reported at the same time

circumduction to move a joint through a circular range of movement

constitutional remedy (the), remedy most appropriate to an individuals constitution

cun a Chinese unit of measurement used to locate the acupuncture points. Sometimes described as 'Chinese inch'. One cun is the width of the inter-phalangeal joint of the patient's thumb, three cun is the width of the four finger together at the level of the dorsal skin crease of the proximal inter-phalangeal joint of the middle finger

cupping A therapy in which a glass cup or bamboo jar is attached to the skin surface by suction to cause local congestion through negative pressure. Cupping has the function of warming and promoting the free flow of Qi and Blood in the meridians in traditional Chinese medicine theory, and to diminish swellings and pain. It is mostly used for conditions such as backache, general musculorskeletal pain, stomachache and asthma

demulcent a soothing substance

de-personalisation a psychiatric term for the symptom which leads a person to complain that she feels unreal

de-realisation a psychiatric term for the symptom which leads a person to complain that the world seems unreal

disease (homeopathy) an alteration in the state of health expressed in morbid signs, the derangement of the life energy trying to correct itself

effleurage a light, superficial massage

emmenagogue encourages menstruation

enfleurage expensive method of extracting essential oils from delicate flowers, e.g. jasmine

erector spinae muscles two large muscles which fill the grooves on either side of the vertabral column. In the lumbar spine belly is a large fleshy mass which gradually diminishes in size in the thoracic spine

galactogue encourages lactation

innervation the nerve supply to any organ or part of the body

Ki the Chinese 'Qi' or 'Chi' or Japanese 'Ki' meaning energy or motive force of life

law of cure (the) an evaluation system to assess decline of disease from above downwards, inside to outside, important to less important organ and reverse order of appearance

law of similars (the) the symptoms caused by too much (overdose) of substance are the symptoms that can be cured with a small dose of that substance

modalities what makes a symptom better or worse, e.g. heat, movement, time of day. This makes a symptom complete and aids differentiation of remedies

moxa the Chinese name for the herb mugwort or 'St John's herb'

moxibustion the burning of moxa to apply heat to an area for therapeutic effect

osteochondrosis non-inflammatory condition affecting the epiphyseal plates in some young people. Necrosis followed by regeneration. Occurs in the ring epiphyses of the dorsal vertabral bodies, leads to reduced mobility and possible kyphosis

posology the study of the quantities in which drugs should be administered

potency medicines produced by potentization on varying scales, e.g. decimal or centessimal

potentization a process used to prepare remedies by dilution and shaking to make more 'potent'

proprioceptive control to be aware of the position, balance and movements of the body due to the reflex action of proprioceptors in muscles, tendons and joints

proving method of ascertaining the curative potential of substances in homeopathic practice

Qi see Ki

Qi-gong Chinese name for the slow-moving, gentle martial art-style exercise, designed to maintain and strengthen health through the building up of Qi

repertory a reference guide to the *Materia Medica*, alphabetically listing symptoms and remedies

sitz bath a means of treating vulval or anal conditions by immersion of the affected area in a container of water to which is often added essential oils or herbs

spasm in piriformis sudden involuntary contraction of the piriformis muscle. This muscle extends from the front of the sacrum, passes out of the pelvis through the sciatic foramen and is inserted into the greater trochanter

synergistic effect when the combined effect of two or more essential oils is greater than the sum of the individual oils

thenar eminence the radial side of the anterior aspect of the hand – the 'ball' of the thumbs

totality of symptoms all principle signs and symptoms experienced, including aetiology and modalities and guides to the selection of a remedy

vermifuge anti-worm property

version the term version is applied when an alteration in the lie of the fetus *in utero* is brought about, or the location of its upper and lower poles reversed. It may occur spontaneously or by manipulation

vital force (homeopathy) the life energy that animates, guides and balances the organism in health and disease

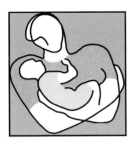

Useful Addresses

Acupuncture Research Association
118 Foley Road
Claygate
Esher
Surrey KT10 0NA
Tel: 0372 64171

Aromatherapy Organizations Council
3 Laymers Close
Bray Carook
Market Harborough LE 16 8LL
Tel: 0455 615466

British Association for Counselling
1 Regent Place
Rugby
Warwickshire CV21 2PJ
Tel: 0788 578228

British Association of Psychotherapists
121 Hendon Lane
London N3 3PR
Tel: 081 346 1747

British Chiropractic Association
Premier House
Greycoat Place
London SW1P 1SB
Tel: 071 222 8866

British Complementary Medicine Association
St Charles Hospital
Exmoor Street
London W10 6DZ
Tel: 081 964 1205

British Council of Complementary Medicine
PO Box 194
London SE16 1QZ
Tel: 071 237 5165

British Holistic Medical Association
St Marylebone Parish Church
Marylebone Road
London NW1 5LT
Tel: 071 262 5299

British Homoeopathic Association
27a Devonshire Street
London
W1N 2RJ

British Homoeopathy Research Group
101 Harley Street
London W1
Tel: 071 580 5489

British Hypnotherapy Association
1 Wythburn Place
London W1H 5WL
Tel: 071 262 8852/723 4443

British Register of Complementary Practitioners
PO Box 194
London SE16 1QZ
Tel: 071 237 5165

British School of Osteopathy
1–4 Suffolk St
London SW1Y 4HG
Tel: 071 930 9254

British School – Reflex Zone Therapy of the Feet
87 Oakington Avenue
Wembley Park
Middlesex HA9 8HY
Tel: 081 908 2201

British Shiatsu Council
121 Sheen Road
Richmond
Surrey TW9 1YJ
Tel: 081 852 1080

British Society for Nutritional Medicine
PO Box 3AP
London W1A 3AP
Tel: 071 436 8532

British Wheel of Yoga
1 Hamilton Place
Boston Road
Sleaford
Lincolnshire NG34 7ES
Tel: 0529 306851

Council for Acupuncture
Panther House
38 Mount Pleasant

London WC1X 0AP
Tel: 071 837 8026

Centre for Autogenic Training
101 Harley Street
London W1N 1DF
Tel: 071 935 1811

Centre for Complementary Health Studies
University of Exeter
Streatham Court
Rennes Drive
Exeter EX4 4PU
Tel: 0392 433828/263263

Council for Complementary and Alternative Medicine
Suite 1
19a Cavendish Square
London W1M 9AD
Tel: 071 409 1440

Centre for the Study of Complementary Medicine
51 Bedford Place
Southampton
Hampshire SO1 2DG
Tel: 0703 334752

**Faculty of Herbal Medicine
(General Council & Register of
Consultant Herbalists)**
Grosvenor House
40 Sea Way
Middleton-on-Sea
West Sussex PA22 7AA

Faculty of Homoeopathy
Royal London Homeopathic Hospital
Great London Street
London WC1N 3HR
Tel: 071 837 8833 ext 85 or 72

General Council and Register of Naturopaths
Frazer House
6 Netherhall Gardens
London NW3 5RR
Tel: 071 435 8728

General Council and Register of Osteopaths
56 London Street
Reading
Berkshire TH1 4SQ
Tel: 0734 576589

Hahnemann Society
Humane Education Centre
Avenue Lodge
Bounds Green Road
London N22 4EU
Tel: 081 889 1595

International Federation of Aromatherapists
Dept. of Continuing Education
The Royal Masonic Hospital
Ravenscourt Park
London W6 0TN
Tel: 081 846 8066

International Journal of Aromatherapy
65 Church Road
Hove
East Sussex BN3 2BD

International Register of Oriental Medicine
Green Hedges House
Green Hedges Avenue
East Grinstead
West Sussex RH19 1DZ
Tel: 0342 313106/7

The International Society of Professional Aromatherapists
41 Leicester Road
Hinckley
Leicestershire LE10 1LW
Tel: 0455 637987

Institute for Complementary Medicine
PO Box 194
London SE16 1QZ
Tel: 071 237 5165

Institute for Optimum Nutrition
5 Jerdan Place
Fulham
London SW6 1BE
Tel: 071 385 7984/8673

ITEC–International Therapy Examination Council
16 Avenue Place
Harrogate
North Yorkshire HG2 7PJ

National Consultative Council for Alternative and Complementary Medicine
39 Prestbury Road
Cheltenham
Gloucestershire GL52 2PT

Osteopathic Information Service
37 Soho Square
London W1V 5DG
Tel: 071 439 7177

Professional Register of Traditional Chinese Medicine
17 Leinster Road West
Rathmines
Dublin 6
Republic of Ireland
Tel: 0001 978906

Register of Traditional Chinese Medicine
19 Trinity Road
London N2 8JJ
Tel: 081 883 8431

Relaxation for Living
29 Burwood Park Road
Walton on Thames
Surrey KT12 5LH

The Shiatsu Society
5 Foxcote
Wokingham
Berkshire RG11 3PG

Society of Teachers of Alexander Technique
10 London House
266 Fulham Road
London SW10 9EL
Tel: 071 351 0828

Index

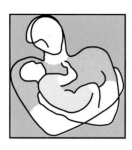

Abdominal breathing, stress reduction, 103
Abortifacients, herbs and oils, 39, 40, 176
Accountability, professional, midwives, 7, 8, 185–186,
    213, 271
Aconite, 202, 210
Acupressure bands, sickness and, 16, 140
Acupuncture, 217–240
  conditions alleviated by, 228–229
    backache and sciatica, 230
    breech presentation, 231–233
    constipation, 19, 231
    haemorrhoids, 237–238
    infertility, 14
    lactation, 238
    nausea and vomiting, 16, 229–230
    overactivity of uterus, 29
    urine retention, 238
  consumers' attitudes towards, 268, 269–270
  diagnoses, 220–221
  history and theories of, 217–218
    Traditional Chinese Medicine, 221–226
    western explanations, 226–227
  in labour, 26–27, 28, 233–237
  midwives' attitudes towards, 272–273
  moxibustion, 219, 220, 231–233
  needles, 218–220
  organisations and associations for, 6, 228, 238–239, 240,
    289, 290–291
  training and regulation, 6, 7, 228, 238–240
Aerobics, pregnancy type, 24
Agnus-castus, postnatal depression, 30
Agrimony, for cystitis, 170
Alcohols, in essential oils, 39
Aldehydes, in essential oils, 38
Alexander technique, 108
  associations and societies of, 111, 293
  backache, 21
  headache, 22
Aloe vera, sore nipples, 173
Anaemia, 19, 168
Analgesia, in labour, 26–29
  acupuncture, 26–27, 28, 234–237
  aromatherapy and massage, 28, 64–65
  herbal medicine, 26–27, 28, 172
  hydrotherapy, 28, 118–125

Analgesia, in labour (*Continued*)
  osteopathy, 256
  reflexology, 28, 84–85
  shiatsu, 28, 145–147
  TENS, 21, 27–28
Anise
  heartburn, 169
  nausea and vomiting, 165
Antacids, heartburn, 17
Anthemis nobilis see Camomile
Anxiety *see* Mood swings and anxiety
Aquanatal exercises, 24, 114, 116–117
Argentum nitricum, ophthalamia neonatorum, 210
Arnica (*Arnica montana*, Leopard's bane), 198–199
  backache, 21
  labour, 28, 202
  perineal care, 30, 198–199
  postoperative recovery, 206
Aromatherapy and massage, 35–68
  administration of essential oils, 44–50
  base (carrier) oils, 42
  blending of essential oils, 41–42
  buying and storage of essential oils, 42–44
  conditions alleviated by
    backache, 21, 57
    breastfeeding and breast problems, 30, 55, 57–58
    constipation, 18–19, 52, 59–60
    cystitis, 24, 53, 61–62
    headache, 21–22, 51, 62
    heartburn, 18, 62
    hypertension, 62
    infertility, 55
    insomnia, 22, 53, 62–63, 110
    labour, 25, 28, 64–65, 66
    mood swings and anxiety, 23, 28, 52, 53, 56–57
    nausea and vomiting, 63
    nipple tenderness, 29, 58
    oedema, 20, 21, 54, 63
    perineal care, 30, 65
    postnatal blues and depression, 30, 43, 52, 55, 56, 66
    retained placenta, 29, 66–67
    stress reduction, 110
    striae gravidarum, 66–67
    vaginal infections, 24, 54, 67
    varicosities, 20, 49, 60, 61

Aromatherapy and massage (*Continued*)
  constituents and properties of essential oils, 37–39
  consumers' attitudes towards, 268, 269
  contraindications, 20, 40–41
  definition, 35
  essential oils for midwives, 50–56
  history of, 35, 36–37
  midwives' attitudes to, 276
  neonates, 31
  organisations and associations for, 6, 41, 68, 289, 292
  training and regulation, 6, 7, 36, 68
Arsenicum
  anaemia, 19
  carpal tunel syndrome, 200
  haemorrhoids, 201
Association of Reflexologists, 90
Attar of roses *see* Rose (*Rosa centifolia/damascena*)
Autogenic training, 291
  stress reduction, 106, 111

Babies *see* Neonates and babies
Bach Rescue Remedy
  labour pain control, 28
  mood swings and anxiety, 23, 56
  perineal care, 30
  postnatal depression, 30, 66
  sore nipples, 29
Backache, 21
  acupuncture, 230
  aromatherapy and massage, 21, 57
  osteopathy, 21, 251–252, 255, 258–259
  reflexology, 21, 83
  shiatsu, 142
Barley water, cystitis, 170
Base (carrier) oils, 42
Basil
  constituents and properties, 38, 39, 40
  stress reduction, 110
Baths, essential oils in, 49
BCMA (British Complementary Medicine Association), 6, 7, 289
Belladonna
  breastfeeding and breast problems, 196, 208
  in labour, 202
Bellis perennis, postoperative recovery, 206
Bergamot oil
  anxiety, 56
  constituents and properties, 38, 39
  cystitis, 60–61
  onset of labour, 25
  postnatal blues, 66
Birth root, labour pains, 28
Black cohosh (Cimicifuga)
  contraindications, 176
  inefficient uterus, 29
  labour, 203
Black haw bark, miscarriage, 166
Black horehound, sickness in pregnancy, 16

Blessed thistle bitter, mood swings and fatigue, 171
Blue cohosh (Caulophyllum), 199
  contraindications, 176
  inefficient uterus, 29
  labour, 28, 199, 203
BMA (British Medical Association), 6, 156–157, 227–228, 265
Borage, lactation, 173
Bran, contraindications, 167, 168
Breastfeeding and breast problems, 21, 29–30
  acupuncture, 238
  aromatherapy, 30, 55, 57–58
  back and shoulder pains with, 21, 87, 258–259
  garlic and, 173
  herbal medicine, 172–173
  homeopathic remedies, 196, 208–209
  osteopathy, 258–259
  reflexology, 29, 78, 87
  shiatsu, 148
Breathing control, stress reduction, 102–103, 106
Breathing difficulties
  osteopathy, 253, 259
  reflexology, 85
  shiatsu, 134, 135
Breech presentation, moxibustion, 231–233
British Complementary Medicine Association (BCMA), 6, 7, 289
British Medical Association (BMA), 6, 156–157, 227–228, 265
Bryonia
  breastfeeding and breast problems, 208
  constipation, 18
Burdock
  herpes, 170
  mood swings and fatigue, 171

Cabbage leaves, engorged breasts and oedema, 21, 29, 58, 172
Caesarean section
  reflexology, 19, 85, 86
  water births, 122
Calcarea
  breastfeeding and breast problems, 208
  ophthalmia neonatorum, 210
Calendula *see* Marigold
Camomile (*Matricaria chamomilla*), in homeopathy, 199
  breastfeeding and breast problems, 208
  colic, 211
  labour, 195, 199, 203
  postoperative recovery, 206
Camomile (*Matricaria chamomilla/Anthemis nobilis*) oil and tea, 53
  backache, 57
  constituents and properties, 38, 39, 52–53
  cystitis, 24, 25, 53, 60–61
  heartburn, 18, 62, 169
  hypertension, 62
  insomnia and, 22, 53, 62–63, 110

Camomile (*Matricaria chamomilla/Anthemis nobilis*) oil and
    tea (*Continued*)
  mood swings and anxiety, 23, 53, 57–58
  nausea and vomiting, 16, 63, 163
  onset of labour, 25
  pruritis, 67
  safe use of, 39, 53
  sore nipples, 29
Camphor, constituents and properties, 39, 40
Candida *see* Thrush
Caraway seeds, heartburn, 169
Carcinogenic oils, 40
Carpal tunnel syndrome
  homeopathic remedies, 200
  osteopathy, 255
  shiatsu, 134–135
Carrier (base) oils, aromatherapy, 42
Catnip, labour pains, 172
Caulophyllum *see* Blue cohosh
Causticum, postoperative recovery, 206
Cephalopelvic disproportion, reflexology, 29, 85
Chamomilla *see* Camomile
Chasteberry
  infertility, 15
  threatened miscarriage, 166
Chickweed, 164
  herpes, 170
  infused oil of, 177
China, acupuncture training colleges, 239, 240
Chinese medicine, traditional
  acupuncture, 221–226
  Professional Register of, 293
  Register of, 293
  shiatsu, 128, 133
Chiropractic
  British Association of, 289
  headache, 22
  osteopathy differentiated, 260
  training and regulation, 6, 260
Cimicifuga *see* Black cohosh
Citrus bigaradia/aurantium see Neroli
Citrus reticulata see Mandarin (tangerine) oil
Clary sage (*Salvia sclarea*) oil
  constituents and properties, 38, 39, 40, 55–56
  labour pains, 28, 56, 64
  onset of labour, 28, 56, 65
Clitoral stimulation, onset of labour, 26
Coccydinia, osteopathy, 255
Colic, 31, 59
  fennel seeds, 173
  homeopathic remedies, 211
  shiatsu, 149–150
Colocynthis, colic, 211
Colostrum, sore nipples, 29
Colour therapy, stress reduction, 110
Comfrey, 164
  anaemia, 168
  breast engorgement, 172

Comfrey (*Continued*)
  herpes, 170
  infused oil of, 177
  lactation, 173
  perineal care, 172
  sore nipples, 173
  varicosities and constipation, 167, 168
Complementary therapy
  attitudes to, 1–4, 265–282
  research into, 4–5, 279–280
Compresses, aromatherapy, 50
Constipation, 18–19
  acupuncture, 19, 231
  aromatherapy and massage, 18–19, 53, 59–60
  diet, 18, 167
  herbal medicine, 18, 167, 168
  iron and, 19
  neonatal, 31, 82, 150
  reflexology, 19, 82
  shiatsu, 19, 136
Contractions *see* Labour
Coughs, shiatsu, 134
Counselling, stress reduction, 99–101
Crab apple, 23, 30
Crampbark, miscarriage, 166
Cramps, 20–21
  herbal remedies, 167
  miscarriage and, 166
  shiatsu, 137
Cranberry juice, cystitis, 25
Craniosacral therapy, neonates, 31, 259
Cypress oil
  perineal care, 30
  toxic effects, 40
  varicosities, 20, 60, 61, 168
Cystitis, 24–25
  aromatherapy, 24, 53, 60–61
  diet and, 25, 60–61, 169, 170
  herbal medicine, 24, 162, 169–170
  reflexology, 24, 83–84

Damiana, herpes, 170
Dandelion, 164
  constipation, 168
  herpes, 170
Decoctions, making of, 177
Depression *see* Mood swings and anxiety; Postnatal
    depression and blues
DHAs, complementary therapy, 280–281
Diabetes, osteopathy and, 255
Diaphragmatic breathing, stress reduction, 103
Diet
  anaemia, 19, 168
  breastfeeding, 173
  constipation, 18, 167
  cystitis, 25, 60–61, 169, 170
  following miscarriage, 167
  food additives, 17, 22

Diet (*Continued*)
  headache, 22
  heartburn, 17, 168–169
  herbs as food, 40–41, 158–159, 163–164
  infertility, 15, 163
  iron in, 19, 167, 168, 179–180
  mood and, 171
  nausea and vomiting and, 15–16, 165
  oedema, 20
  perineal care, 30, 171–172
  postnatal depression, 30
  thrush, 24, 169
  varicosities, 20
  Vitamin B sources, 179–180
  zinc supplementation, 15, 19, 30, 171–172
  see also Herbal medicine
Dill seeds, heartburn, 169
Disproportion, cephalopelvic, 29, 85
District Health Authorities, complementary therapy, 280–281
Drama therapy, infertility and, 15

Echinacea *see* Purple coneflower
Eczema, neonatal, 31, 52
Education *see* Training and regulation
Electro-acupuncture, 219
  see also Acupuncture
Emmenagogue herbs and oils, 39, 40, 176
Essential oils *see* Aromatherapy and massage
Esters, in essential oils, 38
Eucalyptus oil, constituents and properties, 38, 39
European Union, 7–8
  aromatherapists, 36, 68
  herbalists, 157
  osteopaths, 260
Exercise
  aquanatal, 24, 114, 116–117, 167
  mood swings and tension, 23–24
Exeter University, 4, 6, 291

Family Health Service Authorities, complementary therapy, 280–281
Feet, massage of, 49
  see also Reflexology and reflex zone therapy
Fennel
  breastfeeding and breast problems, 29, 58, 172–173
  constituents and properties of oil, 38, 39, 40
  heartburn, 169
  nausea and vomiting, 165
Fenugreek, lactation, 173
Ferrum met., for anaemia, 19
Fetal education, shiatsu, 133
Feverfew, retained placenta, 29
FHSAs, complementary therapy, 280–281
Floradix, 19, 168
Folic acid, 179

Food additives
  headache, 22
  heartburn, 17
Garlic
  breastfeeding, 173
  constipation, 167
  cystitis, 61, 169
  following miscarriage, 167
  heartburn, 17
  thrush, 24, 169, 170
  varicosities, 20
Gelsemium, labour, 204
General Adaptation Syndrome (GAS), 91–92
General practitioners, complementary therapy, 276–279, 280–281
Gentian, postnatal depression, 30
Geranium (*Pelargonium odorantissimum*) oil and leaves
  backache, 21
  breast engorgement, 58
  constituents and properties, 39, 54–55
  herpes, 170
  mood swings, 23, 66
  oedema, 20, 21, 54, 63
  onset of labour, 25
  sore nipples, 29, 173
German chamomile *see* Camomile
Ginger
  constipation, 168
  exhaustion in labour, 171
  heartburn, 18, 62, 169
  nausea and vomiting, 16, 63, 165
Ginseng
  exhaustion in labour, 171
  labour pains, 28
Golden rod, thrush, 170
Golden seal
  contraindications, 176
  following miscarriage, 167
  perineal care, 172
  varicosities, 20
GPs, complementary therapy, 276–279, 280–281
Greenwich University, 6, 68
Ground ivy, 164, 170
Gynaecologists, complementary therapy, 279–280

Haemorrhoids, 20
  acupuncture, 237–238
  aromatherapy and massage, 20, 60, 61
  herbal medicine, 20, 167–168
  homeopathic medicine, 201
  reflexology, 83, 87
  shiatsu, 137, 138
Hamamelis virginica *see* Witch hazel
Hawthorn, varicosities, 20, 167

Headache, 21–22
    aromatherapy and massage, 21–22, 51, 61–62
    diet, 22
    reflexology, 22, 75–76
    shiatsu, 22, 142
Heartburn, 17–18
    aromatherapy and massage, 18, 62
    diet, 17, 168–169
    herbal medicine, 17, 18, 169
    osteopathy, 18, 256
    reflexology, 83
    shiatsu, 17, 138, 139
Helionas root, miscarriage, 166
Herbal medicine
    botanical names of herbs, 177–179
    buying and storing herbs, 176
    conditions alleviated by, 164–173
        anaemia, 19, 168
        breastfeeding and breast problems, 29, 172–173
        constipation, 18, 167, 168
        cystitis, 24, 162, 169–170
        heartburn, 17, 18, 169
        heavy bleeding, 173
        herpes, 170
        inefficient uterine action, 29
        infertility, 15, 163
        insomnia, 22, 23
        miscarriage, 166–167
        mood swings and anxiety, 23, 170–171
        nausea and vomiting, 16, 165
        nipple tenderness, 173
        oedema, 20
        perineal care, 30, 171–172
        postnatal depression, 30
        thrush, 24, 169, 170
        urinary tract infections, 161–162, 169–170
        urine retention, 31
        varicosities, 20, 167–168
    considerations for pregnancy, 160–161
    decoctions, 177
    as food or medicinal meals, 158–159
    herbs to avoid, 176
    history of, 153–157
    infused oil, 177
    infusions, 177
    labour and, 25, 26–27, 28, 172 171
    mechanisms of, 159–160
    midwives' attitudes to, 274–275
    neonates, 31
    preconception care, 15, 160, 162–164
    reasons for, 157–158
    tinctures, 177
    training and regulation, 6, 157, 174
    women as midwives and herbalists, 153–157,
        274–275
Herpes, herbal remedies, 170

Homeopathic medicine, 181–216
    aetiology of disease, 193–194
    antidoting substances, 17–18, 43–44, 197–198
    case taking, 194–196
    common remedies, 198–199
    conditions alleviated by, 200–211
        anaemia, 19
        backache, 21
        breastfeeding and breast problems, 196, 208–209
        carpal tunnel syndrome, 200
        cystitis, 24
        depression, 24
        heartburn, 17–18
        infertility, 14–15
        insomnia, 23
        irritability and oversensitivity, 199
        labour, 26–27, 28, 199, 202–205
        perineal care, 30, 198–199
        postnatal depression, 30
        postoperative recovery, 198, 206–207
        prenatal depression, 23
        retained placenta, 29
        sickness and, 16
        thrush, 24
        urine retention, 31
        varicosities, 20, 60, 201
    consumers' attitudes towards, 268–269, 270
    essential oils and, 43–44
    expectations of, 198
    Faculty of Homeopathy, 16, 184, 212, 213, 291
    history of, 183–184, 187–188
    microdoses, 187–188
    neonates, 31, 199, 210, 211
    potency scales, 189–90
    potentisation, 187–188
    prescribing, 190–191, 194, 196–197
    principles of
        law of cure, 193
        law of least quantity, 188–189
        law of Similars, 183–184, 191–192
        minimum dose, 192
        prescribing, 190–191, 194
        provings (drug tests), 192–193
        single remedy, 192
    quantity determines quality, 188–189
    release of medicinal properties, 187
    remedy sources, 186
    as 'scientific' medicine, 215–216
    training and regulation, 6, 7, 184, 185–186,
        212–213
Hops
    lactation, 173
    mood swings and fatigue, 171
Horseradish
    anaemia, 19
    toxicity, 40

Hydrotherapy, 113–125
    aquanatal exercise, 24, 114, 116–117
    organisations involved in, 125
    water for labour and delivery, 28, 118–119
        facilities required, 119–120
        preparation of mothers, 120–121
        protocols, 121–124
        research and audit, 124–125
        selection criteria for mothers, 121
Hyperactivity, neonatal, 31
Hypericum *see* St John's wort
Hypertension, aromatherapy and massage, 62
Hyperventilation, reflexology, 85
Hypnotherapy, 109
    anxiety, 23
    associations and organisations for, 111, 290
    consumers' attitudes towards, 270
    insomnia, 22
    pain control in labour, 27
    sickness, 16
Hyssop, constituents and properties, 39, 40

Iceland moss, heartburn, 169
Indigestion *see* Heartburn
Induction of labour *see* Labour, onset of
Infants *see* Neonates and babies
Infertility, 14–15
    aromatherapy, 55
    herbal medicine, 15, 163
    osteopathy, 15, 250
    reflexology, 81
Infused oil, making of, 177
Infusions (tea), making of, 177
Ingestion, essential oils, 50
Inhalation, essential oils, 49–50
Insomnia, 22–23
    aromatherapy and massage, 22, 53, 62–63, 110
    reflexology, 84
    shiatsu, 22, 139, 150
Ipecachuana, sickness in pregnancy, 16
Iron, dietary
    anaemia, 19, 168
    following miscarriage, 167
    sources of, 179–180

Jasmine (*Jasminum officinale*) oil, 55
    breastfeeding, 30
    buying and storage, 43
    labour onset, 65
    lactation, 30, 55
    postnatal depression and blues, 30, 43, 55, 66
    retained placenta, 66
    toxic effects, 40, 55
Juniper
    constituents and properties of oil, 38, 40
    toxic effects, 176
    varicosities, 60, 61

Kali carbonicum, labour, 204
Kali phosphoricum, labour, 196, 204
Ketones, in essential oils, 38–39
Ki *see* Qi

Labour, exhaustion in
    herbal medicine, 171
    homeopathy, 195–196
    shiatsu, 145
Labour, onset of, 25–26
    acupuncture, 26, 233–234
    aromatherapy and massage, 25, 65
    herbal medicine, 25, 26
    homeopathy, 26–27, 199
    reflexology, 26, 84
    shiatsu, 143–145
Labour, pain control in, 26–29
    acupuncture, 26–27, 28, 234–237
    aromatherapy and massage, 28, 64–65
    herbal medicine, 26–27, 28, 172
    homeopathy, 28, 199, 202–205
    hydrotherapy, 28, 118–125
    osteopathy, 256
    reflexology, 28, 84–85
    shiatsu, 28, 145–147
    TENS, 21, 27–28
Lactation *see* Breastfeeding and breast problems
Lady's mantle, heavy bleeding, 167, 173
Lavender (*Lavandula augustifolia/officinalis*) oil
    backache, 21, 58
    constituents and properties, 38, 39, 40, 51–52
    cystitis, 60–61
    haemorrhoids, 61
    headache, 21–22, 51, 61–62
    herpes, 170
    hypertension, 62
    insomnia, 62–63
    labour, 25, 28, 51, 64, 66
    mood swings and anxiety, 23, 56–57
    perineal care, 30, 172
    pruritis, 67
    retained placenta, 66
    safe use of, 39, 51–52
Law of cure, homeopathy, 193
Law of least quantity, homeopathy, 188–189
Law of similars, homeopathy, 183–184, 191–192
Leg cramps, 20–21
    herbal remedies, 167
    shiatsu, 137
Lemon balm (melissa)
    heartburn, 169
    herpes, 170
    nausea and vomiting, 165
    threatened miscarriage, 166
Lemon oil
    constituents and properties, 38, 39
    haemorrhoids, 61

Leopard's bane *see* Arnica
Lime blossom
   constipation, 168
   threatened miscarriage, 166
Linseed, constipation, 167
Liquorice root, cystitis, 170
Liverpool University, 6
Lycopodium
   carpal tunel syndrome, 200
   ophthalmia neonatorum, 210

Manchester University, 6
Mandarin (tangerine, *Citrus reticulata*) oil, 51
   anxiety, 56
   constipation, 18–19, 52, 59
   hypertension, 62
   onset of labour, 25, 64
   postnatal blues, 66
   safe use of, 39, 51
   storage of, 43
   stress reduction, 110
Marigold (Calendula)
   cystitis, 25, 170
   herpes, 170
   perineal care, 30, 172
   postoperative recovery, 206
   sore nipples, 29, 58, 173
   thrush, 24, 170
   varicosities and constipation, 167
Marjoram oil
   backache, 21
   constituents and properties, 38, 40, 176
   insomnia, 22
   onset of labour, 25
Marshmallow
   breast engorgement, 172–173
   cystitis, 170
   herpes, 170
   varicosities and constipation, 167
Massage *see* Aromatherapy and massage; Reflexology and
     reflex zone therapy
Mastitis
   herbal medicine, 172–173
   homeopathic remedies, 196, 208, 209
Materia Medica, homeopathy, 192–193, 194, 200
Matricaria chamomilla see Camomile
Meadowsweet
   heartburn, 169
   nausea and vomiting, 165
Media, complementary therapies and, 281–282
Meditation, 104–105
Melaleuca alternifolia see Tea tree
Melissa see Lemon balm
Meralgia parasthetica, osteopathy, 255
Metamorphic technique, reflexology, 74
Microdoses, homeopathy, 187–188
Micturition *see* Urination problems

Middlesex University, 6, 174
Midwives
   attitudes to complementary therapy, 9–11, 271–276
   professional accountability, 7, 8, 185–186, 213, 271
   women as herbalists and, 153–157, 274–275
Miscarriage
   emmenagogue oils, 39, 40
   herbal medicine, 166–167, 176
   reflexology, 79
Mood swings and anxiety, 23–24
   aromatherapy, 23, 28, 52, 53, 56
   herbal medicine, 23, 166, 170–171, 172
   homeopathic approach, 193–194, 195, 197, 199, 200
     breastfeeding and breast problems, 208–209
     carpal tunnel syndrome, 200
     haemorrhoids, 201
     in labour, 202–205
     postoperatively, 206–207
   reflexology, 23, 84, 87
   see also Postnatal depression and blues; Stress
Morning sickness *see* Nausea and vomiting
Motherwort
   contraindications, 176
   labour pains, 172
   mood swings and fatigue, 171
Moxibustion, 41, 219, 220, 231–233
Mugwort
   constituents and properties, 38
   moxibustion, 41, 219, 220, 231–233
   toxicity, 40, 41, 176
Mustard, 21, 30, 40, 221
Myrrh, 29, 38, 40, 170

Natrum mur.
   anaemia, 19
   constipation, 18
   labour, 28, 204
   prenatal depression, 24
Nausea and vomiting, 15–17
   acupuncture, 16, 229–230
   aromatherapy and massage, 63
   diet and, 15–16, 165
   herbal medicine, 16, 165
   neonates, 63, 150
   osteopathy, 251
   reflexology, 16, 82
   shiatsu, 139–141, 150
Needles, acupuncture, 218–220
Neonates and babies, 31
   acupuncture, 220
   candida in, 170
   colic, 31, 58–59, 149–150, 173, 211
   constipation, 31, 82, 150
   eczema, 31, 51
   homeopathy, 199, 210
   hyperactivity, 31
   ophthalmia neonatorum, 210

Neonates and babies (*Continued*)
  osteopathic care, 31, 259
  shiatsu, 148–150
  sleeplessness, 150
  vomiting, 63, 150
Neroli (orange blossom, *Citrus bigaradia/aurantium*), 52
  constipation, 18–19, 52, 60
  hypertension, 62
  insomnia, 62–63
  mood swings and anxiety, 52, 57
  postnatal blues, 52, 66
  storage of, 43
Nettles, 164
  anaemia, 168
  constipation, 167
  cystitis, 25, 170
  heavy bleeding, 173
  lactation, 173
Nipple stimulation
  onset of labour, 25–26
  retained placenta, 66
Nipple tenderness, 29–30
  aromatherapy, 29, 58
  herbal medicine, 173
  homeopathic remedies, 208, 209
Nutrition *see* Diet
Nux vomica
  backache, 21
  colic, 211
  constipation, 18
  haemorrhoids, 201
  sickness in pregnancy, 16

Oak bark
  perineal care, 172
  varicosities and constipation, 167
Oats, herpes, 170
Obstetricians, complementary therapy, 279–280
Oedema, 20–21
  aromatherapy and massage, 20, 21, 54, 63
  carpal tunnel syndrome and, 134–135, 200, 255
  osteopathy, 255–256
  reflexology, 21, 83
  shiatsu, 134–135, 141–142
Oestrogen-stimulating oils, 40
Ophthalmia neonatorum, homeopathy, 210
Oral administration, essential oils, 50
Orange blossom oil *see* Neroli
Orange peel, mood swings and fatigue, 171
Osteopathy, 243–262
  after delivery, 257–258
  aims and concerns of, 245
  chiropractic differentiated, 260
  conditions alleviated by
    backache, 21, 251–252, 255, 258–259
    breastfeeding and breast problems, 258–259
    breathing problems, 253, 259

Osteopathy, conditions alleviated by (*Continued*)
    carpal tunnel syndrome, 255
    coccydinia, 255
    constipation, 19
    cystitis, 24
    headache, 22
    heartburn, 18, 256
    infertility and, 15, 250
    labour pains, 256
    meralgia parasthetica, 255
    nausea and vomiting, 251
    oedema, 255–256
    postural, 252–253
    round ligament pain, 256
    sciatica, 254
    swallowing problems, 254
    symphysis pubis pain, 255
    weight gain, 251, 252–3, 254
  consumers' attitudes towards, 269
  diabetes and, 255
  history of, 244–245
  initial consultations, 246–249
  neonatal care, 31, 259
  physiotherapy differentiated, 260
  postnatal period, 258–259
  preconception care, 250–251
  research into, 261–262
  training and regulation, 6, 7, 244–245, 246, 260–261,
      262, 263
  treatment plans, 249–250
Oxides, in essential oils, 39

Pain control, in labour *see* Labour, pain control in
Panic attacks *see* Mood swings and anxiety
Parsley
  anaemia, 168
  breast engorgement, 172
  constipation, 167
Passiflora, contraindications, 23
Pearl barley water, cystitis, 170
Pelargonium odorantissimum see Geranium
Pennyroyal, constituents and properties, 39, 40, 176
Peppermint oil
  breastfeeding and breast problems, 30, 58
  constituents and properties, 39, 40
  headache, 62
  storage of, 44
Peppermint tea
  anaemia, 168
  mood swings and fatigue, 171
  nausea and vomiting, 165
Perineal care, 30
  aromatherapy and massage, 30, 65
  diet, 30, 171–172
  herbal medicine, 30, 171–172
  reflexology, 87
Phenols, in essential oils, 38

Phosphorus, postoperative recovery, 207
Physical exercise, 23–24, 167
    aquanatal, 24, 114, 116–117
Physiotherapy, osteopathy differentiated, 260
Phytolacca, breastfeeding and breast problems, 209
Pilewort cream, haemorrhoids, 167–168
Pituitary gland reflex zone, 81, 82
Placenta, retained, 29
    aromatherapy and massage, 29, 66
    reflexology, 29, 85–86
    shiatsu, 147
Plantain
    cystitis, 170
    heavy bleeding, 167
    thrush, 170
    varicosities and constipation, 167
Possetting
    aromatherapy, 63
    shiatsu, 150
Postmaturity
    aromatherapy and massage, 65
    shiatsu, 143
Postnatal depression and blues, 30, 98
    aromatherapy and massage, 30, 43, 52, 55, 56, 66
    diet, 30
    reflexology, 84, 87
    shiatsu, 147–148
Potato, varicosities and, 20, 167
Potency scales, homeopathy, 189–190
Potentisation, homeopathy, 187–188
Preconception care
    dietary supplements, 15
    folic acid, 179
    herbal medicine, 15, 160, 162–164
    osteopathy, 250–251
Professional accountability, midwives, 7, 8, 185–186, 213, 271
Provings (drug tests), homeopathy, 192–193
Pruritis, aromatherapy, 67
Puerperal psychosis
    aromatherapy and massage, 66
    reflexology, 87
Pulsatilla (wind flower), 199
    anaemia, 19
    breastfeeding and breast problems, 209
    labour, 195, 205
    ophthalmia neonatorum, 210
    retained placenta, 29
    varicosities and, 20, 60, 201
Purple coneflower (echinacea)
    labour pains, 28
    thrush, 170

Qi (Ki)
    acupuncture, 221–224
    shiatsu and, 128, 132–134
    see also Acupuncture, conditions alleviated by; Shiatsu, conditions alleviated by

Raspberry leaf
    exhaustion in labour, 171
    heavy bleeding, 173
    inefficient uterus, 29
    labour pains, 28
    miscarriage, 166, 167
    mood swings, 171
    morning sickness, 165
    onset of labour, 25
Red raspberry leaf
    labour pains, 28
    sickness in pregnancy, 16
Reflexology and reflex zone therapy, 71–90
    conditions alleviated by
        backache, 21, 83
        breastfeeding and breast problems, 29, 78, 87
        cephalopelvic disproportion, 29, 85
        constipation, 19, 82
        cystitis, 24, 83–84
        depression, 84, 87
        haemorrhoids, 83, 87
        headache, 22, 75–76
        heartburn, 83
        hyperventilation, 85
        infertility, 81
        insomnia, 84
        labour, 26, 28, 84–85
        mood swings and anxiety, 23, 84
        nausea and vomiting, 16, 82
        oedema, 21, 83
        perineal care, 87
        retained placenta, 29, 85–86
        subinvolution, 86–87
        urine retention, 31, 85
    consumers' attitudes towards, 268, 269
    contraindications to, 78–79, 82
    difference between, 76
    history of, 71–77
    midwives' attitudes to, 276
    pituitary gland reflex zone, 81, 82
    process and technique of, 75–78
    reactions to, 80–81
    research into, 87–88
    tools for, 77
    training and regulation, 7, 88–90
        organisations, 90, 290
Relaxation exercises, 103–104
    breathing control, 102–103
    contraindications to, 106
    insomnia, 22
    meditation, 104–105
    visualisation, 105–106
Repertory, homeopathy, 193, 194
Rescue Remedy *see* Bach Rescue Remedy
Retained placenta, 29
    aromatherapy and massage, 29, 66
    reflexology, 29, 85–86
    shiatsu, 147

Rhubarb leaves, breast engorgement and oedema, 21, 58
Roman camomile *see* Camomile
Rose (*Rosa centifolia/damascena*) oil
    anxiety, 57
    buying and storage of, 43
    constituents and properties, 39, 40, 54–55
    onset of labour, 25, 64
    postnatal depression, 55, 66
    safe use of, 39, 55
Rosemary
    constituents and properties of oil, 39, 40, 57, 63
    exhaustion in labour, 171
    labour pains, 28
    mood swings and fatigue, 171
    oedema, 20, 63
    stress reduction, 110
Rosewood oil
    constituents and properties, 39
    hypertension, 62
Round ligament pain, osteopathy, 256
Royal College of Midwifery, 271
    acupuncture and, 239
    BCMA membership and, 7
    homeopathy and, 185, 213
Royal College of Nursing, BCMA membership and, 7
Rue, toxicity, 40, 176

Sage, 38–39, 40, 176, 177
St John's wort (hypericum)
    herpes, 170
    infertility and, 15
    infused oil of, 177
    labour pain control, 172
    postoperative recovery, 207
Samphire, 164
Sandalwood (*Santalum album*) oil, 54
    anxiety, 56
    constituents and properties, 38, 54
    cystitis, 60
    postnatal depression, 66
Savory
    anaemia, 19
    toxicity, 40
Sciatica
    acupuncture, 230
    osteopathy, 254
    shiatsu, 142
    TENS, 21
Scullcap
    labour pains, 172
    mood swings and fatigue, 171
    threatened miscarriage, 166
Secale
    colic, 211
    labour, 205
    postoperative recovery, 207
Senna, 18, 176

Sepia
    backache, 21
    carpal tunel syndrome, 200
    haemorrhoids, 201
    labour, 205
    postnatal depression, 30
    sickness in pregnancy, 16
    thrush, 24
Sexual intercourse
    for onset of labour, 26
    postnatal resumption of, 55, 98–99
Shepherd's purse, heavy bleeding, 167, 173
Shiatsu, 127–151
    benefits of, 132–134
    conditions alleviated by
        backache and sciatica, 142
        breathlessness, 134, 135
        carpal tunnel syndrome, 134–135
        chronic coughs, 134
        constipation, 19, 136
        haemorrhoids, 137, 138
        headache, 22, 142
        heartburn, 17, 138, 139
        insomnia, 22, 139, 150
        labour, 28, 142–147
        lactation, 148
        leg cramps, 137
        nausea and vomiting, 139–141
        oedema, 134–135, 141–142
        postnatal depression, 147–148
        retained placenta, 147
        tiredness, 143
        vaginal discharge, 139
    contraindications, 130–131, 134
    diagnosis, 127–128
    neonates, 148–150
    Traditional Chinese Medicine, 128, 133
    training and competence, 150–152
        organisations, 152, 290, 293
    western explanation of, 128–129
Shizuto Masanaga, 134
Sickness *see* Nausea and vomiting
Silica, breastfeeding and breast problems, 209
Sleeplessness *see* Insomnia
Slippery elm
    heartburn, 18, 169
    perineal care, 172
    sickness, 165
Sorrel, 164
SOS technique, breathing control, 103
Spearmint tea
    mood swings and fatigue, 171
    nausea and vomiting, 165
Spiritual healing, 110, 111
Squaw vine
    labour, 28
    toxicity, 176

Staphysagria, postoperative recovery, 207
Stress, 91–111
  of carers, 101–102
  with changes in pregnancy, 94–99, 101
  reduction techniques, 23–24, 99, 102
    Alexander technique, 108
    autogenic training, 106
    breathing, 102–103, 106
    contraindications, 106
    counselling, 99–101
    environmental methods, 110
    hypnotherapy, 109
    meditation, 104–105
    reflexology, 87
    relaxation, 103–104
    t'ai chi ch'uan, 109–110
    training organisations, 111
    visualisation, 105–106
    yoga, 107–108
  symptoms, 93–94, 101
  women at risk of, 101
  see also Mood swings and anxiety
Striae gravidarum (stretch marks), aromatherapy and
    massage, 67
Subinvolution, reflexology, 86–87
Swallowing difficulties, osteopathy, 254
Swimming, aquanatal, 24, 114, 116–117
Symphysis pubis pain, osteopathy, 255

T'ai chi ch'uan, 24, 109–110, 111
Tangerine oil *see* Mandarin (tangerine) oil
Tansy, constituents and properties, 38, 40, 176
Tea tree (*Melaleuca alternifolia*) oil, 53–54
  constituents and properties, 38, 39, 54
  herpes, 170
  thrush, 24, 53, 67
  verrucae, 78
Teas (infusions), making of, 177
TENS (transcutaneous electrical nerve stimulation), 21,
    27–28
Terpines, role in essential oils, 37–38
Thrush, 24
  aromatherapy and massage, 24, 54, 67
  diet, 24, 169
  Floradix contraindicated with, 168
  herbal medicine, 24, 169, 170
Thyme, 19, 24, 170
  herpes, 170
  thrush, 170
Thyme oil, constituents and properties, 38, 40
Ti tree *see* Tea tree
Tinctures, making of, 177
Tiredness
  herbal medicine, 170–171
  shiatsu, 143
Toxicity, essential oils, 39, 40–41

Training and regulation, 6–8
  acupuncture, 6, 7, 228, 238–240
  aromatherapy and massage, 6, 7, 36, 68
  consumers' attitudes towards, 270
  European Union and, 7–8, 36, 68, 157, 260
  GPs' attitudes towards, 276–277, 278–279
  gynaecologists' and obstetricians' attitudes to, 279
  herbal medicine, 6, 157, 174
  homeopathy, 6, 7, 184, 185–186, 212–213
  midwives
    attitudes towards, 271–273, 275, 276
    professional accountability, 7, 8, 185–186, 213, 271
  organisation addresses, 111, 289–293
  osteopathy, 6, 7, 244–245, 246, 260–261, 262, 263
  reflexology, 7, 88–90
  shiatsu, 150–151
Transcutaneous electrical nerve stimulation (TENS), 21,
    27–28
Tubs, water births, 119–120

UKCC
  approval of TENS, 21
  membership of BCMA and, 7
  midwives' professional accountability, 7, 8, 185, 271
  TENS approval, 27–28
  water births, 118
Urinary tract infections, 24–25
  aromatherapy, 24, 53, 60–61
  diet and, 25, 61, 169, 170
  herbal medicine, 24, 161–162, 169–170
  reflexology, 24, 83–84
Urination problems, 31
  acupuncture, 238
  reflexology, 31, 84, 85
  shiatsu and, 139
Uterine action
  aromatherapy, 65, 66
  overactivity, 29
  regulation by reflexology, 85
  see also Labour, onset of
Uterine bleeding, emmenagogue oils, 40
Uva ursi, cystitis, 170

Vaginal discharge, shiatsu, 139
Vaginal infections, 24
  aromatherapy and massage, 24, 53, 67
  diet, 24, 169
  Floradix contraindicated, 169
  herbal medicine, 24, 169, 170
Valerian
  anxiety, 23, 166
  insomnia, 22, 23
Varicosities, 20
  acupuncture, 237–238
  aromatherapy and massage, 20, 49, 60, 61
  herbal medicine, 20, 167–168
  homeopathy, 201

Varicosities (*Continued*)
  reflexology, 83, 87
  shiatsu, 137, 138
  yoga, 20, 167
Verrucae, 78
Vervain, herpes, 170
Visualisation, stress reduction, 105–106
Vitamin B, dietary sources of, 179–180
Vitamin B{U}6{u}
  perineal care, 30
  postnatal depression, 30
  sickness in pregnancy, 15
Vitamin C
  anaemia, 19, 168
  constipation, 18
  cystitis, 169
  perineal care, 30
Vitamin E, infertility, 15
Vomiting *see* Nausea and vomiting

Water birth *see* Hydrotherapy
Weight gain, osteopathy, 251, 252–253, 254
Wild indigo, thrush, 170
Wind flower *see* Pulsatilla
Witch hazel (hamamelis virginica)
  herpes, 170
  perineal care, 30
  varicosities, 20, 167
Women
  as consumers of complementary therapy, 266–270
  as midwives and herbalists, 153–157, 274–275
World Health Organization
  acupuncture, 217
  pain control in labour, 27
Wormwood, toxicity, 40, 176

Yarrow
  cystitis, 170
  sore nipples, 173
  varicosities, 20, 167
Yin and Yang, theory of, 222–223
Ylang ylang oil
  constituents and properties, 38, 39
  hypertension, 62
  insomnia, 62–63
  onset of labour, 25, 56–57
  postnatal depression, 66
Yoga, 107–108
  constipation, 19
  heartburn, 18
  mood swings, 23
  oedema, 20
  pain control in labour, 27
  regulation, 7
  sickness, 16–17
  training and competence, organisations, 111, 290
  varicosities, 20, 167
Yoghurt, thrush, 24

Zinc
  anaemia, 19
  dietary sources of, 171–172
  infertility, 15
  nausea and vomiting, 15
  perineal care, 30, 171–172
  postnatal depression, 30